Osteopathic Diagnos

Emanuel A. Sammut
DO (Hons), MRO

Sammut & Sammut Associates, West Molesey, Surrey, United Kingdom

Patrick J. Searle-Barnes
MA (Cantab.), DO (Hons), MRO

West Parade Osteopaths, Lincoln, Lincolnshire, United Kingdom

First published in 1998 by:
Stanley Thornes (Publishers) Ltd

Reprinted in 2002 by:
Nelson Thornes Ltd
Delta Place
27 Bath Road
CHELTENHAM
GL53 7TH
United Kingdom

05 06 / 10 9 8 7

A catalogue record for this book is available from the British Library

ISBN 0 7487 3296 9

Page make-up by Northern Phototypesetting Co. Ltd

Changed To Digital Printing 2006

Dedication

To the British School of Osteopathy, considered by the authors to be the centre of excellence of Osteopathic Studies and to its students, past, present and future.

Contents

Foreword

As in all medical systems, diagnosis is as much an art as it is a science. However, artistic flair is no substitute for sound reasoning. This book will help all those who wish to use sensible, anatomical knowledge and logical thinking to help their patients. The authors have brought their considerable teaching experience to bear to record the current thinking used at the British School of Osteopathy (BSO), in the subject.

Technique has generally been taught separately from diagnosis and treatment has been taught in a clinical setting. Although there have been several books on technique, books describing diagnosis and treatment have been very rare. For the first time, a book on diagnosis with some aspects of treatment, has been written to help bridge the inevitable gaps in the system. Emanuel Sammut and Patrick Searle-Barnes have managed to encapsulate a great deal into a small space. Although there is no substitute for data accumulated by the hard knocks of clinical practice, this book will help smooth the path for all those interested in practising osteopathy or furthering their knowledge of it.

Conventional medicine uses diagnosis as a basis for prescription. Osteopathy is similar, but the choice of approach can vary widely according to the practitioners' aims in treatment. This book will achieve its objective if you are encouraged to think about diagnostic criteria in a slightly different way. As in all professions, there are differences in opinion on many matters. These differences should be a source of strength, not of weakness. Having catalogued the BSO approach in such a logical fashion, the authors have given the profession a head start in exposing some aspects of current thinking to a wider audience.

Professor Laurie Hartman

Preface

This book has been written primarily with the osteopathic student in mind. Both authors have lectured for some years in osteopathic diagnosis at the British School of Osteopathy and are aware of the lack of textbooks within the field. Therefore, we hope that this book will help to fill this gap. The book will also be of interest to those working in allied professions as it explains osteopathic theory and an approach to diagnosis and evaluation.

We would like to thank our wives for their patience over the past two years and our children who have been long suffering during their fathers' distraction! Our thanks go also to Nicola Sammut, Ian Whyte and Stephen Tyreman for their reading of various drafts and their helpful comments. Derrick Edwards and Jill Berthon are thanked for their advice and support. Finally, we must pay tribute to Robert Searle-Barnes whose painstaking proof-reading has been invaluable.

Introduction

The art of manual treatment for the aches and ills of the human frame has been practised for many centuries. Indeed it has been used in China for thousands of years. Osteopathy, on the other hand, has been around for little more than a century in America and arrived in Britain in the early 1900s. In the past two decades there has been a rapid growth in the number of practising osteopaths, which reflects the fast-changing attitudes of the medical profession and the general public towards the osteopathic profession.

Osteopathy is a system of diagnosis and treatment that is concerned primarily with mechanical problems of the body framework. These are principally within the musculo-skeletal system. However, disturbance in the viscera may cause secondary changes within the muscles and joints.

Osteopathic philosophy emphasizes that alteration of the structure of musculo-skeletal tissues (for instance as a result of injury, misuse or disease) may cause a change in mechanical function. Normal physiological activity of cells and tissues requires an adequate blood supply to bring appropriate nutrition, and drainage to remove waste products. Tissue function may also be influenced by blood-borne hormonal factors and neurological control. As we shall explain, both the circulation and the control systems may be affected by disturbances of mechanical function.

The aims, therefore, of osteopathic diagnosis are two-fold:

- *To identify the site of the source of the symptoms and the nature of the tissue disturbance*. It is important that we understand the pathophysiological state of the disturbed area and its effect on the body because this will have a bearing on the expectations of the effects of treatment and also on the types of manipulative techniques used. However, the nature of the tissue disturbance does not lead to a prescribed osteopathic treatment. For example, with an intervertebral disc injury, it may be inappropriate to use forceful manipulative techniques since these may aggravate the situation. Also there are certain types of tissue disturbance that may contraindicate manual treatment or be helped more by other forms of treatment, for example severe infection, cancer, gross vascular or endocrine disease.
- *To assess the mechanical structure and function of the body*. How the body has physically responded to the problem (in the short term particularly by inflammation and muscle spasm and in the longer term by structural changes of both soft tissue and joint structures) is assessed, since it is the results of this that we shall attempt primarily to alter and

improve by manual treatment. In addition, other factors that may have predisposed the person to the problem in the first place are established. These may involve all parts of the person: body, mind and spirit.

The first aim is similar to that of a medical diagnosis. Indeed, the word diagnosis means to identify a disease or condition on the basis of the observed symptoms and signs. It is perhaps the second aim that differentiates the osteopathic approach, both in evaluation of the patient and, consequently, in treatment. It emphasizes the importance not only of the local tissue damage or disturbance but also the interaction with the rest of the body. This is a two-way process; the local dysfunction has an impact on the rest of the body but equally the local response will be affected by factors in other parts. It is ultimately our purpose to assist the person to cope with and, where possible, overcome the problem so long as it is amenable to an osteopathic approach.

The book divides naturally into two parts. Part 1 deals with the general approach of the osteopath to the patient. The theoretical aspects are discussed in Chapters 1–4. These include the philosophy (Chapter 1) and possible mechanisms underlying the clinical findings that are discovered on physical examination (Chapter 2). The significance of postural abnormalities is explored (Chapter 3) and types of treatment and their possible effects are explained (Chapter 4). Part 1 concludes with an overview of the analysis of the case history and of the osteopathic examination (Chapters 5 and 6).

Part 2 deals with more specific clinical aspects. Chapter 7 considers the practical implications of various problems associated with spinal curvature. It draws together many of the principles discussed in Part 1 and also how the effects of myofascial adaptation cause interaction of each body area. The following chapters then look at each region of the body in turn and explore in detail the osteopathic assessment of the area while placing it in the context of the rest of the body. The clinical presentation of the more common problems seen in osteopathic practice within each region of the body is discussed, particularly considering the involvement of the muscles and other soft tissues as well as the presence of joint dysfunction. Underlying these chapters is the appreciation of the interrelationship of structure and function. *Although it is principally the function of an area that we assess and attempt to change, we are aware that this will be influenced by structural changes as well as by alterations of the neurological control of muscles in the area.*

Disturbed mechanical function may have a significant effect on the health of a person, but it is not the only factor in disease. Therefore the scope of manual treatment is limited to dealing with patients where there is a significant mechanical component to the problem.

Osteopathic practice is a complex art with an understanding of the scientific basis that is steadily growing. Much has been learned over the past century but there is much yet to be discovered. Of course we have to be specific in our local diagnosis but there are times when we are uncertain as to the importance of the various factors contributing to the presenting problem. This is of course true of any therapy dealing with complex human beings. A working hypothesis has to be developed which is then tested by treatment. Scientific research will provide greater clarity in the coming years, but it should be recognized that every person is unique and thus brings the osteopath a unique set of problems. Our diagnostic model and approach needs to be flexible to cope with this individuality.

Note: As osteopathy is generally practised on a one-to-one practitioner-to-patient basis, in the text we have used the first person masculine for the practitioner and the first person feminine for the patient, to avoid the clumsy use of he/she and him/her in these instances. No sexism is implied – this is purely a means of making the text more readable.

Osteopathic Overview

Osteopathic concepts

1

HISTORY

Osteopathy was developed by A.T. Still in the latter half of the nineteenth century in the mid-west of America in the years following the Civil War. Still had from youth been an observer of current medical practice and had at one stage spent some time at a medical school. He was unimpressed by the available remedies of the day, which commonly consisted of alcohol, mercury salts or opium. It was out of his disillusionment with orthodox medicine that his ideas developed. He reasoned that God made man perfect. Therefore, seen from a mechanical viewpoint, if the body structure was in correct alignment and functioned normally, with no impairment to the flow of blood or nervous impulses, then full health would follow. He therefore sought to understand the body framework and contents and how they worked, using what was known of anatomy and physiology at that time.

He started to explore ways of treating people suffering from a broad range of problems by assessing how their body framework was misaligned or functioning abnormally. He used his hands to free joints and loosen muscles. He would often also give specific exercises, aiming to prevent recurrence and help the body to remain healthy. Treatment would involve dealing with distant as well as local parts of the body in order to deal with, as he saw it, the cause or causes of the presenting problem. He scolded those of his later students who attempted merely to treat the symptoms without addressing the underlying cause.

Still did not envisage osteopathy as dealing with only musculo-skeletal problems. He did indeed take on some difficult 'mechanical' problems, but he would also take on patients with a wide range of diseases. During a diarrhoea epidemic [1] he dealt with many sufferers and his reported success suggests that he was rather more helpful than his medical opponents (he was viewed as an outsider by them). This success may well have owed more to his philosophy of using no drugs and simple hygiene measures. Given that the local doctors would almost certainly have used arsenic, mercury and alcohol, iatrogenic death may have been quite high!

Still opened a college of osteopathy in 1892 in Kirksville and trained a rapidly increasing number of students. Some crossed to Britain in the early twentieth century. In 1917 the first osteopathic school opened in Britain, named the British School of Osteopathy.

Osteopathy has developed along rather different lines in Britain than the USA.

In Britain osteopaths currently practise separately from the orthodox profession whereas in the USA all osteopaths effectively train as doctors as well as osteopaths. American osteopaths therefore may use allopathic drugs and surgery whereas British osteopaths are primarily manual therapists. Discussion of osteopathy in this book will focus on its practice in Britain.

The 'osteopathic lesion'

In the early days osteopaths identified areas in the spine which were restricted in mobility, associated with changes in soft tissue texture and at times apparently misaligned. Still himself described these areas as dislocations or strains. As the profession developed, the term osteopathic lesion was used to describe such an area. Implicit in the definition was the belief that the osteopathic lesion was amenable to osteopathic treatment. It was therefore diagnosed by palpation and treated by manual therapy.

A further belief of Still was that these areas of spinal lesions could lead to disturbance of blood flow or nervous impulses in related structures. Thus, for example, if there was a lesion in the mid-thoracic spine then the flow of blood in vessels that were controlled by nerves from these segments would be impaired. Organs such as the stomach supplied by such blood vessels would then be more vulnerable to disease. The inference was that internal disease might be caused primarily by spinal osteopathic lesions. This was a highly controversial hypothesis and with hindsight somewhat naive. Scientific study has now identified a multitude of factors that can contribute to the development of disease. The relevance of the presence of spinal lesions will be discussed in more detail in the following chapters.

Positional lesion diagnosis

In the first half of this century an osteopathic lesion was analysed according to the relative position of one vertebra to the next. Therefore, if on palpation the upper vertebra appeared slightly rotated and side-bent to the right, then it might be described as a right side-bending rotation lesion (a form of positional lesion). In theory the treatment for this would then be some form of manipulative technique that 'corrected' the lesion to bring 'normal' alignment. However it became apparent that improved function could be achieved by other techniques, which might even involve exaggeration of the lesion. Associated with any abnormal alignment of a spinal segment were abnormalities of tissue texture and restricted mobility. The emphasis in diagnosis, therefore, moved from identifying abnormal alignment to abnormal tissue texture and mobility. It was also accepted that the normal position of a vertebra may be in a position that is rotated or side-bent because it is compensating for some structural or functional asymmetry in an adjacent or distant area. For example, if there is some difference in leg length due to asymmetrical growth then the spine may form a C or S curve to support the head so that the eyes and ears are naturally held in a horizontal plane. It had been suggested by some osteopaths that the body's natural posture needs to be maintained in symmetrical alignment, but this is a controversial hypothesis that is not accepted by the authors.

In the 1960s the term 'osteopathic lesion' was changed to 'somatic dysfunction' for two reasons. First, the sense of exclusivity that the term engendered was unhelpful since it implied that only osteopaths could diagnose or treat it. Second, the emphasis on 'the lesion' was causing some osteopaths to concentrate purely on lesion recognition and lose sight of the relationship of the identifiable lesions to the rest of the body. The term somatic dysfunction was initially used to describe altered function of a specific spinal segment. This definition has now been widened to include the more widespread effects that segmental dysfunction may have, since somatic dysfunction may be a complex reaction of a series of different parts of the body. This will be explored in more detail in Chapter 2.

Recent developments

In the 1970s Audrey Smith developed this concept further by attempting to analyse the spinal lesion in terms of what tissues may be involved within the segment and beyond and the pathophysiological states affecting those tissues. For instance, it is widely accepted that damage to a variety of tissues within a segment may cause pain and dysfunction. These include the intervertebral disc, the apophyseal joint capsule, spinal ligaments and muscles. Damage to various tissues may also cause secondary problems in spinal nerve roots. At times it is helpful to be able to differentiate between these, though in practice this is not always possible. For instance, it may be important to identify whether the primary damaged tissue is the intervertebral disc because it may be unstable and should not be forcefully manipulated. (Other techniques may be used however.) Also from the case history and palpatory examination it may be possible to establish the nature of tissue changes around a joint. The concern here is whether there is inflammation within the joint or surrounding it, whether there is more chronic shortening of the capsule or ligaments or whether there is shortening of the deep or superficial muscles surrounding the spine.

CURRENT CONCEPTS OF OSTEOPATHY

Osteopathy is a system of clinical practice that looks at the person from a mechanical point of view and emphasizes the importance of the musculoskeletal system to the overall function and health of a person. Still's original ideas have been developed at the Kirksville College of Osteopathic Medicine in the eight philosophies shown in Figure 1.1 and described in detail below. These are described as philosophies since they are derived by logical reasoning rather than by empirical findings through scientific experiment.

1 The body is a unit
2 Structure and function are reciprocally interrelated
3 The body possesses self-regulatory mechanisms
4 The body has the inherent capacity to defend itself and
   repair itself
5 When normal adaptability is disrupted, or when
   environmental changes overcome the body's capacity for
   self-maintenance, disease may ensue
6 Movement of body fluids is essential to the maintenance of
   health
7 The nerves play a crucial part in controlling the fluids of
   the body
8 There are somatic components to disease that are not only
   manifestations of disease but also are factors that contribute
   to maintenance of the diseased state

   Implicit in these philosophies is the belief that osteopathic
   intervention can have a positive influence on the above

Figure 1.1 Osteopathic philosophies. [2]

OSTEOPATHIC PHILOSOPHIES [2]

1 The body is a unit

The body is made of many parts which relate to each other in various ways. This usually only becomes apparent when one part is disturbed by injury or disease. Mechanical injury to one area can increase strain on another; for instance, an injured knee may cause abnormal gait and increase strain on the spine. If the spine is already vulnerable to strain for some reason, then the altered gait may be enough to tip the balance: 'the straw that broke the camel's back'.

Disease or dysfunction of viscera may well affect the health of other body tissues; for example, an infection of the lung may reduce oxygenation of the blood which may then reduce perfusion of other body tissues, predisposing them to disease or dysfunction. Likewise hepatic function will be less efficient if the liver is diseased and thus toxins may build up in the blood. Visceral dysfunction may also cause abnormal neurological activity, which may then affect musculo-skeletal function.

This philosophy can also be extended beyond the physical level; the mind, body and spirit are believed to be interdependent (Figure 1.2). For example, if someone is emotionally stressed they may develop physical symptoms such as headaches, indigestion and diarrhoea and there may be physical changes in the body, such as increased blood pressure or altered acid level secretion in the stomach. Conversely, uncertainty aroused by physical symptoms sometimes leads to anxiety or other emotional reactions. Furthermore, if the person is under emotional or physical stress for other reasons, this will have an impact on the body's ability to cope with further imposed stresses. When assessing a patient's body therefore, it is important to be open to the possibility of stresses in a domain other than the physical.

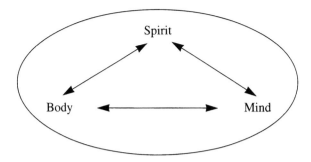

Figure 1.2 Relationship between various domains of a person.

Compensation

Although the interrelationship of different body parts is most apparent when a problem has developed, nevertheless adaptation by one part to another occurs continuously. None of us is 'perfect' in either body, mind or spirit. For instance, very few of us are physically symmetrical and most have areas of abnormal function in either the musculo-skeletal system or the viscera. Generally we are able to adapt to or compensate for these abnormalities. For example, the pelvis of a patient with a short lower extremity will tilt in a lateral plane. The spine therefore will compensate by forming a lateral curve, which will depend to an extent on the anatomical configuration of the vertebrae and the presence of other structural abnormalities. Because this scoliotic alignment will be the patient's natural posture, the soft tissues will adapt by hypertrophy (or sometimes fibrosis, depending on the nature of the postural strain imposed) on the convexity and partial wasting on the concavity. Thus compensation causes long-term changes in the body structure.

Compensation may occur in other ways. If there is a damaged area of the nervous system then the body will, where possible, find a way of adapting to this. If there is weakness of a region or muscle group, possibly resulting from a congenital or developmental problem, the body may adapt by altering a gross movement pattern. For instance, weakness around the shoulder joint may be overcome by using the periscapular muscles to 'throw' up the arm, thus allowing some flexion or abduction of the arm. Within the nervous system, if a nerve pathway becomes damaged, sometimes other parts of the nervous system can actually take over the task. At a chemical level, if there is a chemical or enzyme defect, the metabolic processes may adapt to minimize the impact on the body.

Compensation also occurs at a psychological level. We each develop psychological strategies consciously or, more frequently, unconsciously for coping with situations that may cause us emotional stress. We may have learned these strategies in early life but they affect how we respond even as adults. We learn ways to cover up our emotional vulnerability. We also develop various ways of coping with stress.

So what then is the 'aim' of the compensation? Its (unconscious) purpose is to minimize the effect of any internal abnormality since potentially this may reduce the body's efficiency and ultimately its ability to survive. This does not necessarily mean that compensation always provides maximum efficiency. We are highly adaptable and resilient creatures and thus will cope with a large combination of stresses. The onset of illness or disability, however, indicates that our ability to cope has been overwhelmed.

The concept of compensation is extremely complex and requires more detailed analysis than is possible here. It is an implicit aim of osteopathic practice to maximize the patient's ability to compensate.

2 Structure and function are reciprocally interrelated

During fetal development, body tissues differentiate into highly specialized forms. Their structural development dictates the function they are able to perform throughout life. If during life the structure of a tissue is altered, then its function will be altered also. For instance the bowel wall is adapted to allow absorption of nutrients passing along it. If the bowel is damaged in some way the function of absorption may be impaired. Here the term function is used to describe both the purpose or activity of the bowel wall and also the efficiency of this activity.

Changes in musculo-skeletal structures often lead to disturbance of mechanical function. For example, minor damage to tissues at the base of the spine may lead to altered protective muscle tension. This altered muscle tension disturbs the normal mechanical behaviour or 'function' of the area and is part of the body's response to injury that is described as 'somatic dysfunction'. If this dysfunction is prolonged then secondary connective tissue shortening may develop in the local area and there may be further effects in more distant parts occurring as a result of both mechanical and neurological mechanisms. These are described in Chapter 2.

3 The body possesses self-regulatory mechanisms

The study of human physiology presents an almost endless list of examples of homeostatic mechanisms. For example, under normal circumstances the internal environment is controlled both by neurological reflexes where there is continuous feedback, plus the endocrine system with constant chemical feedback of hormonal levels. Blood flow to the kidney is controlled predominantly by chemical feedback at a local level. There is feedback from neural receptors in the musculo-skeletal system that allows the body to maintain a vertical (or any other) static posture or allows the body to move in a controlled manner.

4 The body has the inherent capacity to defend and repair itself

The discussion on compensation has so far focused on internal abnormalities that impose a strain on the system. However, the internal environment of the body may be threatened by mechanical, chemical, microbial or psychological factors from without as well as within (see Table 1.1). In Selye's model of stress [3] both internal and external factors are known as stressors. These may occur individually though more often a variety of stresses are experienced simultaneously.

Various defence mechanisms have developed in the body which are able to cope with most stressors. The first of these is a tough external layer of skin and dermis, and if the outer surface of the body is breached there are a number of cellular responses by the immune system. A specific physical insult such as a trauma or an infection will initiate a local inflammatory reaction. With a psychological trauma, however, there is no local inflammatory reaction since there is no local site of damage. With all forms of stressors though there may be a more *general* body response which will involve the neurological, immune, and endocrine systems in a much broader response. The extent of the general body response will vary according to the degree of stress imposed.

Table 1.1 External stressors

Mechanical	Trauma, lifting, sports injury, occupational repetitive action, postural strain, poor ergonomic design of workplace, excess body weight
Chemical	Food, air pollutants, e.g. smoking (poison or allergy)
Microbial	Bacteria, virus, fungus
Psychological	Extrinsic: excessive workload, relationships, perceived threat by other(s)

Internal stressors may also have an impact. For example, previous emotional trauma may have led to altered behaviour patterns; past physical trauma may have left residual scar tissue, abnormal joint mobility or abnormal movement patterns. Other internal stressors include functional conditions such as asthma and irritable bowel syndrome. Indeed anything that causes abnormal function of a tissue in theory may have an influence on another part by increasing the functional demand on that part. In practice though the significance of any particular factor needs to be weighed carefully. This is often a matter of clinical judgement and may sometimes only be assessed by a 'trial of treatment', i.e. by changing the factor involved we discover whether it is of importance.

An individual's response to any particular threat will depend on a variety of factors. There are many factors that will slow the recovery rate from injury or illness, such as poor nutrition or poor housing conditions which may be damp or where infection may breed. Although the emphasis when evaluating patients may be on their somatic and visceral function, attention must also be given to external factors such as the stresses they may be under, the environment that they work in and the demands made on them by their occupation and general lifestyle. For instance, a postal worker presented with a persistent low back problem which was aggravated by his work. When asked what his work involved he explained that he spent up to 4–5 hours in the back of a security van that delivered money to sub-post offices. He worked on his feet but was unable to stand up inside the van. This clearly had a bearing on the understanding and prognosis of his problem. Factors such as the strain imposed by this man's occupation are known as *maintaining factors* since the strain affects the rate of recovery.

When discussing stress many tend to emphasize the negative effects. However, there are certain factors that enhance health and the body's stress responses. A positive psychological state of mind is probably the most important of these. Rehabilitation and nursing care has long attempted to enhance this by encouragement and the setting of goals. Good eating habits and regular exercise will also stimulate the body's normal defence mechanisms.

Table 1.2 Negative and positive stress factors that may affect the body's ability to cope with dysfunction and disease

	Negative factors	*Positive factors*
State of general health	Poor nutrition Excessive/inadequate exercise Infection, endocrine imbalance State of general fatigue Smoker, excess alcohol consumption	Good nutrition Appropriate regular exercise Regular sleep
State of mind	Emotional stress levels: unstable relationships, insecurity of occupation, pressure of exams, etc. Intrinsic: anxiety, depression, psychosis	Stable relationships Able to deal with stress appropriately
Environment	Poor physical environment, e.g. home/working conditions	Well-designed workplace that minimizes physical stress
State of body	Musculo-skeletal: poor posture, poor muscle tone, localized or widespread somatic dysfunction, degeneration Visceral: visceral dysfunction, degeneration in viscera, e.g. cirrhotic liver, obstructive airways disease, scarring of bowel, arteriosclerosis	Good muscle tone and flexibility

According to Selye, the effect of stressors is accumulative. For example, one person may succumb to a chest infection while another may not, despite being exposed to the same bacteria. The latter person is able to deal with the infecting agent, whereas the first person's body is vulnerable to the infection because a number of factors have already stressed them to the point where they are unable to tolerate and overcome any further stress. These might include previous chest infections, with scarring within the lungs, depressed immune function due to the use of steroids for asthma or other 'allergic' condition, poor spinal and thoracic spinal mobility due to inadequate exercise, postural fatigue or chronic overwork of the spinal muscles in manual work. (Poor rib cage mechanical function can lead to reduced gaseous exchange and thus poorer tissue health in the lungs, thus increasing the chance of infection.) Psychological factors might include stress at work or in personal relationships, or clinical depression which is not necessarily directly related to the immediate circumstances surrounding the patient. Conversely, positive psychological enhancement may occur; the patient may have some exciting event coming up which they do not wish to miss (Table 1.2)!

Given this inherent capacity, the aim of osteopathic treatment is to enhance the body's healing response by removing any barriers to the restoration of normal physiological function and improving the body's ability to compensate for any irreversible structural or functional abnormalities.

5 When normal adaptability is disrupted, or when environmental changes overcome the body's capacity for self-maintenance, disease may ensue

It is not unusual to see people who have quite significant abnormalities for which they have compensated for many years without developing any symptoms. However, because the abnormality imposes greater demands on the body tissues, it predisposes the system to strain and the person is potentially more vulnerable to injury (Figure 1.3). These internal stressors are described

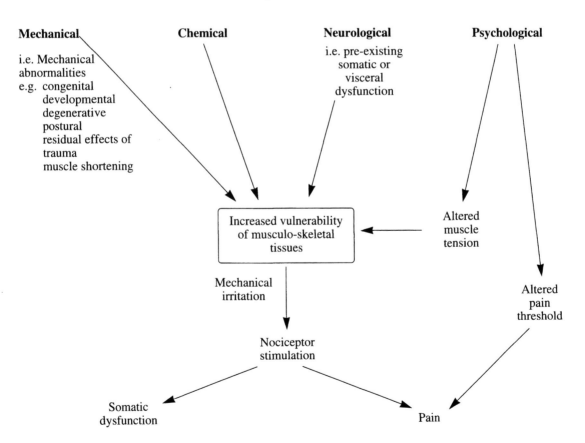

Figure 1.3 Factors predisposing to somatic dysfunction.

as predisposing factors. As we have seen, whether the compensation 'breaks down' (when symptoms develop) will depend on a wide variety of factors. It is likely that in many patients with pain and disability there are various predisposing factors to the problem. Where there has been significant external trauma imposed on the body in a sporting injury or a road traffic accident these are less likely to be important, since the intensity of the force involved meant that the damage would have occurred regardless of any predisposing factors. In this case predisposing factors may still influence the recovery rate or may prevent full resolution. Though initially treatment might be best directed to the local dysfunction, a plateau is sometimes reached in the progress. This may well be because there are other factors, including dysfunction at different sites in the body, which are preventing further improvement.

However, commonly, people develop symptoms for apparently relatively trivial reasons and often no physical trauma is recalled at all. This may be due to the result of the type of tissue that has been injured (e.g. a disc injury may occur but not cause symptoms until the inflammation spreads to other surrounding tissues). It may also be because the affected area was already vulnerable for some reason and it required an insignificant trauma or even a repeated minor stress to 'tip the balance' and cause symptoms to develop. This then requires a full evaluation of the person's body since it is unlikely that there are no predisposing factors other than locally.

As can be seen in Figure 1.4, the breakdown of compensation may occur suddenly or slowly. This will depend mainly on the environmental stresses

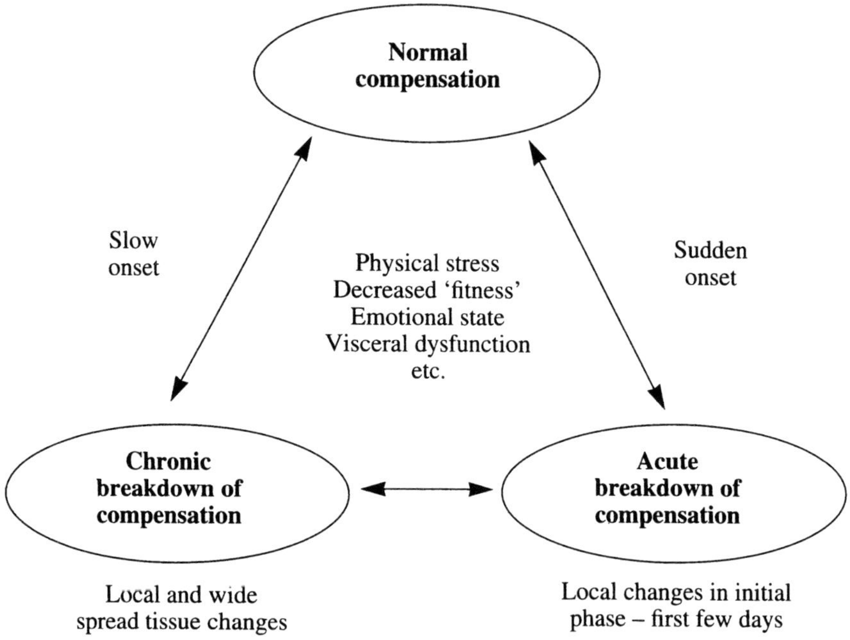

Insidious O/S, or O/S from trivial event = wide investigation necessary to find pre-disposing factors

Figure 1.4 Possible pathways of compensation breakdown.

imposed on the system. If the static compensation is poor, such that strain is caused, for example, by sitting, if the patient works at a desk for many hours at a time, then it is likely that this may lead to a chronic breakdown. When the patient eventually seeks help, because the problem has developed over a period of time, then secondary effects may have developed elsewhere in the body and these may need treatment.

However it is conceivable that this patient may just bend down to pick up a piece of paper from the floor and precipitate the onset of acute low back pain. Sometimes it is a chance movement at the wrong time when the body is already vulnerable that finally triggers the symptoms. Notice too that the patient may develop mild symptoms gradually over a period of weeks or months but then precipitate an acute episode. Here a chronic breakdown then develops into an acute breakdown.

6 Movement of body fluids is essential to the maintenance of health

If there is stasis of fluid in any part of the body then this can lead to poor tissue health because of lack of oxygen and a build up of waste products. Excessive swelling and oedema resulting from tissue damage and consequent inflammation may then slow up the natural healing response. So, for example, in the case of an acute ligament or muscle injury it is advantageous to minimize the oedema that develops by resting with the leg raised for the first 1–2 days. Passive movement of the affected part should be encouraged at an early stage.

Often fluid movement from tissues and through venous and lymph channels depends on muscular contraction and relaxation associated with joint movement. Thus if there is excessive sustained muscle tension this can contribute to poor drainage of an affected area. This excessive muscle tension may develop as a result of the injury and may initially be an appropriate response. However if it is prolonged then it may actually maintain the problem and treatment is helpful to enhance the body's healing.

7 The nerves play a crucial part in controlling the fluids of the body

The sympathetic nervous system is the vasomotor system and therefore fluid movement through blood vessels is influenced by sympathetic neurological tone in the smooth muscle surrounding the vessels. Blood flow is primarily governed by local control mechanisms within an organ or tissue. However, there is resting neurological tone which may be modified according to the needs of the body-part supplied by the arteries or drained by the veins. There is evidence to suggest that autonomic control may be modified by dysfunction in a related part of the musculo-skeletal system through altered nervous reflex activity [4]. This may be observed as increased skin temperature locally, moisture (because of increased sweat-gland activity), tenderness and oedema. Osteopathic treatment aims to improve mobility and reduce the reactivity of muscle tension, and also alter other abnormal reflexes that are initiated by somatic dysfunction and result in the above signs. The neurological reflex interaction involved in somatic dysfunction is an important mechanism (though by no means the only one) by which dysfunction in one area may influence another. A specific implication of this philosophy is that when there is damage in the body it is relevant to consider the related areas in which dysfunction might alter the autonomic regulation. For example, healing of tendonitis in the arm might in theory be slower if there were dysfunction in the upper thoracic spine, where the sympathetic control of the circulation of the upper extremity is mediated.

8 There are somatic components to disease that not only are manifestations of disease but also are factors that contribute to maintenance of the diseased state

Traditionally the term somatic refers to the body structures to differentiate it from the psyche and thus includes internal viscera. However, here 'somatic' is defined as relating to neuro-musculo-skeletal structures only.

The effects of disease affecting an organ will not be confined to that organ alone. Because of the neurological interconnections of a organ there will be reflex effects in other tissues. For example, when there is an inflamed organ such as an acutely inflamed appendix or gall-bladder, muscle spasm and tenderness develop in the abdominal wall. There are also more subtle changes that occur in segmentally related spinal tissues, including muscle tension and superficial oedema. Thus there may be dysfunction of one or more segments of the spine as a result of visceral disturbance.

It is also believed by many that the presence of somatic dysfunction in the spine may be more than purely secondary to the visceral disturbance but may act as a factor contributing to the causation of the visceral disturbance. Currently there is no strong evidence to substantiate or refute this. It is possible that the presence of somatic dysfunction may have the effect of focusing the effects of other stresses on the involved area of the body. Korr [5] described an area of somatic dysfunction as acting as a 'neurological lens' because it amplifies the response to any reflex activity within the segment and may thus modify the autonomic nervous tone to a viscera.

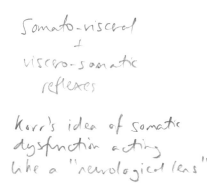

Case study 1.1 may illustrate some of the above philosophies:

Case study 1.1

Mr P is a 33-year-old man who presented with a 9-year history of recurrent lower neck ache which sometimes radiated into the left arm. The pain was affected by different postures and sometimes turning the head might cause sharp pain. The pain was originally caused by an injury while playing rugby, though he had since given this up some 5 years ago. He also reported having developed asthma about 4 years ago. This was controlled reasonably well by taking Ventolin and Becotide inhalers, though he still had occasional attacks.

When asked about abdominal symptoms he denied any problems, but he later admitted that he was prone to indigestion when he was under pressure at work. He explained that he used to do manual building work, but about 5 years ago he moved into a management post, running a small building firm for a friend. Because of a slump in the building trade he had at times been under considerable pressure with a heavy workload and the threat of losing his job. This had also affected his relationship with his wife.

On examination there was marked tightness across the shoulder girdle on both sides. There was an exaggeration of the normal upper thoracic kyphosis and lower cervical lordosis. There was significant restriction of movement in his cervico-thoracic region, particularly when turning to the left. There was restriction of rib cage excursion especially in the lower ribs and the rib cage was held relatively in inspiration; there was also poor diaphragm excursion. In the mid-thoracic spinal area there was tenderness and the muscles were more reactive on palpation and on gentle thoracic rotation.

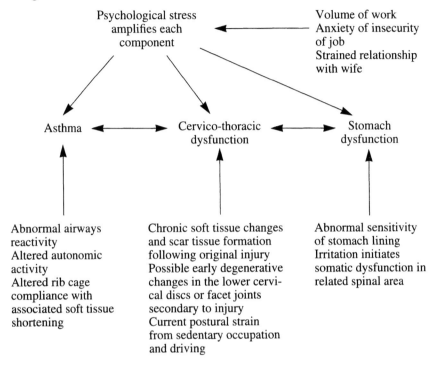

Figure 1.5 Interaction of various components of the problems of Mr P.

The main components of Mr P's problem are shown in Figure 1.5 and include the cervico-thoracic joint disturbance, asthma and the stomach irritation causing indigestion. The details of the specific problems are not the concern at this point. This case illustrates how the osteopath views the interrelationship of the various components of the problem. The osteopath seeks to understand each component by assessing the localized tissue disturbance, including what tissues are damaged or are involved in the dysfunction, and then attempts to understand the relationship between the parts. In this case there is persistent cervico-thoracic somatic dysfunction with chronic soft tissue changes. The prolonged sitting at a desk and in the car adds a further postural strain; this acts as another predisposing factor to future episodes of pain.

The asthmatic state that has become symptomatic over recent years may also further predispose the neck to strain because of soft tissue changes that have resulted from altered thoracic function. Conversely the soft tissue changes associated with the neck problem may affect the upper thoracic function. There may also be reflex interconnections (see Chapter 2). In addition, there are signs of somatic dysfunction in the mid-thoracic spine, initiated by the stomach condition, which may have been triggered in turn by the psychological stress.

The reflex changes potentially caused by the dysfunction of both of the viscera may also affect the neurological behaviour of somatic dysfunction in the cervico-thoracic region. Thus each of the components is seen as interlinked. The mechanisms between them will be explored later in this chapter and in Chapter 2. There are probably many further factors involved and many other interactions occurring.

Although this man had a musculo-skeletal problem that would respond to local manipulation, by assessing the various components contributing to his state of health or dysfunction, we observe a broader picture that will lead to a better understanding and thus hopefully a clearer prognosis and treatment plan. This does not, however, mean that the osteopath will then treat all components of a problem. Some factors are amenable to treatment and others may not be or will require a different form of treatment, either instead of or in addition. For instance, in the case of Mr P, if the relationship with his wife deteriorates because of the work pressure then specific marriage guidance counselling might be helpful. Alternatively, if the stomach problem develops into an ulcer and if perforation occurred then osteopathic treatment would be entirely inappropriate at that stage, though it might still be appropriate in the rehabilitation phase to help restore more normal reflex behaviour. Thus osteopathic treatment may complement other forms of treatment.

In this case osteopathic treatment is appropriate because there are areas of the musculo-skeletal system where there is dysfunction or soft tissue abnormalities that are contributing to the problem and these changes in the musculo-skeletal system are reversible.

Although within the above eight philosophies there is emphasis on the importance of the body framework and its potential significance to the maintenance of health, they do not present the scope of osteopathy as a system of therapeutics. Most osteopaths would agree that its scope is wider than musculo-skeletal pain and disability, but there is less agreement about the breadth of problems that can be helped by osteopathic intervention. This uncertainty is explained by the paucity of strictly controlled clinical trials. The question remains, therefore, whether individual successes can be repeated under controlled circumstances.

DIFFERENT CONCEPTUAL MODELS

The eight osteopathic philosophies form a framework for a complete conceptual model. Thus in principle we need to understand the whole person in each case. In theory this is desirable but it is also time consuming. There are times therefore when a more localized model, concentrating on perhaps only the local area, may be adequate to resolve the presenting problem. This may well be appropriate with a localized traumatic injury that has occurred only a few days previously. The same patient might present some months later when the problem has improved but not yet resolved. A broader model will be more appropriate since the body will have adapted and compensated for the secondary changes that have been imposed by the effects of the injury. Treating only the local area will probably be less effective in the medium term than dealing also with the more distant effects of the original injury, since these may inhibit the restoration of function in the symptomatic area.

Even within an osteopathic context different models may be appropriate. With pain that is mainly related to sustained posture a 'biomechanical' or 'postural' model may be particularly helpful. This would emphasize the postural balance of the body and attempt to improve the body posture to minimize the strain placed on the muscles. With a problem where there is significant swelling secondary to inflammation or stasis, then a diagnostic model emphasizing factors that might affect the fluid drainage of an area might be more helpful. This might be useful for instance with a patient presenting with sinusitis or where there is marked swelling secondary to injury as may occur with an ankle or knee strain. Alternatively, where there may be both visceral and somatic sources of dysfunction a model may be applied where the emphasis is on relating the various structures involved by neurological mechanisms. None of these models is exclusive. They are in fact merely different ways of viewing the same problem. We may apply them to improve our understanding and therefore effectiveness.

As mentioned above, the importance of a conceptual model is not merely academic as it also helps in rationalizing the therapeutic approach; this will be developed further in Chapter 4.

IMPORTANCE OF 'FUNCTION'

Osteopaths are principally concerned with body function, particularly when it deviates from the expected 'normal'. It is by alteration of function that osteopathic treatment aids the recovery from pain and disability. From a knowledge of anatomy, physiology and biomechanics, the role or action that a body tissue or region may perform is known. For example, one biomechanical action of the hip joint is that it allows movement between the lower extremity and the pelvis during ambulation. However, when we discuss function we are concerned more with the behaviour of the joint rather than its role within the body. Is it able to perform its normal action or is it in some way impaired? Within the musculo-skeletal system the term 'function' describes, therefore, both range and ease of movement of the joint within its normal range rather than its biomechanical 'role' or action. So within the context of this book, hip 'function' would be considered 'normal' if it had a range of movement typical of a person of the patient's age and build and if there were no particular abnormal resistance to movement in any range.

Normal function is therefore a *relative* term. What is normal for a 65-year-old would be considered abnormal in a teenager. It is therefore important for a practitioner to develop a working knowledge of the 'normal' range that we might expect at a given age, sex, and body build. With paired joints (e.g. hips, shoulders, etc.) it is often helpful to compare one with another.

Function is therefore measured by assessing range of movement and quality or ease of movement by observation of active movement (performed by the patient) and by palpation of passive movement (performed by the practitioner). Assessing the passive range of movement is relatively easy in peripheral joints since it is fairly straightforward to isolate the movement to only one joint by preventing movement in adjacent joints. Measuring passive range by palpation is more difficult in spinal and pelvic joints and takes considerable practice to build up the tactile and proprioceptive awareness – it is a manual skill and, as with any skill, it requires persistence and regular practice to develop (compare for instance learning to play a musical instrument).

Quality or ease of movement will be affected principally by the muscle tone surrounding a joint. If there is any structure that is injured or disturbed (with or without resulting inflammation) nociceptive activity will cause an alteration in the behaviour of local muscles to protect the area. Therefore in certain directions of movement there will be an increase of resistance to passive movement (see Figure 4.1). With experience it is the recognition of increased resistance within the range that is perhaps the most important feature in identifying dysfunction.

It is of course not enough to be able to identify abnormal function in an area of the body, since there may be a wide range of possible causes that will require different management. For instance, altered hip function may be the result of a congenitally unstable acetabulum, traumatic muscle damage, a pelvic joint disturbance, hip capsule irritation or degeneration of the hip joint itself, pelvic fracture, or a tumour in the upper femur or ilium, etc. Before proceeding with treatment it is necessary to establish that there is no serious pathological process present that would require either urgent medical treatment or further tests to clarify the nature of the problem. It is our aim to establish the cause of the abnormal function, since this will determine whether and how much we may alter the function of the disturbed area through osteopathic treatment and management. Treatment may then be compared to the tuning of a car engine; the structural effects of damage and degeneration cannot be reversed but the body can be helped to optimize the available function.

Although the emphasis in the above discussion has been on *joint* function, it must be stressed that assessment is made of not only the joint structures, i.e. the capsule, synovium and cartilage, but also the surrounding structures, including the muscles and fascia, since they are integrally related and will be involved, and may even be the major factor in the function of the joint. *Function* is emphasized because it is this that we palpate and may alter with treatment.

CAUSES OF ABNORMAL FUNCTION

Movement is important to tissue health. Reduction of movement within and around a tissue may reduce tissue perfusion. On a grosser scale, reduced joint mobility may cause increased mechanical strain on surrounding or distant structures. There are a number of reasons why the function of an area may be abnormal.

Congenital

Mobility of a joint or body area may vary according to the genetically governed body tissue type and shape. Some people are by nature more flexible than others; for example, generally the aesthenic person is more flexible than the pyknic. There may be more localized restriction of movement resulting from abnormal development of a body part; the lower lumbar spine is an area prone to developmental anomalies, such as incomplete separation of the last lumbar and first sacral vertebra leading to partial fusion. Mobility may also be altered because of asymmetry of the facet planes of the spinal joints in this area.

Developmental

Certain conditions may develop which cause altered mobility which have prolonged biomechanical effects, e.g. osteochondritis, organic scoliosis. These are probably due to problems during the growth phase; scoliosis may be idiopathic and develop *in utero*, in early childhood or even in teenage, or may be secondary to some other disorder such as polio affecting the spinal muscles asymmetrically during the early years. Spinal curvature is discussed in more detail in Chapter 7. Spinal osteochondritis also tends to develop during the teenage growth phase.

Degenerative

A common, though not inevitable, effect of degeneration of a joint is the reduction of movement. As we will see in Chapter 2, joint degeneration may involve a number of tissues in and around the joint. Most joints will allow movement in a number of directions and when degeneration develops, restriction commonly occurs in predictable ranges of movement. For instance, hip degeneration tends to affect internal rotation and abduction early on while external rotation and flexion may be affected later. In the later stages of degeneration all ranges will be affected.

Soft tissue adaptation

The structure of muscles alters according to the stresses placed on them. Persistent postural stress will cause shortening of the affected muscle and associated fascia and fibrosis may occur. Muscle shortening may also result from occupational strain or through particular hobbies, sporting or otherwise.

'Dysfunction' resulting from injury or other body insult

Somatic dysfunction is the result of the body's response to injury in both local and in more distant tissues. It involves a local inflammatory reaction and more widespread neurological responses to the trauma to the body. It may be short-lived but, if there are any barriers to resolution, then somatic dysfunction may be persistent. It may involve alteration in both musculo-skeletal and in related autonomic function. Because of increased muscle tension there is usually reduced joint mobility. As well as external trauma causing injury, dysfunction may be secondary to visceral disturbance. Somatic dysfunction is discussed in more detail in Chapter 2.

Our aim as osteopaths is primarily to enhance the body's attempt to overcome the body insult. Treatment is therefore directed at improving function, which includes both range of movement and ease of movement within the range by removing any barriers to resolution.

Visceral function

Viscera may be considered in the same way as musculo-skeletal structures. First it is necessary to know the action or role of the various visceral organs and systems and then be able to recognize symptoms and signs of abnormal function which may or may not be caused by serious disease. Visceral function may be disturbed as a result of serious structural pathology (e.g. serious cardio-vascular disease with disturbance of blood flow within the heart, or a cancer in the gastro-intestinal tract, etc.). We must be open to this possibility at all times and refer immediately if there is cause for suspicion, since there are more effective treatment measures that may be used.

However dysfunction may occur in viscera also. Asthma is an example of a condition where the function of the viscera is not normal and yet the structure is not (necessarily) pathologically damaged. Here the control of the airway diameter is aberrant and reacts in an exaggerated or inappropriate fashion, thus producing an acute episode which involves both inappropriate narrowing and excessive secretion of mucus. Because the changes are reversible this may be described as a functional disorder as opposed to structural or pathological. There are probably both neurological and local tissue mechanisms involved with the exaggerated reactivity of the lungs.

A further example of a functional visceral disorder is irritable bowel syndrome. This results from hyperirritability of the gut. It involves irritation of the gut wall and resulting abnormal gut motility. Again this does not result in bowel pathology and is a reversible state. It is a good example of a multifactorial condition since it is affected by a wide range of stressors which may be in different domains; for example, emotional stress, general fatigue, diet and possibly mechanical dysfunction also.

There are times when osteopaths may be able to help people with visceral problems. This will depend on whether there are 'mechanical' factors affecting the visceral function that are amenable to treatment.

INTERACTION OF DIFFERENT PARTS OF THE BODY

As discussed in philosophy 1 above, a problem in one part of the body may interfere with the functioning of another part and thus predispose the second area to strain or dysfunction. There are a number of mechanisms by which parts of the musculo-skeletal system may interact.

Neurological interaction

When there is local injury, as will be seen in the next chapter, there are both local tissue responses and also reflex reactions within the neurological system. This may involve reflex changes in muscle tone locally in the damaged area but it may also involve more widespread effects within the musculo-skeletal system and at times in the autonomic system.

Somato-somatic interaction

Sensory information may be transmitted by nociceptors (and other receptors) from damaged tissue. When reaching the spinal cord, if the intensity of the total input reaches a significant level, it may then facilitate other neurones that would not, under normal circumstances, react to a given stimulus. These will particularly occur within the local spinal segment but they may spread further through the spinal cord and to higher centres. The most obvious effect at a higher level is, of course, the perception of pain but there may be effects on muscle tone in other areas where there is already dysfunction present for other reasons. It is as if dysfunction in one area makes it more reactive to other reflex activity.

Viscero-somatic interaction

There are three possible relationships:

1 Pain is referred from a somatic structure to a visceral area and the pain is misinterpreted as originating from the viscera

In the past there have probably sometimes been errors of interpretation when pain from somatic structures has mimicked visceral disturbance. The patient has been treated by manipulation for intense chest pain which may even have been ascribed by their doctor to angina pain. When relieved of their chest pain by treatment the patient then erroneously believes that the manipulation has 'cured' their heart problem. Regrettably, cases of misdiagnosis of this kind do indeed occur.

2 Nociceptor stimulation from a visceral structure may cause somatic dysfunction within the neurologically related segment or segments

In the same way as in somato-somatic reflex interaction there are neurological pathways between visceral and somatic structures. Thus as well as causing referred pain in somatic regions there may also be signs of somatic dysfunction including increased muscle tension and mobility of the spinal joint, and altered soft tissue texture in the spinal area also.

3 An area of somatic dysfunction may modify autonomic output to related viscera

It is likely that the thresholds for these pathways are higher than local and even distant reflex routes within the musculo-skeletal system, but nevertheless they may well lead to interaction. The higher threshold is probably highly significant in reducing the impact of the somatic system on the viscera. Thus not all somatic dysfunction will cause abnormal visceral function; even if there are abnormal autonomic impulses to a viscera this will not necessarily cause any symptoms or signs. However, the effects of the autonomic reflex changes may combine with other stress factors to precipitate symptoms. For example, mid-thoracic somatic dysfunction may cause altered sympathetic tone to the stomach. It is known that the bacteria *Helicobacter pylori* predisposes the stomach to ulceration but that its presence does not always initiate the breakdown of the gut wall. It is conceivable that the abnormal autonomic impulses may also be one factor that predisposes the stomach to *H. pylori*.

The autonomic nervous system influences not only the internal viscera but also has a major role in the control of blood flow throughout the body and the body temperature by sweat gland activity. It was an early observation by osteopaths that, when mechanical dysfunction was present, changes in the soft tissues were sometimes visible and palpable in areas that were related by having a nerve supply associated anatomically at the spinal cord level. Often the tissue was more puffy due to tissue oedema and warmer due to increased blood flow. (See also 'Autonomic response' in Chapter 2.)

Extra-segmental interaction

The previous neurological interactions tend to occur within one spinal segment. However, as will be described in Chapter 2, there are also neurological responses that extend throughout the nervous system. Therefore dysfunction in one area may affect another area.

Static mechanical strain

Where there is abnormal function for some reason in the musculo-skeletal system this may cause increased static or dynamic strain on adjacent or distant areas. Some of the examples given above that cause abnormal mobility also cause alteration in shape. An osteochondritic area in the spine will be stiff. In addition, when it occurs in the thoracic spine there will be an increased kyphosis and when in the lumbar spine there will be a flattening of the normal lumbar lordosis. Because of the alteration of shape and because there is loss of flexibility, the local area is unable to conform to the normal body shape. Therefore other areas of the body have to adapt or 'compensate' for the abnormality. For example, with lower thoracic osteochondritis there is commonly an increase in the lumbar lordosis. This adaptation usually involves changes in the soft tissues, particularly the muscles and fascia. This will be discussed further in Chapter 3.

Dynamic mechanical strain

Abnormalities of shape put increased strain on adjacent and distant areas, causing static or 'postural' strain. However, any of the causes of reduced mobility listed above will increase strain on adjacent and distant areas of the body when movement occurs.

Many of these conditions cause loss of mobility as well as alteration of shape. For example osteochondritis causes increased relative flexion in the spine but it also leads to restriction in all ranges. This imposes dynamic strain on surrounding areas.

With both dynamic and static stress other areas of the body cope with the increased strain placed on them; they 'compensate' for the abnormality. The areas that have to cope with the increase in strain may eventually become symptomatic due to accumulated stress. This is then described as a breakdown of compensation.

Mechanical interaction of somatic and visceral structures

Disturbance of visceral activity may cause changes in the musculo-skeletal system. Abdominal pain may lead to altered posture involving a slightly stooped position to relieve abdominal pressure. This may cause an aggravation of an already poorly adapted posture. This may then lead to symptoms of postural fatigue in addition to the abdominal symptoms.

Conversely, with marked distortion of the spinal column, visceral function may be impaired because of the resulting deformation of internal organs. Thus lung capacity may be reduced in a patient with a severe thoracic kyphosis and abdominal organs such as the stomach may have reduced capacity because of the encroachment of the lower rib cage to prevent normal movement of the hollow viscera. It is probable that this mechanism operates with only marked asymmetry or distortion of the musculo-skeletal system.

With a condition such as asthma there are commonly persistent alterations of somatic function, particularly with chronic or frequent acute attacks. Narrowing of the airways makes exhalation particularly difficult requiring an increase in the work of breathing by the muscles of respiration. Prolonged hyperactivity of these muscles may lead to shortening. This then causes a decrease in the mechanical compliance of the rib cage which further increases the effort of breathing; this may by itself aggravate the asthmatic condition. On an emotional level, the resulting feeling of tightness of the chest may lead to increased anxiety of the patient about their condition. Anxiety is a known stress factor for asthmatics; treatment aimed at releasing soft tissue tension and improving thoracic cage function is often of help in alleviating (though not curing) the asthmatic condition.

WHEN IS OSTEOPATHIC TREATMENT APPROPRIATE?

Osteopaths aim to alter the mechanical function of the body by manual treatment. This may have an impact indirectly on other parts of the body. It may also have an impact on the mind and the spirit; on a simplistic level by merely touching a patient we may comfort them. Touch is a powerful tool and not to be underestimated. However, we must be conscious that problems of the mind and the spirit may be deep rooted and need more direct intervention, using counselling or some other form of psychological help. Similarly, problems in both the somatic and visceral systems may be caused by serious pathology that is beyond the influence of manual treatment. Here, also, referral to other agencies is therefore appropriate. From this it can be inferred that osteopathy is not an all encompassing system of therapy, as Dr Still originally believed, but has parameters within which osteopaths work. It will be clear by now that osteopaths do not treat 'conditions', diseases or syndromes such as a disc prolapse, stomach ulcer or asthma. Appropriateness of osteopathic treatment may be determined from the following questions.

- Is there somatic dysfunction or abnormal musculo-skeletal function present?
- Is this dysfunction related to the symptoms either as a result of or as a predisposing or contributing factor to the immediate cause of the symptoms?
- Is it considered that the dysfunction can be improved or eliminated by treatment?
- Are there any contraindications to treatment?

If so, then osteopathic treatment is appropriate either by itself or in conjunction with other approaches; Case Studies 1.2–1.6 may help to explain this.

Case study 1.2

Mrs A has strained her shoulder while playing tennis without warming up. She appears to have an inflamed supraspinatus tendon with associated palpable marked tightness in her rotator cuff muscles. Here there is a recognizable area of dysfunction with a physical cause which on the basis of experience we can be confident will respond to osteopathic treatment.

Case study 1.3

Mr B has persistent low back pain with severe unilateral leg pain. He has marked weakness of his foot dorsiflexion. He has just started to develop problems with his bladder, with mild incontinence. Here there is probably a serious disc injury, a physical problem with mechanical dysfunction. However, there are serious signs that the disc injury is unstable and bladder incontinence can be a medical emergency that unless dealt with may lead to permanent damage to bladder control. This patient should be referred urgently.

Case study 1.4

Mr C complains of central low back pain which is a constant nagging ache, that is unaffected by any particular posture or movement. When examined there are no signs of local dysfunction in the low back and he has a full range of movement without aggravating the pain. On further questioning he explains that he has been under a great deal of emotional stress and is feeling very down. The absence of physical signs in this patient is important, suggesting that the symptoms are psychosomatic. Since there are no physical signs of dysfunction there is nothing to be treated and therefore, while acknowledging that Mr C's symptoms are as real as any mechanical problem, he would be best advised to seek some psychological rather than physical treatment.

Case study 1.5

Mrs D also has central low back pain which is fairly persistent. She too has been under a great deal of emotional stress and is feeling rather low. However, her pain tends to be worse in the mornings and she is stiff when rising from her bed. She can stand with little pain but sitting for more than 15 minutes aggravates the pain. On examination pain is caused by active flexion and there are signs of dysfunction in the lower lumbar spine. Mrs D has signs of a mechanical problem with identifiable dysfunction which is likely to be amenable to treatment. There may, in fact, be two elements to her problem, a physical back problem and an emotional problem also. At times it may be hard to know how effective treatment may be if the cause of the emotional stress is continuing. However, although the stress may be a contributing factor, by reducing the back pain osteopathic treatment may help Mrs D to cope better with the ongoing stress, because she is no longer in pain.

Case study 1.6

Mrs E has a chronic wheeze as a result of her asthma, which is particularly bad in the autumn. The problem started 4 years ago and has been fairly persistent since, with occasional acute attacks which are controlled by Ventolin and Becotide. On examination there is persistent tightness in the scalene muscles and signs of upper thoracic somatic dysfunction, and the chest is held in a state of relative inspiration. It is controversial to suggest that the reactivity of the airways may be reflexly influenced by somato-visceral reflexes from the upper thoracic area. However, using a purely mechanical model the effect of chronic soft tissue changes may have a detrimental effect on the breathing pattern of the asthmatic patient. Because of the presence of abnormal musculo-skeletal function that is amenable to change, osteopathic treatment is appropriate in this case; the aim is both to reduce the exaggerated musculo-skeletal reaction and also to reverse the chronic soft tissue changes that are now reducing the total expiratory range. Improving the mechanical function of the rib cage reduces the effort of breathing. This may complement other interventions, for instance removal of environmental or dietary allergens. This approach may then allow, with the general practitioner's consent, a reduction of the asthma drugs taken.

SUMMARY: AIM OF THE OSTEOPATH

Where possible the aim is to understand the anatomical and physiological breakdown and the resulting dysfunction in the context of the whole person. The osteopath should attempt to discover where and what the cause of the symptoms are, and also why the dysfunction has occurred, considering aetiological, predisposing and maintaining factors. The purpose of osteopathic treatment and management is then to enhance the body's response by encouraging the restoration of normal function and also to remove or reduce the person's predisposition to the problem.

2 Theoretical aspects of dysfunction

Early osteopaths observed that pain and disability seemed to be associated with areas of palpable restricted joint mobility and abnormal soft tissue texture, and at times apparent bony malposition both in peripheral and spinal joints. By treatment to these areas they produced a reduction of symptoms and restoration of mobility. One or a number of treatments were required to resolve the problem. They described such an area as an 'osteopathic lesion' believing it to be the cause of the symptoms. A. T. Still himself never used this term, preferring to describe problems as strains or dislocations. He also attempted to understand the local problem in the context of the rest of the body.

With the increasing emphasis on the osteopathic *lesion* some practitioners became absorbed with finding the 'lesion' only. The term gradually lost favour and it was eventually replaced by the term 'somatic dysfunction'[6]. The change was prompted for two reasons: first, it lessened the emphasis on the localized lesion since as will be seen in this chapter somatic dysfunction involves a much wider reaction in the body rather than being purely local to the region of a joint. Second, the use of 'osteopathic' in the term inferred a sense of exclusivity. It is not the case that these lesions are only present in the patients of osteopaths, nor that they can only be identified by osteopaths. Spinal segmental dysfunction is also recognized and treated by physiotherapists, chiropractors, manipulating doctors and others, though they may use different terms to describe it. There are differences of opinion as to the underlying mechanisms causing the observed dysfunction.

The aim of this chapter is to consider some of the possible mechanisms that may explain the observed mechanical clinical findings and thus provide a rationale for mechanical treatment.

DEFINITION OF SOMATIC DYSFUNCTION

In the USA the term has been registered as a classified disease. It is defined as: 'Impaired or altered function of related components of the somatic (body framework) system; skeletal, arthrodial, and myofascial structures and related lymphatic and neural elements.'

'Somatic'
Within conventional medical circles the term somatic refers to the body structures to differentiate it from the psyche and thus includes internal viscera. In

the above definition, somatic is defined as relating to neuro-musculo-skeletal structures only. As we shall demonstrate, this is an artificial differentiation, since somatic dysfunction may be initiated by visceral disturbance and somatic dysfunction may affect visceral structures.

Notice that the above definition does not restrict somatic dysfunction to spinal structures but includes any part of the somatic system. Thus dysfunction may occur around the hip, knee shoulder or any other part of the neuro-musculo-skeletal system.

'Impaired or altered function'

As was seen in Chapter 1, in this context the term function is used to refer to the mobility and ease of movement of a part of the neuro-musculo-skeletal system. It is the altered behaviour of the joint and its surrounding tissues that we are concerned with rather than the actual 'role' of the joint. Function may be altered by many factors (see Chapter 1). However somatic dysfunction occurs when a body part is stressed beyond its normal capacity. This then leads to damage in one or more tissues. Somatic dysfunction is initiated by the body's response to an excessive or abnormal demand on the body. At a tissue level, dysfunction is therefore an *appropriate* response and not an aberrant one, at least in the initial phase. However from an observer's viewpoint a problem is apparent and the sufferer may well experience pain. Thus the body's appropriate response is perceived as dysfunction.

The body's normal response will proceed through a sequence of events which should lead to healing and resolution of the problem. Therefore any therapeutic intervention is directed to promoting and enhancing this process. Our aim is to accelerate the process where possible or to remove barriers to recovery, and encourage the maximum restoration of normal function. The nature of such barriers will be discussed later in this chapter.

Vertebral somatic dysfunction

The osteopathic lesion was initially described according to its characteristic features [7]. These are altered range and quality of joint movement, altered tissue texture in the surrounding tissues, and sometimes apparent asymmetry of one vertebra in relation to its neighbour. Quality of movement refers to the ease with which movement can be passively initiated and continued. There is often increased resistance to movement in an area of somatic dysfunction. Altered tissue texture may include muscle that is increased in tone and more reactive to small movements, palpable congestion of the superficial tissues, changes in the skin temperature and moisture (due to altered autonomic activity involving blood vessels and sweat gland activity). These may vary according to whether the dysfunction is acute or chronic (Table 2.1).

One vertebra may appear to be slightly side-bent or rotated in relation to the next, giving the appearance of an alteration of the 'normal or resting position'. However this is rarely of diagnostic value since it is now appreciated that the body is rarely aligned in perfect symmetry anyway. In the absence of other features of somatic dysfunction vertebral misalignment is of no significance.

Table 2.1 Features of acute and chronic somatic dysfunction [8]

Feature	Acute	Chronic
Temperature	Increased	Slight increase or decrease
Texture	Boggy, more rough	Thin, smooth
Moisture	Increased	Dry
Tension	Increased, rigid, board-like	Slight increase, ropy, stringy
Tenderness	Greatest	Present but less
Oedema	Yes	No
Erythema test[1]	Redness lasts	Redness fades quickly or blanching occurs

[1] Erythema test involves firmly stroking the skin parallel to the spine and observing any skin colour change.

Somatic dysfunction in other parts of the neuro-musculo-skeletal system

Injury to one or more tissues around any other part of the musculo-skeletal system will lead to a similar response. For example, a tear or irritation of one of the muscles or tendons of the rotator cuff surrounding the gleno-humeral joint will cause not only local inflammation but also palpable altered muscle tension in the rotator cuff muscles and also often in the periscapular muscles. Limitation of movement as a result of pain is usually obvious in one or more ranges. Hyperaesthesia is usually present in both the muscles and over the tendons involved.

Secondary dysfunction

With the above example of a tendonitis in the rotator cuff muscles there may also be reflex changes in related spinal areas. The sensory supply from the shoulder region principally enters the dorsal horn in the C5–6 region. It is therefore most likely to affect reflex behaviour in other tissues with their motor control in this part of the spinal cord, i.e. spinal muscles controlled by the C5–6 segment.

Often it is easier to establish which specific tissue is damaged when a peripheral joint is involved, but it is important not to lose sight of the effect that the local lesion has had on the function of the region affected and on the body as a whole. Thus a muscle or tendon injury in the hip area will alter muscle tone in other muscles around the hip, as well as the involved muscle. It may also, therefore, affect the sacro-iliac mobility. Because of altered gait more strain may be imposed on the spine. This may lead to further dysfunction with or without symptoms at a number of sites, particularly if there is already predisposition due to previous strain or pre-existing dysfunction.

Similarly dysfunction in part of the spine may have an effect on another part via altered reflex behaviour. These neurological effects will be described later in this chapter.

Visceral dysfunction

Dysfunction is not a process restricted to the somatic structures. Indeed there are many examples of abnormal function in visceral structures in the absence of structural pathology such as heart arrhythmia, irritable bowel syndrome, asthma, migraine and hypertension. In the past some osteopaths have attempted to infer that all disease results from the presence of spinal lesions. This is a highly simplistic contention and has no validity. In the examples of visceral disturbance listed above the cause of the problem is not within the musculo-skeletal system. However visceral dysfunction may interact with the musculo-skeletal system via the mechanisms discussed later in this chapter. The systems should not be viewed in any sense as mutually exclusive; on the contrary, they are highly integrated. Thus visceral disturbance may be modulated by the presence of somatic dysfunction and in theory osteopathic treatment may influence visceral dysfunction by reducing or removing the somatic dysfunction.

POSSIBLE MECHANISMS OF SOMATIC DYSFUNCTION

There are a number of possible mechanisms that may be involved in the generation and maintenance of an area of somatic dysfunction. These include:

- Altered neurological reflex responses affecting muscle tone and reactivity around a joint.
- Prolonged oedema in injured tissues causing altered tissue elasticity.
- Formation of intra-capsular adhesions causing loss of mobility.
- Facet joint 'locking' involving the trapping of an intra-capsular villus between opposing surfaces and consequent restriction of movement.

It is conceivable that at different times even in the same patient one or more of these mechanisms may play a part. To see how, first explore the body's normal response to any damage that occurs. Then it is possible to explore how the somatic dysfunction may develop.

In addition to the effects of tissue damage, somatic structures may also change as a result of adaptation for everyday stresses, as described in Chapter 1. For instance, muscles subjected to prolonged postural strain may become hypertrophic or fibrotic. This may be an appropriate adaptation but it may still lead to altered mobility of an area which then predisposes the person to injury either in that or another area. Depending on the cause, adaptive changes usually develop in a large area and involve a group of myofascial tissues. These adaptive changes are not due to dysfunction but may predispose to it.

RESPONSE TO A BODY INJURY

The body framework may be damaged by excessive mechanical strain. This may be due to one sudden trauma such as a car accident or an awkward body movement when a joint is under considerable load, for instance twisting on one knee while kicking a football. Smaller forces involved in repetitive movements may lead to gradually increasing irritation of muscles or joints, perhaps while performing a task sitting at a desk which requires twisting to a drawer to one side of the desk. Prolonged postural stress imposed by sitting at a poorly adapted computer workstation may also eventually cause soft tissue strain.

When the body is injured in some way a number of defence mechanisms are initiated. There are two important components to this response (described below), involving local tissue inflammation and a neurological response, which occur both locally and further afield within the nervous system.

It must be emphasized that the components of the body's response are non-specific with regard to the nature of the tissue damage. Thus the dysfunction resulting from a disc injury will be similar to that resulting from irritation of other structures in the spine. There may be differences but these are rarely enough to provide confident differential diagnostic criteria. This will be explored in more detail later in this chapter.

Tissue inflammation

If trauma causes tissue damage then a chemically mediated inflammatory response is initiated. This will cause a degree of hyperaemia in the local tissues, leading to swelling in the immediate area. The swelling will contribute to the altered tissue texture if the damage is near to the body surface. In addition, swelling in or around a joint will alter the viscosity of the joint and the elasticity of the peri-articular region, and consequently mechanical function will be altered. This may contribute to the palpable finding of altered 'quality of movement' by the osteopath. Quality of movement refers to the resistance to movement within the natural range.

The release of chemical mediators will stimulate local nociceptors and if the stimulus is great enough this will cause pain. The perception of pain is not the result of a simple sensory stimulus (as is light touch or temperature) but a very complex process. This will be discussed later in this chapter.

The inflammatory response is an ongoing process (Figure 2.1). After the initial hyperaemia and swelling the tissues become gradually more organized by the white blood cells which lay down granulation tissue consisting of random collagen. This occurs within 5–7 days. Over the following 14 days this is then remodelled to form more organized scar tissue which is laid down in response to the physical stresses placed on the tissues. Prolonged tissue oedema leads to inappropriate scar tissue resulting in decreased tissue elasticity. The local tissue effects may play a significant part in the maintenance of localized dysfunction because of their effect on the mechanical function of the area and may contribute to secondary mechanical effects elsewhere in the body. This has implications for rehabilitation; encouraging a patient to rest most of the time to avoid pain in this phase of recovery is unwise since it will reduce the formation of appropriate scar tissue and result in a weaker repair of the damaged area [9].

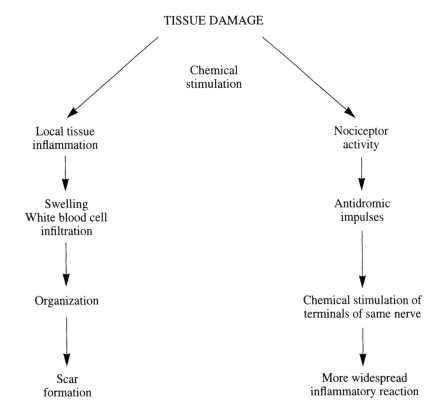

Figure 2.1 Response of local tissues to trauma.

Altered nervous reflex patterns

The neural mechanisms described below were first postulated by Richard L. Van Buskirk in 1990 [10].

As mentioned above, the local chemical reaction caused by the products of tissue damage stimulates particular receptors called nociceptors. These nociceptors are either small myelinated (A delta or type III) and unmyelinated (C or type IV) neurones. They have free nerve endings in the periphery and are found in all connective tissues of the body except the interstitial spaces of the brain, i.e. in periosteum, muscle, fascia, tendons, ligaments, joint capsules, subdermis and dermis, all blood vessels except capillaries, in meninges and in viscera [11].

These nociceptors respond to a variety of stimuli including strong mechanical force (enough to damage or deform the nerve endings), temperature greater than 45°C, the presence of a variety of chemical irritants in the vicinity of the terminals including prostaglandins, histamine, bradykinin and lactic acid. (These are known as *noxious* stimuli.) If the stimulus is great enough the signalling of nociceptors may cause the *perception* of pain by the CNS. However the absence of pain does not mean that nociceptors are inactive. They may still activate reflex responses without causing consciously experienced pain.

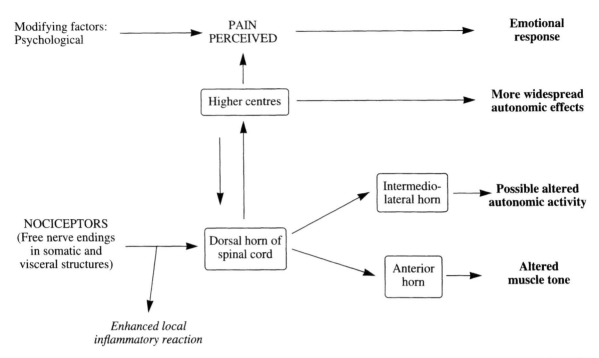

Figure 2.2 Summary of possible reflex responses resulting from nociceptor stimulation. These depend on the degree of sensitization of the dorsal horn both by nociceptors and also by influences from the higher centres.

The emphasis above on the free nerve endings being nociceptors is not to infer either that this is the only function of free nerve endings nor that the perception of pain may only be mediated by these receptors; high levels of stimulation of other receptors are also believed to contribute to pain. In addition, pain may be generated within the CNS without any peripheral stimulation.

Nociceptor stimulation causes responses in related local nociceptor terminals, in related areas of the same segment of the spinal cord and in supra-segmental reflexes including the higher centres (Figure 2.2).

In local related nociceptor terminals

Each nociceptor nerve cell body has a number of fibres passing from the dorsal root horn to the periphery and these fibres may divide further, supplying quite closely related areas of a tissue (Figure 2.3).

There are important implications to this anatomical arrangement. When a nociceptor is stimulated, this generates action potentials which travel to the CNS (see below). However, it has long been recognized that the action potentials will also travel in an antidromic fashion to the related nerve terminals. It has been observed also that this triggers release of chemicals from these related terminals which stimulate a further inflammatory reaction in these areas. This appears to be the basis of the 'flare' response to a surface skin insult and is a demonstration of the body's second phase of the inflammatory response.

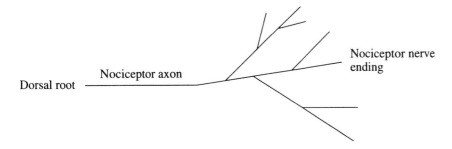

Figure 2.3 Branching of nociceptor axons.

As well as stimulating and potentiating inflammation in the region, the increase of chemical mediators in the area, such as substance P and 11-amino acid neuropeptide, causes a further decrease in the threshold of the nociceptors [12]. If there is damage to somatic tissues that results in inflammation, then the inflammatory chemical cascade may cause persistent nociceptor stimulation. This may lead to a cycle of muscle spasm and hyperalgesia that results in persistent pain [11].

In 'segmentally' related areas

In the early days of research by Korr and others into the neurological mechanisms that might underlie the observed findings of the osteopathic lesion, emphasis was focused on the spinal segment. A spinal segment includes two vertebrae, the intervening disc and associated tissues. A segment also has a nerve root that emerges on either side of the spine and supplies a multitude of structures in more distant parts of the body.

Segmentation of the spine occurs in the first few weeks of intrauterine life. As the fetus grows each part of the body draws with it its nerve supply. For example, branches of the nerve roots C3–5 not only supply the neck region but also reach down as far as the diaphragm. If a nerve root is compressed, in theory all the tissues supplied by this nerve root will be affected. Fortunately, serious nerve root compression is relatively rare and even when it does occur often only partial compression occurs. However, it is the proximity of the synapses of the entering afferent fibres in the dorsal horn that are equally important with regard to segmentation.

The dorsal root area is not segmented but is a continuous region along the length of the spinal cord. Thus for instance the information entering from the T4 root may overlap with the territory of the dorsal horn that receives input from the T5 root. Although often one spinal segment appears to be affected, the effects almost certainly will spread into adjacent segments, though to a lesser degree. Thus muscle hypertonia and reactivity may be increased in segmentally related muscles, but this may also extend into other associated areas.

When damage occurs in the periphery a barrage of nociceptor activity causes 'sensitization' of the dorsal horn. (This is known as central sensitization [13].) This causes reduced thresholds, increased spontaneous discharge, an increased response to afferent input (hyperalgesia), increased response to repeated stimulation and an expansion of receptive fields.

It has been demonstrated that neurones from different somatic structures may converge on the same interneurones. Thus in experiments on cats a single neurone in the dorsal horn may be stimulated by mechanical pressure on the skin, facet joint, ligament or muscle [14]. There is also convergence of axons entering separately from visceral and somatic structures. This means that they may synapse on the same or adjacent interneurones in the dorsal horn and that they may also sensitize pathways from the other type of tissue. The dorsal horn therefore receives a mass of information which it then processes.

This may also have implications for the threshold of pain experienced from internal viscera since pain pathways from visceral structures may be facilitated by somatic nociceptor excitation. It is conceivable, therefore, that affecting the somatic system with manual treatment may at the least alter the pain experience from internal organs. This does not imply necessarily that osteopathic treatment improves the visceral disturbance, though it may bring pain relief while the natural healing response proceeds. Clinical experience suggests that often pain relief can be achieved, if only as a temporary effect. Further clinical research is required to study the impact of manual treatment on visceral conditions.

The convergence of peripheral neurones in the dorsal root may contribute to the phenomenon of referred pain; nociceptors synapse in the dorsal horn from a range of sites and due to facilitation of other pathways the brain misinterprets the area from which the pain originates (but see section on 'Pain' below). Nociceptors from somatic structures therefore may refer to other somatic structures; for example, a noxious stimulus in the lumbar spine may refer to the leg without any actual damage or dysfunction in the leg. (See Figure 5.2.) Grieve has written a review of referred pain mechanisms [15]. Similarly, a noxious stimulus from the heart synapses in the upper thoracic region and the brain interprets the pain as generated in the related somatic structures in the medial arm.

A further consequence of this convergence is that the character of pain is rarely helpful in establishing the cause of pain. An exception to this seems to be pain resulting from nerve root irritation. This is characteristically sharp, shooting in a narrow dermatomal distribution when in a limb. However, nerve root pain does not always present like this, nor is all sharp pain due to nerve root pain.

Axons pass from their ganglia in the dorsal roots and synapse at a number of sites in the spinal cord and brainstem, mainly at the segment of entry, but also they may travel up to five segments cephalad or caudal before synapsing in the dorsal horn [16]. Interneurones may then project to motor neurones in the anterior horn producing segmental reflex muscle responses, to the intermediolateral horn causing autonomic arousal, and to the brainstem and thalamus causing the perception and the affective response to pain.

Altered muscle tone

Any 'protective' motor response is most likely to occur to minimize the stretch of the damaged tissue. This may be in the synergists, in overlying muscles or in the muscle itself by contracting the non-damaged fibres. However, since there may be more than one tissue damaged, the body seems to 'protect' itself by minimizing the total nociceptor input to the spinal cord. With increasing nociceptor stimulation, the neurological segment becomes more highly facilitated and effectively the threshold is lowered in more reflex pathways. This may lead to other muscles supplied from the motor horn of the segment becoming excited. For instance, when there is facet joint irritation in the lower lumbar spine, there may be reflex hamstring spasm which reduces straight-leg raising (SLR). This is not due to nerve root irritation because the hamstring spasm and restricted SLR may be eliminated within 5 minutes by anaesthetic injection of the inflamed facet joint [17].

The overall result at the segmental level of the nociceptor activity is that the spinal cord is *facilitated* and appears to be more reactive to most stimuli.

Even with a mild level of facilitation, a small movement causes an excessive response in the local muscle, commonly greater in one or more ranges but not usually all. Stimuli from any sensory receptors within the segment may contribute to increasing the exaggerated reaction in the related muscles. Also nociceptor stimulation in more distant areas of the body has been shown to cause a muscular reaction in the disturbed segment, demonstrating the hyper-reactivity of the segment [7].

Non-neural influence on muscle tone
Prolonged muscle tension may also be maintained by non-neural mechanisms. The tone of a muscle is proportional to the force required to stretch it. There are two components in a muscle that contribute to this (Figure 2.4): the passive connective tissue including the intramuscular fascial supporting structure and the fascia that surrounds the muscle itself, and the contractile fibres of the muscle. At rest the muscle usually is electrically inactive [18], thus any resistance to stretch is due to the connective tissue element. This is important when considering the palpation of muscle states. However it must also be noted that manual palpation causes an immediate electrical response. When there is dysfunction present the muscle is more reactive electrically in the involved area than in adjacent areas.

If a muscle is maintained in a contracted state for a sustained period there will be shortening of the non-contractile connective tissue by cross-bridging of collagen fibres. (This is potentially reversible with sustained stretching.) This will occur as a result of sustained postural muscle tension or from hypertonia secondary to dysfunction. Although the hypertonic muscle may and frequently does become neurologically inactive when the person lies horizontally, as soon as they become vertical there is increased tension compared to their normal state and thus sustained shortening occurs. When lying down it is unlikely that they will lie in a position that stretches the muscle and thus the shortening is maintained by connective tissue. In addition persistent oedema in muscle and other soft tissues may also add to the reduction of elasticity and a consequent increase in apparent muscle tone.

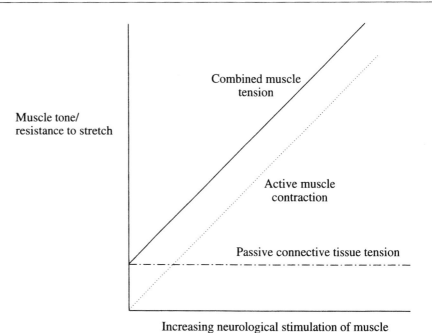

Muscle tone/
resistance to stretch

Combined muscle
tension

Active muscle
contraction

Passive connective tissue tension

Increasing neurological stimulation of muscle

Figure 2.4 Components of muscle contributing to myofascial tone. When a muscle is neurologically inactive there is residual passive connective tissue tension. As a muscle is stimulated by nervous impulses the passive tissue tension becomes of less significance. Persistent active contraction may lead to shortening of connective tissue within the muscle, thus increasing passive tissue tension.

In addition, according to Stoddard, segmental restriction of movement may theoretically be limited by intra-capsular adhesions that may develop within 7–10 days within the joint [19].

Autonomic response
Interneurones from the dorsal horn project to the intermedio-lateral horn which produces the motor output for the sympathetic nervous system (SNS). Most viscera are controlled by local autoregulatory mechanisms, but may be modulated by the autonomic nervous system as the needs of the whole body vary; thus, for example, in a stressful situation visceral function is modified to prepare the body to cope – the 'fright or fight reflex'. Thus high level stimulation of the dorsal horn may lead to reflex activity in the SNS. Since the sensory neurones may project up to five segments either way from the point of entry, then the SNS response is unlikely to be restricted to only one segment. Prolonged stimulation by the SNS can cause alteration of function of a number of body tissues and organs [20]. Thus somatic dysfunction may be one factor of many that contributes to the modulation of visceral function.

In addition to its effects on the viscera, the SNS also sends out branches to all spinal nerve roots. These branches form the vasomotor control system throughout the body. Thus somatic dysfunction may also modulate vascular control in related parts of the body (Figure 2.5).

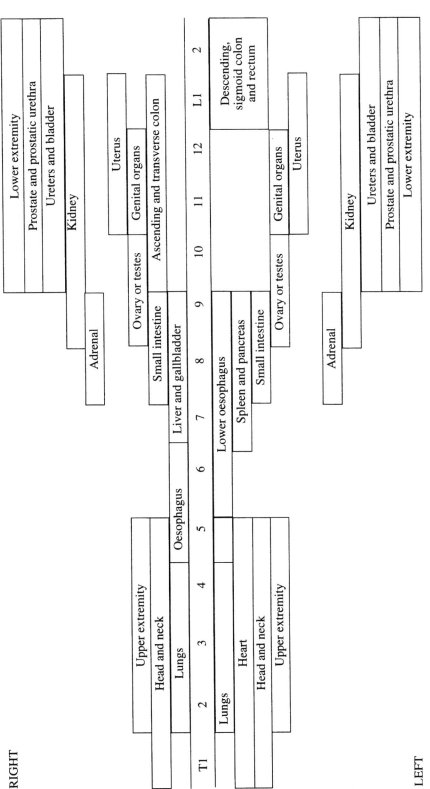

RIGHT

LEFT

Figure 2.5 Sympathetic nervous supply to organs and limbs. The segmental levels given are those from which the sympathetic motor control for the organ or viscus is derived. There is variation between authors as to the exact levels. These should therefore only be used as a guide.

Supra-segmental reflex changes

Depending on the level of stimulation, autonomic responses may include altered heart rate, blood pressure, vasodilatation, gastro-intestinal stasis or bronchodilatation. There have also been reports of temporary alteration in immune function, but the significance in the generation of actual disease has yet to be established.

Persistent alteration of neurological reflexes

It is important to note that although the nociceptor activity appears to be the primary stimulus which triggers off the dysfunction, and may also act to maintain it, Patterson and Steinmetz [21] observed that the resulting somatic dysfunction may be more lasting even if the nociceptive input is eliminated. After a stimulus of only 45 minutes the exaggerated reflex response may last for more than 72 hours. This suggests that the reflexes that are activated are not 'hard-wired' but are 'plastic' and can be altered by stimulation. This has implications for treatment because if the reflex patterns have been changed by injury then treatment of persistent problems will need to address these neurophysiological patterns rather than just the connective tissue changes.

Pain

Pain is commonly perceived when there has been injury within the body. This has led in the past to the mistaken belief that we have simple sensors for pain throughout the body which then 'report' the sensation to the brain via direct pain pathways. It is now well recognized that pain is a most complex phenomenon of which at best we have a partial understanding and which at worst remains in many cases an enigma.

Nociceptor stimulation by injury may cause pain if the degree of injury is great enough. However the perception of pain will be affected by a number of factors. Pain is modulated by higher centres [22], both by regulating descending inhibitory pathways and by the release of endorphins [23]; these centres are in turn influenced by higher centres for attention, emotion and concentration [24]. So, for example, the sportsman playing a contact sport may play on with a serious injury with no conscious sensation of pain, and the pain threshold may be raised in a soldier on the battle-field. Conversely, the threshold may be lowered by social and cultural influences.

Pain can be generated in the CNS without peripheral stimulation. This is common in mental illness. A significant proportion of psychiatric patients complain of pain for which there is no physical cause identifiable; this is known as somatization. The behaviour of pain generated centrally rather than through peripheral nociceptor stimulation is usually different; for example, though the pain may be felt in the limb of a patient, it is not affected by movement or use of the limb or of the neck (which may often cause referred pain in the arm). It is the inconsistency with expected patterns of presentation that should provoke caution in the diagnosis.

Patients with centrally generated pain are not malingerers. These sufferers experience pain that is as 'real' as pain initiated in the body periphery and should be acknowledged as such. There is indeed a problem causing the symptoms which deserves as much care and attention as any other form of pain and disability, but it requires a different therapeutic approach.

Referred pain

The nature of pain as a perception by the CNS as opposed to a peripheral sensation is further emphasized by the experience of phantom limb pain by amputees. This suggests that pain does not happen in hands or feet but in the conscious image of hands or feet. This helps in the understanding of referred pain. When a person experiences pain in the arm that is aggravated by neck movements it is probable that the pain is referred to the arm. Thus the brain perceives the pain as 'in the arm' though there is no actual tissue damage or functional disturbance of the arm. Some have described this as a misinterpretation by the brain. The underlying assumption is that pain perceived as in the arm *should* be caused by local tissue damage. This is presumably based on our early experience where for example if we hit our arm or damage the skin then we clearly associate the pain we feel with the obvious local lesion. Therefore if the heart then causes pain due to ischaemia we assume that pain should be felt in the region of the heart.

Localization of the cutaneous sensation appears to be directly related to the cells in the post-central gyrus of the cortex. Any damage to the skin can therefore be accurately localized. Localization of deeper tissue damage is much poorer; it is reasonable to assume this is because localization is of less importance with internal structures, since the required response will be different.

Various areas of the body have typical referral patterns (Table 2.2). Patterns of pain referral from spinal joints are described in more detail in Chapter 5 (see Figures 5.1–5.5).

Table 2.2 Common examples of referred pain

Site of irritation	*Site of pain experienced*
Cervical joint	Headache
Neck, shoulder	Arm
Heart muscle	Anterior chest wall, medial arm
Thoracic joint	Pectoral, costo-chondral
Gallbladder	Epigastrium, posterior body wall, right shoulder
Lower thoracic osteoporosis	Lower lumbar spine
Lower lumbar spine	Lower limb, groin
Sacro-iliac joint	Posterior thigh and calf, groin
Hip	Anterior thigh and knee, groin

Apparent joint locking

Some patients report that their symptoms commenced not when they experienced sudden significant physical trauma but while performing an otherwise trivial movement such as bending down, not necessarily to their full range, or while performing a slightly awkward movement, for example involving twisting. Pain frequently is initiated as they return to the vertical position and they may then find that their active movements are markedly and immediately limited. In this case it is impossible for the effects of the inflammatory reaction to have developed. There are three main theories to explain this sudden locking:

- Movement of a fragment of inter-vertebral disc material moving and putting pressure on another pain-sensitive structure causing secondary muscle spasm.
- Primary acute muscle spasm. Korr [25] postulated a mechanism of apparent joint locking or restriction resulting from sudden unexpected shortening of muscle spindle receptors which then causes secondary increase in alpha motor unit excitation. This leads to an inappropriate level of neurological stimulation of the muscles surrounding a joint.
- Intra-capsular locking from meniscoid entrapment (Figure 2.6). Meniscoids have been identified in spinal joints by Tondury [26] and in extremity joints by Kos [27]. Kos and Wolf [28] observed that meniscoids have a soft base and a hard edge that does not compress easily. They may therefore be trapped between the opposing joint surfaces thus preventing movement of the joint. This theory does not deny that the reflex phenomena described earlier in the chapter occur, but suggests that they are precipitated by the meniscoid entrapment. There are many instances when a spinal joint appears very restricted or may even feel locked. If then the joint is manipulated, movement may return to normal virtually instantly. It is posited that a trapped meniscoid has been released by the manipulation.

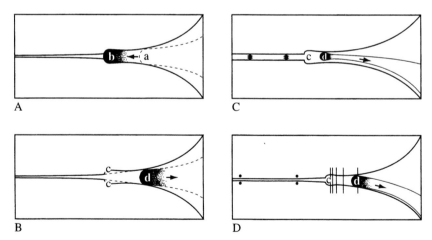

Figure 2.6 A, B. Entrapment of a meniscoid at the edge of a joint space, according to the joint blockage theory of Kos and Wolf [28]. A. The meniscoid normally lying in position (a) has moved between the joint facets and its hard edge has impinged (b). B. It has returned to normal position after treatment. A groove (c–d) remains for a short time, but being flat it offers only minor resistance to slipping back. C, D. The effect of therapy. C. Gapping of the joint by high-velocity thrust, making it possible for the meniscoid to slip back. D. Repetitive mobilization enabling the meniscoid to move back into its original position, first by small degrees and then more rapidly. (From Lewit [49]. Copyright © 1991 Butterworth-Heinemann. Reproduced with permission.)

In practice it is likely that each of these mechanisms may play a part in different patients.

Table 2.3 Summary of responses to trauma

Local inflammation	Palpable tissue changes from oedema and congestion within the damaged tissues and related tissues, i.e. muscles Altered sensitivity of nociceptors
Joint 'locking'	Acute restriction of joint movement
Neurological reflex changes at the segmental level	Increased muscle tone at rest (if asymmetrical then there may be altered joint alignment) Increased muscle reactivity on movement because stimulation from mechanoreceptors is amplified by facilitation at the level of the spinal cord Tenderness due to altered threshold of nociceptors and facilitation Altered autonomic reflexes, e.g. sweat gland activity, microcirculation
Extra-segmental reflex changes	Pain experienced (not inevitable) Secondary changes of behaviour that have been learned previously Interaction with other areas of somatic dysfunction; pre-existing areas of dysfunction may become symptomatic More widespread autonomic disturbance

RESOLUTION OF SOMATIC DYSFUNCTION

Dysfunction is the term used to describe the outward manifestation of the body's attempt to deal with internal injury of some kind (Table 2.3). Under normal circumstances in the absence of any barriers to resolution, the inflammatory process proceeds within the disturbed tissues. Any damaged tissue is removed by white blood cells including neutrophils, macrophages and lymphocytes and repair is achieved by formation of scar tissue. Pain will reduce as chemicals that were previously a source of nociceptor stimulation are removed by fluid drainage of the affected tissues. In addition, nociceptors will normally slowly adapt under chronic stimulation and therefore will not cause persistent spinal cord stimulation.

Depending on the degree of damage caused initially, this normal process may take a matter of a few hours to a few weeks. At what stage does this 'normal' process become dysfunction? If dysfunction is considered to be the manifestation of the body's attempt to deal with internal injury, then even normal healing should be described as dysfunction. The majority of acute dysfunction is indeed self-limiting and resolves spontaneously. It is clear though from clinical experience that dysfunction often does not resolve entirely and may indeed persist for months and even years.

Barriers to resolution

In principle the body's own self-healing mechanisms should resolve the symptoms and restore normal flexibility and function in the musculo-skeletal system. However this is commonly not the case. Quite often, although the symptoms gradually ease, even without treatment, normal function may not be recovered and some symptoms may remain. There are a number of possible reasons for this which are detailed below.

Chronic tissue congestion

Prolonged inflammation sometimes occurs which may lead to the production of inappropriate connective tissue and sustained congestion of interstitial fluid. This will prevent the restoration of normal mechanical behaviour.

One cause for the chronic tissue congestion is an inappropriate level of physical activity. The outcome of a musculo-skeletal injury will be significantly affected by the patient's own management of the problem. The swelling of the inflammatory response tends to peak by 48 hours. If the symptoms are very acute, the patient is best to rest in a comfortable position for 2–3 days while the inflammatory process may still be increasing in intensity. After this time 'controlled activity' is more appropriate. This involves moving the affected part in a cautious and non-traumatic way to ensure that the area is not allowed to stiffen unnecessarily. This is particularly important when there is marked inflammation because, as the swollen area becomes more organized by connective tissue repair, unless it is stretched, it will become less mobile and rehabilitation will take considerably longer. Stretching the affected area may be uncomfortable but not necessarily painful if performed slowly and progressively.

Lack of movement may lead to prolonged stiffness. This may then predispose to further injury later, since the tissues are not able to function as they were before the injury and may then be more vulnerable to physical stress.

Conversely there are patients who will carry on regardless! Attempting to ignore the problem may, especially in the initial phase, lead to excess swelling and this can lead to similar complications as with lack of movement. Excess swelling leads to excess scar tissue formation and shortening of tissues. However, overzealous stretching in the recovery phase may also lead to hypermobility in the affected area. For instance with a ligament injury of a joint, the joint may be less stable because of the ligament damage. If scar tissue that forms to repair the ligament is stretched excessively, then the joint becomes unstable and is predisposed to further acute or chronic injury.

Persistent structural changes

The initial dysfunction may have been triggered by tissue damage that has not resolved; for example, a residual disc prolapse may cause chronic irritation to surrounding tissues. This will, in turn, maintain abnormal nociceptor activity and alter other reflex patterns. Where there has been persistent swelling there may be excessive connective tissue laid down, causing an alteration of mechanical behaviour. There may also be intra-capsular adhesions which cause persistent reduction in the range of movement.

Prolonged altered reflex response within the nervous system

As was discussed above, if there has been persistent stimulation of a reflex pathway for more than a few hours it appears that the threshold of this pathway will become lowered (due to central sensitization) and therefore, even as the stimulus reduces, the motor output of this pathway will be overreactive; this may result in prolonged abnormal muscle tension or, if a visceral reflex, there may be prolonged autonomic stimulation.

Other reflex influences preventing restoration of normal function

Nervous stimuli may be additive due to facilitation in the same segment or even at different levels. So another stimulus such as a minor visceral disturbance may contribute to the maintenance of overactive pathways of nervous activity

Inappropriate movement patterns

On a larger scale because of altered neurological stimulation gross motor patterns may be disturbed. Professor Janda [29] studied the initiation patterns of groups of muscles that are involved in a particular movement and found that 'normally' muscles will contract in a typical order to achieve the movement. If dysfunction existed the muscles would often contract in an abnormal pattern. It appears that these patterns can be retrained, first by restoring normal length of the muscles involved and then by exercises to improve the co-ordination of complex movements.

Persistent joint locking

If a meniscoid becomes trapped, then joint restriction may be persistent. Initially this will be painful but over a period of time the pain may subside with only the joint restriction remaining.

Distant primary dysfunction

A dysfunction may not resolve because it has been predisposed or aggravated by a dysfunction in a different part of the body. For instance, there may be a problem at the lower lumbar spine leading in some way to an increased compensation in the cervical spine. It has been observed by many authors that treatment may be required to the distant area before the local dysfunction is resolved adequately to allow the problem to settle down [15, 19 and 30]. This is an empirical observation; the mechanism behind this may be due to mechanical or reflex phenomena.

Psyche changes

It has long been appreciated that the mind and the body are integrally linked by various physiological mechanisms. If a person is stressed in some way then the muscles tend to be held in a state of hypertonia. This is in addition to any localized muscle tension from dysfunction and therefore compounds any dysfunction present in the body.

The increased muscle tension may also have an effect on the co-ordination of movement patterns. This leads to an inappropriate muscle control; the joint is inadvertently overstressed, leading to further excessive muscle reaction. This is the first step in the development of a new dysfunction.

If a person has been chronically stressed then they may reach a state of adrenal exhaustion. At this stage, because of altered hormonal levels, inflammation and tissue healing may be impaired, leading to slow or inappropriate scar tissue formation.

Long-term effects of dysfunction

Persisting dysfunction will therefore involve:

- Altered mobility of an area.
- Altered soft tissue tension.
- Abnormal stresses on the local joints.
- Increased stress on other areas of the body.
- Altered reflex thresholds in the segment involved.

This may lead to the dysfunctioning area becoming more vulnerable to further problems or if the dysfunction is sufficiently serious, to chronic pain and disability.

Dysfunction may, in theory, predispose to problems in other parts of the body both as a result of mechanical strain secondary to the altered mobility of the segment(s) involved and also because of the altered reflex patterns both within a segment and beyond, in other parts of the nervous system. So, for example, an area of persistent somatic dysfunction in the thoracic area may interfere with the normal reflex behaviour of other areas of somatic dysfunction, for example in the lumbar spine. Therefore the co-ordination of the lumbar joint may be altered such that it becomes less efficient in its movement pattern. It is possible that this altered co-ordination may be a part of the reason why a somatic dysfunction develops in a segment suddenly without any significant trauma.

Another possible interaction would be between somatic dysfunction in a lumbar segment affecting an area of dysfunction in the thoracic area which may have been triggered by a visceral disturbance. The lumbar dysfunction therefore might exaggerate or highlight the visceral problem.

The significance of the effect of persistent somatic dysfunction on autonomic function has long been a controversial issue. In the past it has been suggested that sustained somatic dysfunction may, by itself, lead to visceral dysfunction as a single causative factor. This simplistic belief is not supported by clinical experience. A reasonable comment on this subject comes from Kunert:

> We have no evidence that lesions of the spinal
> cord can cause genuine organic disorders. They

are however, perfectly capable of simulating, accentuating, or making a major contribution to such disorders. There can, in fact, be no doubt that the state of the spinal column does have a bearing on the functional status of the internal organs. [31]

As well as influencing internal organs the sympathetic nervous system has an important role in the modulation of the cardio-vascular system. Theoretically, somatic dysfunction may interfere with normal reflex control and thus affect the blood supply and drainage of areas of the body. The circulation is important in the process of inflammation; any alteration of blood flow resulting from somatic dysfunction, therefore, may affect the repair process. For example, the sympathetic nervous supply to the arm comes from T1–4. Somatic dysfunction in this area might affect the blood supply to the arm. Damage around the elbow for instance, as a result of a musculo-tendinous tear ('tennis elbow'), may heal less quickly if there is somatic dysfunction in the upper thoracic region, and, by implication, treatment to the upper thoracic area should influence the recovery rate. Though this is commonly the experience of osteopaths there is not, as yet, research data to verify this.

Because of increased mechanical stress on a joint, degeneration may be accelerated. These structural changes in turn will have a further effect on function. First there will be a brief discussion on the most significant changes that occur and then the mechanical and clinical implications will be considered.

SPINAL DEGENERATIVE CHANGES

Circumferential and radial tears and fissures develop in the intervertebral disc as early as the teenage years and become increasingly common with age. The nucleus becomes less turgid due to an alteration of the collagen matrix; consequently the disc height may reduce and it deforms more easily and more shearing of the disc can occur [32]. The nuclear pulp becomes more fibrous and the nuclear/annular border becomes less well defined. Any tears in the outer part of the annulus will trigger an inflammatory reaction. This may stimulate scar and vascular tissue to be formed in the outer annulus, which may accelerate further tissue breakdown. Osteophytes may form at the border of the disc, especially at areas of mechanical stress. These may encroach on surrounding structures (Figure 2.7).

Minor trauma causes inflammation of the synovial membrane and capsule, which may lead to reorganization with thickening and fibrosis. Decreased vascularity may result in altered secretion and also loose body and meniscoid formation. There may be a loss of connective tissue and weakening of the spinal ligaments as a result of scar tissue. This may contribute to spinal instability.

Typical osteoarthritic changes may occur in the joint cartilage, initially with minor cracks and later with thinning and breakdown of the cartilage. With more advanced degeneration there is osteophyte formation around the edges of the joint.

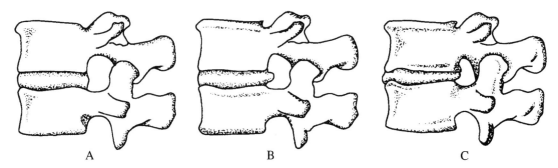

Figure 2.7 Three progressing stages in the degeneration of an intervertebral segment. A. A young intact intervertebral disc. B. The disc height reduces and there is bulging of the annulus fibrosis. As the disc reduces in height there is altered alignment of the posterior joints. C. The disc is further narrowed and the disc bulging is now accompanied by osteophyte formation. There are degenerative changes in the posterior joints also. These combine to cause marked narrowing of the lateral (and central) intervertebral foraminae, which is further compounded by thickening of the soft tissues adjacent including the joint capsule and ligaments.

Effects of degenerative changes on function and dysfunction

The loss of disc height leads to altered segmental stresses [33] and may accelerate degenerative changes of the facet joints. It is common, though not inevitable, to find osteoarthritic changes in the facet joints at the levels where there is disc thinning.

The increase of the possible shearing within the segment, because of disc and ligament changes, reduces its stability. This therefore results in inappropriate strain on other tissues including the muscles and ligaments in the region. This may predispose a spinal segment to intra-capsular locking. This does indeed appear to become more frequent in some patients.

As the instability increases in the late stage there may be encroachment of structures in the spinal canal. This may clinically present in the neck as cervical myelopathy (see Chapter 8) and in the lumbar spine as spinal stenosis (see Chapter 11).

With disc height reduction there will be narrowing of the vertical dimension of the root foramen. This foramen will be further reduced horizontally by osteophyte formation from both disc and facet joint. This may be further complicated by disc bulging. These structural changes do not necessarily cause symptoms of nerve root encroachment, since it has also been observed that the spinal nerve roots reduce in size with ageing by loss of their surrounding connective tissue. However the nerve roots may be more vulnerable because of this and therefore, if traumatized, may become inflamed and cause intense nerve root pain.

Fibrosis and consequent shortening of the facet capsule and synovium and of the spinal ligaments may combine to reduce the flexibility of a segment. This may have mechanical implications for adjacent or distant parts of the body which have to compensate for this loss of function. At a local level the loss of movement may have a detrimental effect on the nutrition of the tissues of the particular segment, since movement of the tissues has an important role in fluid exchange which enhances nutrition.

Since dysfunction also causes a reduction of mobility, chronic dysfunction may theoretically lead to a reduction of local tissue nutrition. In association with other mechanical effects resulting from a dysfunction it is conceivable that degeneration will be accelerated. Clinical observation appears to bear this out.

Clinical significance of signs of degeneration on X-rays

There are frequently mild to moderate degenerative changes seen on X-rays taken of patients over the age of 40 and sometimes below. Although we may assume that this is an indication that there is increased mechanical strain being absorbed by these areas, research has demonstrated that there is little correlation between the X-ray observations and the patient's experience of symptoms, except where there are signs of gross degeneration [34].

It is important therefore not to assume that the symptoms are merely due to 'arthritis'. There may be either dysfunction that is primary or is secondary to degenerative changes which may be amenable to manipulative treatment (Figure 2.8).

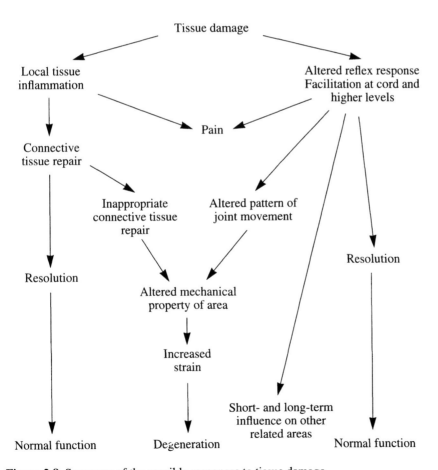

Figure 2.8 Summary of the possible responses to tissue damage.

DIFFERENTIATION OF THE CAUSE OF PAIN AND DYSFUNCTION

Tissue disturbance may result from chemical and infective irritation as well as mechanical irritation. Each will potentially cause dysfunction of the local and also related tissues as discussed above. Thus the manifestation of the disturbance from various causes may have similarities. For example, back pain may be caused not only by irritation of spinal tissues as a result of mechanical strain but also by a multitude of other causes including disease of bone, spinal cord or internal viscera. These may all initiate signs of somatic dysfunction. However it is usually possible to differentiate that the cause is not a benign mechanical cause because the 'pain behaviour' is different and with visceral disturbance there may be other symptoms of altered function of the viscera itself; for example, dysuria and frequency with a kidney infection, diarrhoea with bowel irritation, altered menstrual pattern with a gynaecological cause. It is important to establish the nature of the problem in these examples because, although osteopathic treatment may be able to help, in many cases there are often better, more effective, treatments that are available. In some problems, such as cancer, osteopathic treatment is inappropriate and, if forceful techniques were used, potentially harmful. It is therefore essential to establish whether the problem is primarily due to strain of musculo-skeletal tissues, or to a dysfunction involving a viscera or other non-somatic tissue (e.g. migraine, asthma, irritable bowel) where there is not irreversible pathological change or whether there is a more serious underlying cause. This does not mean that osteopathic treatment can only deal with purely musculo-skeletal dysfunction. Often non-musculo-skeletal problems may have a somatic component that is amenable to treatment (see philosophy 8 in Chapter 1).

Pain resulting from mechanical irritation of spinal structures may cause local and possibly referred pain in the legs and signs of somatic dysfunction in the low back region. The manifestations of joint restriction and other tissue texture changes will not necessarily be specific to the particular tissue damaged and thus it is not easy to differentiate for instance between a disc and an apophyseal joint injury. How important is this to the osteopath? Since we principally aim to treat the effects that have occurred in the tissues, and thus how the body has responded to the tissue damage rather than the actual damaged tissue, it is not necessarily essential to differentiate between these two mechanical causes. This may be possible by considering the details of the clinical presentation, using information in both the history and examination. This will be discussed in Chapters 5 and 6.

However, where possible it is important to ascertain the nature of the tissue breakdown because this may have a bearing on the prognosis. For instance a serious disc injury is likely to take considerably longer than a minor facet joint disturbance. Prognosis will, of course, be influenced also by many factors in the body, mind and spirit.

In addition, the nature of the tissue breakdown may be relevant to what particular technique is used. For instance if there is a disc injury, there is the possibility that the disc material may be unstable, and forceful manipulation might therefore aggravate the situation. If there is a possibility of a disc injury, even though we are not sure on clinical examination, it is wise to use a more gentle technique to encourage normal function rather than risk further irritation of the problem.

WHAT THEORETICAL EFFECTS MAY TREATMENT HAVE?

Manipulative treatment has a number of theoretical effects on the body. (Specific techniques are discussed in Chapter 4.)

Fluid movement

Fluid movement is essential to maintain normal tissue activity since it provides transport of oxygen and other nutrients and removes waste products. The movement of fluid through tissues is particularly important when damage has occurred.

Fluid movement is primarily initiated by the heart pumping arterial blood around the cardio-vascular system. This produces fluid pressure gradients within interstitial spaces and this is a significant force in driving fluid on into the venous system. However fluid movement is also enhanced by the pumping action of muscles which occurs when there is movement of joints. Active contraction of a muscle causes an increase of pressure within the muscle and this drives fluid into the venous and lymphatic systems. These both have valves within their vessels, particularly in the lower extremities. Within the torso the action of the diaphragm has a significant effect on the intra-thoracic and intra-abdominal pressure, as well as a direct massaging effect on the internal viscera, causing a pumping action within these cavities.

Techniques such as gentle articulation, efflurage or soft tissue massage may enhance tissue drainage, by encouraging excess fluid in inflamed tissues into the lymphatic circulation. However if techniques are applied too vigorously then the inflammation may be further irritated. With very acute tissues, techniques are best employed in a gentle rhythmic fashion within the pain-free range.

Neurological reflex response

It is believed that a range of osteopathic techniques have an effect on the reflex behaviour that has been altered in somatic dysfunction. Wyke [35] has described the effect of passive movement on type 1 and 2 mechanoreceptors (which are mainly found in joint capsules). Stimulation of these receptors acts to modulate the transmission of nociceptive afferent activity in the dorsal horn of the spinal cord thus reducing pain perception. Mechanoreceptors also have a reflex effect on fusimotor neurones which are involved with stretch reflexes via the muscle spindles. The effect is to reduce the excitability of the stretch reflexes. As a result there is a palpable reduction in resistance to movement and an increase in range if the technique has been effected correctly.

Indirectly these techniques may also have an effect on the fluid congestion. This may be worsened because the altered reflex activity may reduce fluid drainage from the damaged area by its effect on sympathetic control of the local circulation. If the manipulative technique alters the neurophysiological response, including the sympathetic supply to the injured area, then fluid drainage may be improved.

These techniques may also have a direct effect on the circulation thus enhancing the reduction of congestion but, particularly with the gentle methods such as functional and counter-strain techniques, this is relatively unlikely, since there is very little movement actually employed in the manoeuvre.

Connective tissue

As the inflammatory exudates start to organize the damaged tissues it is important that the body lays down appropriate scar tissue. During the healing and restoration phase of connective tissue repair it is important that bundles of collagen are formed in the correct orientation, i.e. along the lines of force that the connective tissue has to resist. Controlled activity will help with this as the body part involved is allowed to be used with care. This stimulates scar tissue to be formed along lines of physical stress. However sometimes scar tissue will lead to tissue shortening and altered mobility of an area. Manipulative treatment helps to stretch the joint and surrounding structures and enhances the restoration of normal mobility [36]. It is widely accepted that physical therapy is helpful even at an early stage of rehabilitation, even before active mobilization may be possible.

Myofascial tissue

Myofascial tissues may become shortened, altering the function of the affected area of the body, and thus may predispose to dysfunction. Treatment using stretching techniques such as muscle energy, soft tissue massage and articulation may be of benefit.

Release of joint locking

If there is joint locking, for instance as a result of meniscoid entrapment, then specific manipulation may release this rapidly either with a single high-velocity thrust, muscle energy technique or with careful articulation.

SUMMARY

For a variety of reasons the body may develop an area or areas that are not functioning normally as demonstrated by altered mobility and other tissue changes. This 'dysfunction' may be short lived or persistent. In the early phase the dysfunction involves a local tissue reaction and a more widespread response through related areas of the nervous system. This in turn may cause an alteration of muscle tone and visceral activity as part of the body's response to trauma or stress.

If this dysfunction is maintained then there may be further tissue changes involving organization of the inflamed areas, leading to scar tissue and possibly shortening of the affected tissues, producing local and distant mechanical effects. In the longer term these may predispose to an acceleration of degenerative changes.

Our task in assessing a patient therefore, is to evaluate the functional changes that have occurred by:

- Locating areas of dysfunction, both symptomatic and asymptomatic.
- Where possible assessing the cause of the dysfunction, i.e. discovering the tissues that have been damaged.
- Assessing the state of the tissues by palpation.
- Assessing what factors have predisposed the body to develop or are maintaining the problem.

Based on our understanding of the tissue pathophysiology and dysfunction, our treatment can then be planned to enhance the body's attempts to resolve the problem.

3 | Significance of posture

Musculo-skeletal pain is frequently worse when the patient maintains a particular posture which may be standing, sitting or lying. It is believed by many that poor posture contributes to the likelihood of developing such pain. This chapter explores how and why this occurs and the implications that poor posture has on overall musculo-skeletal function.

WHAT IS GOOD POSTURE?

A good posture is one that uses a minimum of energy to maintain it. This infers that the body is well balanced in both an antero-posterior (AP) and lateral plane. It does not infer any particular shape. However some body shapes have been shown to be predisposed to low back pain, for example excessive lordosis [15], which may cause nipping of ligaments between the spinous processes, and traction stress on the ilio-lumbar ligaments resulting from increased shearing force in the lower lumbar spine, especially when standing and walking.

HOW IS POSTURE MAINTAINED?

Any body position is a posture. It implies a static position, if only temporarily. When standing, the body frame is relatively unstable since it is a tall structure balancing on a small base. The effect of gravity is principally resisted by the bone structure, linked by ligaments and other passive connective tissues. Posture is maintained by a combination of passive connective tissue tension and intermittent muscle tension. If a joint is near the end of its range, for example the hip or knee joint, then for brief periods the body may 'rest' on the ligamentous support of the anterior ligaments of the hip; but, to prevent persistent strain on the ligaments, the anterior hip muscles contract slightly to take the strain from the ligaments. In the spine the joints are held nearer the mid-range and therefore it is less easy to put full stress on the ligaments. However the body may balance for brief periods without muscle activity. If the body sways forward the posterior muscles contract in a controlled manner to prevent the posture becoming unstable and to restore the body to a position of balance. This also occurs in the lateral plane (Figure 3.1). In this way the centre of gravity is maintained within a fairly small range, well within the area of the base formed by the two feet. Nies and Sinnott [37] measured body sway patterns in subjects with healthy backs and those complaining of low back pain and demonstrated a significantly increased body sway pattern in the latter group. The implications of this will be discussed later.

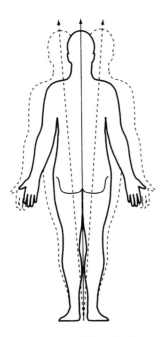

Figure 3.1 Muscle control of body sway. Since the ligamentous spine is inherently unstable when standing, the body is prevented from falling over by highly co-ordinated muscle contractions to bring back the body to a point of more stable equilibrium.

Neurophysiology of posture

Muscle elasticity is the result of passive connective tissue tension and of active muscle fibre contraction. Even when a muscle is electrically inactive there is still some resistance to stretch due to connective tissue elements. The tone of a muscle can only be increased beyond this by active contraction resulting from nervous stimulation. Nervous tone, in turn, is the result of the sum of excitatory and inhibitory influences at the level of the anterior horn synapses which 'drive' the muscle tone. These inputs converge on the anterior horn cells from all levels of the central nervous system.

The maintenance of balance occurs by constant monitoring and feedback through the central nervous system (Figure 3.2). The sensory input comes from proprioceptors in muscles (muscle spindles), ligaments, joint capsules and tendons all over the body, though the upper neck is particularly important in the process. This input is integrated at various levels of the central nervous system (CNS), starting at the segmental level, and then processed at higher levels of the cord, so that the higher centres and cerebellum do not receive direct messages from the individual proprioceptors involved but receive patterns of information regarding body position which it can then process. The

CNS also receives information from the eyes and balance organs in the ears. According to the information received the CNS then initiates motor responses that are required for the immediate maintenance of balance. Simultaneously any changes required in the visceral and vascular systems will be made via the autonomic nervous system, to provide the necessary nutritional support for muscles that are activated. The efficiency with which the CNS affects the change depends to a degree on the conditioning of the neuro-musculo-skeletal system. Perhaps an extreme example is that of the tightrope walker. Here the balance system through practice and repeated training becomes highly tuned. As we will see later, however, there are other factors which can upset these posturing mechanisms.

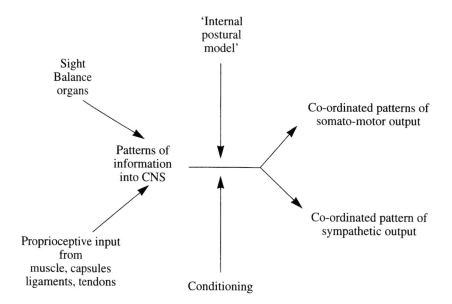

Figure 3.2 Factors influencing control of posture.

Variations in spinal muscle tone when standing

Asmussen and Klausen observed that muscle activity is normally low in the cervical and lumbar spine in relaxed standing [38]. Others, however, have reported that the activity in the lumbar erector spinae muscles varies in different subjects from being continuous in some, intermittent in others and silent in a third group. This probably relates to where the line of gravity lies in relation to the front of the L4 vertebra. If the line of gravity falls through the body of L4 then the erector spinal extensor muscles will be silent, whereas if it lies in front of the body then the muscles will be constantly active to prevent falling forwards. The variation between subjects demonstrates clearly that there are significant differences in posture between members of the 'normal' population. Other authors, however, have reported continuous activity in the longissimus and rotatores muscles during active standing [39].

One factor affecting the AP balance is the tone and length of the abdominal muscles. If the tone is poor the spine may be more extended, with the line of weight-bearing more posterior. Abdominal tone is frequently poor if the patient has excess fat anteriorly or has a sedentary occupation with little physical exercise.

In unsupported sitting, activity appears to be similar to standing in the lumbar spine but is increased in the thoracic spine [40]. Electrical activity in the lumbar spine is reduced, however, if the subject sits with their arms resting on a desk and also if, when sitting, the body is reclined, thus taking the weight of the thorax.

This variation of muscle tension is easily palpated if the osteopath places a hand on the subject's back and gently sways them backward and forward from their point of balance. As the subject sways backwards the muscles will become relaxed as the abdominal muscles contract to prevent falling backwards.

NATURAL POSTURE

It is apparent that an individual tends to have a natural shape or posture that one would recognize even from a distance. This characteristic posture is the result of both physical and psycho-social factors (Table 3.1). It is important therefore to discover during the case history the degree and type of physical activity that the patient undertakes, since this may have a bearing on their posture and the state of their muscles.

Table 3.1 Factors influencing 'natural' posture

Physical factors	Psycho-social factors
Shape of bones	Repeated daily activity, e.g. carrying a heavy bag on the shoulder
Discs	
Sacrum	
Position of the centre of gravity	Lifestyle, e.g. military posture
Body weight/distribution	Training, e.g. model, sway back
Muscle strength/length	Psychological state: depressed, etc.
Structural asymmetry, i.e. short lower extremity	
Osteochondritis causing flexed area in spine	Copying family or friends
Osteoarthritis, e.g. of hip joint	

The physical factors will dictate the range of postures that the body can take up (Table 3.1). For example, if the person has an anomaly such as a hemivertebra then this will have a major impact on the possible configurations of the spine. This will obviously be present from birth. In later years the bones may become softer as a result of osteoporosis and then the spine may gradually flex more, causing increasing strain on soft tissues to maintain a vertical position. The joints may also be modified during life as a result of trauma or degeneration, causing a reduction in the range of postures possible.

Muscle length may limit postural adaptability. Even in children and adolescents muscles such as hamstrings, quadriceps and psoas may be shortened. This will influence the pelvic posture, which has a bearing on the spinal balance also. Muscle length may be further modified by training through excessive use in sport or manual occupations.

The actual natural posture developed will also be significantly affected by the psycho-social factors listed. Barlow [41] discussed the concept of a person's internal postural model based on a number of influences including those factors listed above. He argued that whether the posture is efficient or not, the person will unconsciously correct their posture to conform to their internal model. Any attempt to alter the person's posture by retraining is unlikely to be wholly successful, unless the 'teacher' is able, with the person's co-operation, to alter this internal model. It is the experience of most manual therapists that trying to change a patient's posture just by altering the length or the strength of their muscles is rarely successful.

Another interesting feature of Barlow's work was his observation that the head/neck relationship was very important in affecting the rest of the body's posture. This demonstrates the close functional relationship between different parts of the spine. The effect of dysfunction on postural control is discussed later in this chapter.

A person's state of mind is often reflected in their posture (e.g. compare the posture of two football teams as they come off the pitch!). If the state of mind is prolonged the posture may become relatively 'fixed' because of structural and soft tissue changes which then limit the potential for other, perhaps more efficient, configurations. For example, a person may experience a period of depression which causes them to develop a round shouldered posture. If their lifestyle also becomes less physically active, the soft tissues shorten anteriorly across their shoulder girdle. If and when the depression improves the patient may maintain their previous posture, not because they are still expressing the same emotions but because the body tissues have adapted to this posture.

POSTURAL COMPENSATION

Most of us have less than 'perfect' bodies! The body adapts for various abnormalities in both the body and mind (see Chapter 1). It is rare to see someone who is symmetrical with evenly balanced spinal curves. Indeed, a large proportion of the population have one leg shorter than the other. The body compensates for these 'imperfections' or aberrations from the hypothetical 'norm'. So if there is a pelvic tilt resulting from a short lower extremity then a lateral curvature in the lumbar and possibly to a smaller extent in the thoracic and cervical spine may develop. Postural compensation may also occur when there is a sudden change in the musculo-skeletal system (e.g. a fracture involving the leg) or a slow change such as a progressing osteoarthritic hip that leads to a flexion deformity. With the latter example, compensation will be required in both antero-posterior (AP) and lateral planes, since the flexion deformity not only increases the demand for extension in the lumbar spine but also causes a shortening of the affected leg.

Thus postural compensation is a process of adaptation for asymmetry. In addition to the altered alignment of the bones over a long period, there may be changes of the shape of the joints since they will respond to the effect of asymmetrical strain over a period of time. As we shall see later (see Chapter 7) sometimes quite gross structural changes develop in the joints within an organic scoliosis.

In addition though, even with minor curvature, there may be soft tissue changes. These are also part of the body's compensation and may involve hypertrophy or fibrosis, depending on the level of activity of the person's lifestyle. Where muscles are held in a state of constant contraction, muscle ischaemia and shortening occur, sometimes leading to fibrosis. If, however, the patient is relatively active, by taking part in intermittent exercise, muscle will hypertrophy in areas of the body where the demands on it are greatest.

BREAKDOWN OF POSTURAL COMPENSATION

Compensation may place increased strain on muscles and joints throughout the body. These may be able to tolerate this strain for many years without any problem and this may be considered a successful compensation. However this compensation may be efficient or inefficient depending on how much effort the body requires to adapt. So in the example of a person with a short lower extremity there will be a resulting pelvic tilt. Commonly the lumbar spine may form a gentle lateral curve, which is then balanced by a counter curve in the thoracic spine, thus allowing the centre of gravity to remain in the midline in the lateral plane. An alternative compensation might involve a lateral curvature that did not bring the centre of gravity into the midline and therefore would require a greater energy expenditure by the spinal muscles to maintain balance. Also there would be increased stress on joints to cope with asymmetrical mechanical strain. This increased stress may lead to acceleration of degenerative changes in the joints and to fibrosis or shortening in the affected muscles. These changes may make the area more vulnerable to further stress – it is *predisposed to develop a problem*. Other factors may also contribute. If the body is unable to compensate adequately then symptoms may occur – this is described as a *breakdown in compensation*. Breakdown occurs when the cumulative strain on an area causes irritation of the tissues that triggers nociceptive activity and thus pain.

ACUTE PROTECTION

As discussed in Chapter 1, breakdown of compensation may be chronic or acute. A patient's posture may be markedly altered when damage has occurred to certain spinal structures (see Figure 7.1). For example, with some disc injuries a marked lateral curvature develops that moves the centre of gravity away from the midline and any attempt to restraighten the spine causes pain.

This is described as a 'protective' posture because it appears to be an attempt to prevent or minimize further damage by resisting any movement that aggravates the tissue damage. The posture is maintained by muscle spasm which is presumably mediated by nociceptor activity in the damaged tissue.

Not all acute injuries cause a protective posture. However if there is a protective posture then we may make no judgements about the patient's normal posture. It cannot be observed since the acute posture has been superimposed upon it.

Assessment of protective posture

As can be seen from Table 3.2 there is no posture that is diagnostic of a particular tissue damage. However it is important to recognize when the patient is not standing (or sitting) in his/her 'normal' posture. Because of the adaptive changes that occur in the myofascial tissues as a result of postural demands, it is often important that, when examining a patient presenting with musculoskeletal pain, we should assess the patient's overall static posture, including any structural and functional changes that have resulted from the patient's natural posture, since this may help us in identifying any postural predisposition to a mechanical problem.

Table 3.2 Typical protective postures caused by various tissue injuries and visceral conditions

Tissue	Possible protective posture
Disc herniation or prolapse	Lateral curvature
	Flexion deformity
Capsular inflammation or apophyseal joint locking	Lateral curvature
	Flexion deformity
Sacro-iliac joint locking or strain	Attempt to avoid weight-bearing on the affected leg
	Lateral curvature
Pelvic/femoral fracture	Attempt to avoid weight-bearing on the affected leg
Visceral structures	
Kidney infection	Lateral curvature. *Note:* Compare musculo-skeletal causes: with kidney, side-bending towards the centre of gravity/straightening the spine is not necessarily painful. Pain may be only in the back
Acute bowel condition	Flexion deformity – associated with acute abdominal pain

Features of a protective posture

- The spine is held in an unbalanced position.
- Muscle spasm is inappropriate merely to maintain balance, i.e. muscle tension actively draws the body away from the centre of gravity.

- When asked to perform active movements the patient is unable to move the trunk back towards the midline comfortably. For example, the patient stands with their trunk leaning to the right. When asked to bend to the left, pain is experienced in the back.

Note: The direction of the protective curvature is not related to the side of the pain. For example the pain may be felt on the right side; the protective curve may be to the left or to the right depending on which direction relieves or minimizes the pain.

A common cause of lateral protective curvature is a disc injury. It has been suggested that when the pain is related to nerve root irritation, the direction of the curvature is related to the position of the nerve root in relation to the disc bulge; if the nerve root is lateral to the disc bulge then the scoliosis will be towards the side of pain, whereas if the nerve root is medial to the disc bulge, then the scoliosis will be away from the side of pain. This, however, has been disputed by Porter [42], who found no correlation in a series of 100 patients with a spinal protective scoliosis. The presumed mechanism behind the protective posture is an attempt to minimize the nociceptive input to the spinal cord.

It must be emphasized that, even when the posture appears balanced, the posturing mechanism may still have been altered. Conversely a posture that is not perfectly balanced may be the person's 'normal' posture.

EFFECTS OF DYSFUNCTION ON POSTURAL CONTROL

An inefficient posture imposes greater stress than necessary because it demands more energy to maintain it. However the efficiency of the posture control mechanism may also be reduced. As mentioned previously, Nies and Sinnott measured body sway patterns in subjects with healthy backs and those complaining of low back pain and demonstrated a significantly increased body sway pattern in the latter group. This indicates that when there is dysfunction in the lower spine, then the posturing mechanism tends to overreact, leading to an increase in the extent of sway. This itself will require more energy than optimum.

Further it has been shown that osteopathic treatment can lead to an immediate improvement in the posturing mechanism [43]. Johnston used the hip shift test to examine the posturing mechanism. To perform this test the practitioner stands behind the patient and places his hands laterally on her hips. He gently attempts to sway the subject's hips laterally and assesses whether there is any difference in resistance to initiation of movement to either the left or right. A positive hip shift is reported if there is greater resistance in one direction compared to the other. (Sway tests performed on the whole body are described in Chapter 6.)

Using this test Johnston assessed the resistance to hip shift of a group of patients presenting with spinal pain. Treatment was then applied to any area where dysfunction was identified in the spine. Hip shift was then retested and commonly found to have changed. It is of particular interest that in some patients the only areas of dysfunction which were treated were in the cervical spine, and yet the hip shift changed palpably, implying an interaction between dysfunction in the cervical spine and the posturing mechanism in a distant area. This presumably involves a neurological mechanism since the change is immediate (Figure 3.3).

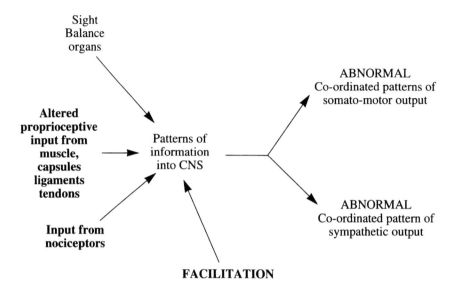

Figure 3.3 Altered neurological control of posture by somatic dysfunction.

Dysfunction therefore causes an alteration in the posturing mechanism. This may not be obvious but may be visible as a result of an acute change in posture. The importance of these observations is twofold. First, it emphasizes the interrelationship of different parts of the body. Second, it provides a different tool by which we can study the whole posturing mechanism of the patient and offers a different and valuable view of assessing musculo-skeletal function rather than simply localized joint assessment.

Chronic postural breakdown

Symptoms may develop gradually, for instance as the result of increasing fatigue of muscles that maintain an inefficient posture. Thus the patient may report that 6 months before she presented, she started experiencing low backache when sitting for more than 4 hours at her desk; by 3 months before, it came on after 3 hours and now it develops after only 10 minutes. The symptom pattern involves the following features:

- Aching or pain that is aggravated by sustaining a particular or a range of postures, e.g. standing, sitting or even lying down.
- The ache gradually builds up while the posture is maintained.

- It is relieved by moving about or changing position.
- Prolonged postural ache is often associated with stiffness when the person moves after a period of inactivity.

What tissues cause the symptoms?

There are a number of tissues that may be involved in the generation of symptoms, including the discs, ligaments, capsules and muscles. If the apophyseal joints have become seriously degenerate, the articular surfaces (or the subchondral bone) may also become pain sensitive. Some or all these may then precipitate nociceptor stimulation. Given that there has been a gradual breakdown, it is highly unlikely that only one tissue is involved. In practice it is not easy to establish which tissues are involved and in terms of treatment it may not be vital to clarify this.

It is not unusual that an underlying area of somatic dysfunction acts to sensitize an area and is therefore more vulnerable to postural strain. As well as altered reflex activity, as discussed above, there may also be chronic connective changes associated with the dysfunction. Frequently, therefore, treatment directed towards improving this localized dysfunction may considerably relieve the symptoms. However it is wise not to deal merely with the localized dysfunction without considering the more widespread changes in postural muscles and fascia that may be involved.

Management of chronic postural breakdown

There are a number of possible approaches to treatment and management:

- Improve local function of the tissues to reduce the fatigue effect that is precipitated by persistent strain imposed by the inability to compensate. This will involve stretching muscles and joints in the local symptom area and enhance fluid exchange to reduce tissue ischaemia.
- Improve muscle stamina by exercises of local muscles.
- Improve postural compensation in other parts of the body. As mentioned above the compensation may have broken down because function in other regions of the body has been altered. It is the task of the osteopath to explore other parts of the body to identify any region where function is less than optimum. Theoretically any body region is linked to any other by a number of mechanisms: these include mechanical, neurological, circulatory and fascial links.

  Some of the more common muscles that may be shortened, and therefore affect the posture because of abnormal muscle balance, are psoas, rectus femoris, hamstrings, lumbar erector spinae and pectoral muscles. It is particularly important to assess these muscles to ensure that they are not limiting the range of postures possible.

  These are not mutually exclusive approaches but may be used together.

EFFECTS OF POOR STATIC POSTURE ON DYNAMIC FUNCTION

Poor static posture can lead to chronic breakdown, commonly commencing with pain that is related to the static posture. However the adaptive tissue changes involving soft tissue shortening may lead to altered dynamic stress on local or distant tissues; thus when undertaking certain movements the body is predisposed to strain and symptoms may therefore be caused on movement *as a result of the postural adaptation* (Figures 3.4 and 3.5). This may therefore present with a chronic or more acute onset.

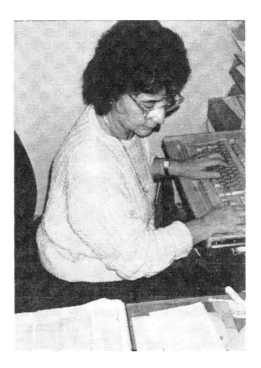

Figure 3.4 Typist with copy always on right side of keyboard.

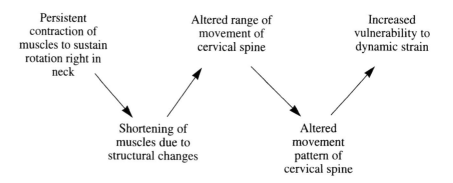

Figure 3.5 Effect of postural strain on dynamic function.

EFFECTS OF POOR POSTURE ON VISCERAL FUNCTION

As discussed in Chapter 2 the viscera may be affected by abnormal reflex activity from facilitation of the spinal cord. However, marked postural asymmetry or increased lateral curvature may lead to altered physical forces on internal viscera. This may then contribute to altered function. In addition, fascial tightness may be transmitted to the thoracic or abdominal contents. This can be palpated and sometimes treated by visceral or cranial techniques.

SUMMARY

Posture is a dynamic process, not a static state.

The range of postures possible is variable within the limits set by a person's structural anatomy. However the posture is psychologically driven, based upon a preconceived mental image. Therefore it cannot be changed purely by stretching and strengthening muscles and soft tissues.

Every person carries imperfections in their musculo-skeletal structure (as well as in other systems and within their genetic makeup). The body will compensate for these abnormalities in an efficient or inefficient way which may be asymptomatic for many years.

As the accumulated stresses build up a breakdown in compensation may occur and symptoms result.

Tissue changes resulting from poor posture may predispose to dysfunction.

Dysfunction in somatic tissues will interfere with neurological control of posture; this appears to be amenable to change by treatment directed at reducing the dysfunction.

Observation of static posture may identify areas of postural abnormalities (e.g. postural asymmetry or exaggerated curvature) which may lead to static or dynamic strain in local, adjacent or distant tissues of the body.

Dynamic strain may result because of restriction of movement of an area of altered curvature (e.g. osteochondrosis or scoliosis).

Even if the posture appears relatively balanced there may still be an abnormal posturing mechanism secondary to somatic dysfunction. This may predispose to dynamic strain as a result of abnormal movement patterns. Thus identification of dysfunction by dynamic postural assessment may help indicate to the osteopath that there are areas distant to the local dysfunction that may be of relevance.

The examination of posture is discussed further in Chapter 6.

4 Approaches to osteopathic treatment

When symptoms occur as the result of irritation or strain of body tissues there is a normal physiological response by the body. The various aspects of this have been considered in Chapter 2. This tissue disturbance will be significantly modified by the state of many other aspects of the person as described in Chapter 1. It is therefore the aim of osteopathic assessment to seek to discover where there is altered function in the body (compared to what is expected in that person), whether musculo-skeletal or visceral, and also what has caused this dysfunction. It is important to establish what tissues are principally involved and also their pathophysiological state.

It is not the intention of the authors to define an 'osteopathic treatment' for any or all of the 'conditions' described later in this book, because treatment is not directed at the 'condition' as much as the resulting tissue dysfunction both locally and in more distant parts of the body.

When discussing osteopathic assessment and treatment, the term 'tissue' is intended to include musculo-skeletal soft tissues, i.e. muscles, their surrounding fascia and dermis and epidermis.

As discussed in Chapter 2, osteopathic techniques are believed to have the following effects on neuro-musculo-skeletal tissues.

- *Fluid movement.* Many techniques enhance the passage of fluid both into and out of tissues and thus help perfusion, particularly when there is congestion resulting from inflammation.
- *Connective tissues.* Inflammation may lead to an increase in connective tissue particularly if congestion is prolonged and tissue shortening may occur. Treatment using passive techniques can help restore normal mobility by gently stretching shortened tissue in a controlled way without further aggravating the inflammation. This is particularly helpful in the early phase, when active mobilization by the patient may irritate the inflamed area rather than help it.
- *Myofascial tissue.* This may become chronically shortened as a result of persistent postural or dynamic strain (as opposed to injury) (see Chapter 3). Various stretching techniques may be useful in reversing these adaptive changes which may have become inappropriate.
- *Release of specific segmental joint locking or restriction.* A number of mechanisms for joint restriction have been discussed. Localized treatment may bring a rapid change in mobility.
- *Alteration of neurological reflex responses.* There appears to be altered (often exaggerated) neurological reflex activity in tissues related to areas

of somatic dysfunction. This includes altered muscle tone and reactivity, which is most marked in segmentally related muscles, altered surface sweating and local tenderness. There may also be altered blood flow in segmentally related tissues, both somatic and visceral. It is believed that a variety of manual techniques may alter these reflex responses, reducing their reactivity towards more normal levels.

- *Reduction of pain.* A consequence of the above effects, particularly the last, will have a beneficial effect on the pain experienced by the patient.

In this chapter various osteopathic manipulative techniques will be discussed and their theoretical effects will be considered.

TISSUE TENSION AND TEXTURE

Palpation of the state of soft tissues as well as the mobility of joints is essential to the osteopath, since most treatment techniques depend on careful positioning of a joint or the sensitive assessment of soft tissue tension and texture. Soft tissue tension refers to whether the tissues feel tight or loose when palpated by directly pressing the muscle. The soft tissue tension may also be palpated by moving a joint and sensing the resistance to movement. Within the range of movement the resistance is mainly from the elasticity of the soft tissues surrounding a joint, whereas at the end of the range the resistance is mainly due to the stretch of ligaments, joint capsule and in some circumstances the direct contact of articulating bones. When the patient under examination is lying down the postural muscles are normally relaxed; if tissue tension is found to be increased this is generally due to increased neurological excitation resulting from facilitation at the spinal cord level (tissue tone and reactivity are discussed in more detail in Chapter 2). However, even a hypertonic muscle may become neurologically inactive when rested, but on palpation the muscle may still feel tighter than normal. This is due to connective tissue shortening, which occurs when a muscle is held in a contracted state for a period of time. This results from increased tension and reactivity of a muscle, as a result of dysfunction which is present when the patient is not resting. In addition, a muscle may be found to be more congested as a result of tissue oedema secondary to dysfunction; this is described as bogginess. This is an example of altered tissue texture; other examples are given in Table 2.1.

The degree and nature of the tissue changes will depend on the cause and the duration of the dysfunction. For instance, after a traumatic injury, the effects of tissue damage and inflammation may be more prominent, with obvious swelling and hyper-reactive muscle. With a dysfunction resulting from repeated minor trauma which has gradually developed, the muscle reactivity may be quite marked, while there is less palpable altered tissue texture resulting from inflammation. With a more prolonged dysfunction passive movement restriction may be the most obvious alteration of function. These different states may be palpable with experience since they affect the tissue texture as well as the range of movement (Figure 4.1).

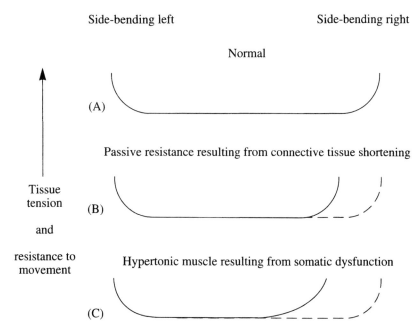

Figure 4.1 Resistance and tissue tension during range of passive movement. As a joint is moved through its range the resistance changes according to the state of the tissues surrounding it. (A) Normal joint; (B) restriction resulting from connective tissue shortening. Notice that the resistance at the end of range is similar to a normal joint but that the range is reduced; (C) restriction associated with joint dysfunction. In addition to reduced range of movement the resistance increases throughout nearly half the range.

Different tissue states may and often do require different techniques or modification of the application of the same technique. For instance, with recent muscle spasm related to underlying joint dysfunction, treatment is probably best directed to restoring the joint mobility specifically, whereas if the dysfunction has been present for some time, there may be shortening of myofascial tissues as well as altered reflex behaviour. These respond well to prolonged stretch techniques.

Specific osteopathic techniques are not routinely prescribed for any particular condition. Techniques are chosen and carefully modified according to feedback received mainly from the practitioner's proprioceptors in his limbs and, to a lesser extent, from direct palpation of the tissues beneath the fingertips.

Wherever possible treatment should be applied in a sensitive way to 'encourage' a change in musculo-skeletal function rather than to impose or force a change. Frequently pressure is applied to tender tissues; if too much force is used the body will react by increasing tension rather than releasing it. If this is palpable to the practitioner then a change in the force or even the technique is necessary. If an inappropriate technique is pursued the patient may well experience an adverse reaction to treatment. In all cases it is wise to employ the minimum force that will achieve the required change in tissue state. Unfortunately, for the inexperienced this is perhaps one of the most difficult judgements to make, since without experience one cannot anticipate how the body tissues will react. However, this is all part of learning a new skill and can only be improved with practice. It is prudent therefore during the first treatment to be gentle. If at the next treatment the patient has made only a little or no improvement, then, so long as there has been no marked reaction to treatment, more forceful treatment may be applied.

MOBILITY RESTRICTION AND 'END FEEL'

When dysfunction is present, as well as an alteration of resistance to movement within the normal range, there is also a reduction in the range of movement in one or more directions of movement. Thus, when the joint is moved passively (and also often when moved actively), the range is restricted in relation to the expected normal (Figure 4.2). This does not necessarily indicate that there is structural pathology present, since the limited range may be predominantly or even solely the result of (reversible) local muscle tension. Conversely there may be relatively irreversible tissue changes, for example adhesions in an adhesive capsulitis or contracture of the connective tissues in a recurrently sprained joint which has healed with repeated scar tissue. It is important to be able to palpate the 'end feel', since this will reflect the type of tissue change that has caused the restriction. The type of tissue state may have a bearing on both the techniques used and the potential change possible, and thus affect the prognosis. An extreme example would be a lumbo-sacral joint that is restricted because it is anomalous or even congenitally fused. In this case there is no possibility of altering the mobility. Given that there is usually more potential for change, the aim of treatment is to improve the mobility towards the normal. The causes of joint restriction and their differentiation are discussed in Chapter 6.

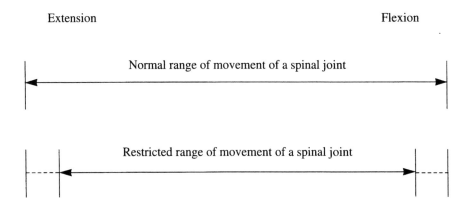

Extension   Flexion

Normal range of movement of a spinal joint

Restricted range of movement of a spinal joint

Figure 4.2 Normal compared with reduced range of movement.

Some muscles may act in only one plane and therefore alteration of mobility resulting from strain, specifically of the muscle, will cause a restriction in that one plane. However, more often, with both spinal as well as peripheral joints, there may be restriction in more than one plane, particularly where the dysfunction involves the whole joint complex. This potentially includes joint ligaments and capsules as well as the surrounding muscles. For some techniques it is important to be able to assess the end point of the range in different planes of movement, since the response to the technique is greater if the end point is localized in a number of planes (e.g. muscle energy technique). For example a spinal joint may move around an axis in an AP (flexion/extension), lateral (side-bending) and axial plane (rotation). In each of these ranges there may be restriction of movement. By placing the joint at the end point in each plane and combining these positions, less force is required to achieve a desired result.

DIRECT AND INDIRECT TECHNIQUE

As suggested above, many osteopathic techniques depend upon finding restricted mobility and in some way increasing it to restore more normal movement. These are known as direct techniques. There are, however, other techniques that involve sensitive palpation of the state of the tissue tension in order to find a point at which the myofascial tissues are most relaxed or 'at ease' rather than finding a barrier which is at a point of tension. These include functional, strain and counter-strain, and cranio-sacral technique. Because they do not require taking a joint to a barrier, patients sometimes feel that 'nothing is being done'. When executed effectively, however, the result can be just as effective and will minimize any adverse after-effects, but there may still be a significant reaction to treatment. These types of techniques, although traditionally applied to musculo-skeletal tissues, may also be applied to visceral structures. Although these visceral structures may be sensitive, they can be approached by such indirect techniques.

APPLICATION OF DIFFERENT MODELS

As discussed in Chapter 1, a clinical model is a particular way of looking at a person and her problem. A psychological model is concerned principally with the mental and emotional behaviour of the person, which would require investigation mainly by verbal discussion or observation. A biomechanical model emphasizes the physical forces involved and the body's ability to cope with them. This may therefore require an examination of the physical properties of the joints of the body, both actively and passively, and of how they adapt to different forces that may be applied. Importance is placed on the mechanical interaction of the various parts of the musculo-skeletal system. Treatment is then directed towards altering the mechanical properties of the muscles and joints by stretching passive structures such as connective tissue and fascia.

An alternative view of this system may consider how the parts of the system are interacting as a result of neurological relationships, as described in Chapter 2 when discussing dysfunction. Here the reflex control of the area involved in the dysfunction is emphasized; the aim of treatment is then the restoration of more normal reflex activity within the nervous system, thus leading to more normal function once more.

It is quite feasible to use different models to understand different patients and also to use different models even while treating the same patient.

EFFECT OF TOUCH

Irrespective of which particular technique is being used, there is a non-specific but very powerful effect of any manual treatment. The experience of being comforted by stroking or rubbing the body surface dates back to our earliest days or even minutes of our lives. Thus careful and caring handling of a patient will have an immediate effect both in reassurance and comfort, which in itself will lead to a lessening of pain. In the past it has been suggested that osteopaths help their patients merely by this psychosomatic mechanism. One should not deny the benefit of touch but it is apparent that if this is the only effect, then the response is temporary for a period of hours or even a few days, but rarely longer. The significance of touch in osteopathic treatment has been explored more fully by Nathan [44].

Table 4.1 Types of osteopathic technique

Rhythmic
  Kneading
    Inhibition
    Effleurage
    Stretching
    Vibration
  Articulation/springing
  Traction
High-velocity thrust
  Combined leverage and thrust
  Combined leverage and thrust with momentum
  Minimal leverage and thrust
  Non-leverage and thrust
  Non-leverage and thrust with momentum
Low-velocity stress
  Muscle energy
  Functional
  Strain and counter-strain
  Cranial
Visceral

SPECIFIC TECHNIQUES

At the British School of Osteopathy, the teaching faculty has defined techniques according to the method of application of force after a classification first proposed by Middleton. These are inevitably arbitrary divisions and some techniques may be included in more than one category. However, this avoids attempting to categorize them on the basis of their perceived effects. Various types of techniques and some of their probable tissue effects will be described briefly here (Table 4.1). The application of these techniques has been discussed in more detailed by Hartman [45].

Rhythmic

Rhythmic techniques involve the application of force to a muscle or joint. The force is most commonly applied until a barrier is met. The pressure is applied in a rhythmic fashion with the intention of moving the barrier back, such that gradually the range of movement and the resistance met decreases. The pressure and the rate of the rhythm used depend on the body's response to the technique; using too much force or too fast a rhythm causes an increase rather than a decrease of resistance.

Kneading

Rhythmic pressure may be applied either parallel to or perpendicular to the length of a muscle. This is the basis of all massage techniques and it has a number of effects. Stretching and massaging a muscle has an impact on the perfusion of the muscle. If there has been prolonged contraction of the muscle, often with resulting muscle ischaemia, then waste products build up; this includes substance P and other chemicals which are mediators in the inflammatory response and in nociceptor stimulation. Massage aids the fluid exchange within the tissues and thus reduces the aching from the muscles. A further effect may be to alter the neurological control from the spinal cord. Slowly stretching a muscle may stimulate the muscle spindles that monitor the length of a muscle. Feedback from these may lead to a reduction of the alpha motor tone to the muscle, leading to palpable relaxation of the muscle. Passively lengthening a muscle may also help to stretch shortened connective tissue resulting from prolonged contraction secondary to dysfunction or postural fatigue. Variations on kneading include inhibition, effleurage, stretching and vibration.

Articulation/springing

Articulation involves rhythmically moving a joint through all or part of its range of movement. It is often used as an examination as well as a treatment technique since the practitioner may assess the range of movement in this way. It may be applied through a long leverage. For example, the lumbar spine may be articulated, with the patient in a side-lying position, by flexing the hips to 90 degrees and flexing the knees also (Figure 4.3). Further flexion of the hips tends then to flex the lumbar spine. If the hips are stiffer than normal, then lumbar spine movement may commence before the hips flex 90 degrees. The movement in the lumbar spine may be monitored by palpating the movement of the spinous processes. Alternatively, a more direct or short leverage may be applied. In the neck the individual movement of intervertebral joints may be palpated by applying force in a medial direction to the articular pillar. This causes a side-bending motion. With practice this gives accurate information about cervical joint mobility. In addition, the resistance to movement throughout the range can be palpated. This can be perceived using a long or short leverage.

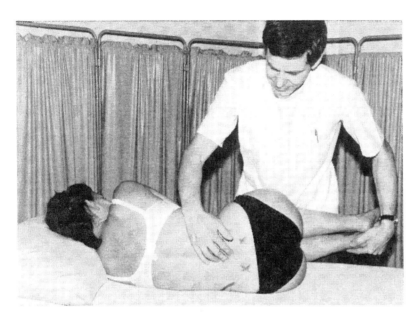

Figure 4.3 Articulation of the lower lumbar spine into flexion. The left hand is guiding the legs to produce flexion at the hips and then in the lumbar spine while the legs are supported by the practitioner's upper thighs. The right hand palpates the movement of the spinous processes and the surrounding muscle response. The crosses mark the position of the posterior iliac spines, the lines mark the level of the iliac crests.

Although these manoeuvres are used for examination of joint mobility, they may also be used therapeutically by rhythmically moving the joint. Movement may be within the midrange of the joint, particularly if there is swelling of the joint or if it is very irritable (Figure 4.4). This aids fluid exchange without stimulating the nociceptors and aggravating the pain. With a chronically restricted joint the technique may be applied close to the end of the range, with

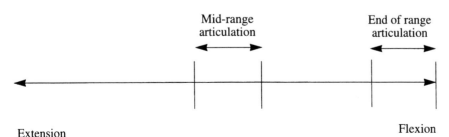

Figure 4.4 Articulation in mid-range and at the end of range.

the intention of gradually increasing the range. Here also the rate of movement will be dictated by the response of the underlying tissues. Since the resistance in this case may be due to chronic connective tissue shortening, the force required may well be greater. Sustained pressure rather than rhythmic articulation is more effective [36]. When connective tissue is first stretched it reaches an elastic limit. If the tension is sustained then there is a 'creep effect' whereby the connective tissue elongation continues over a period of time.

'Springing' is a form of articulation (see Figures 6.10 and 6.11). It involves applying a rhythmic force to a bony point or points. For example, pressure applied to the spinous process in a postero-anterior direction in the lumbar or thoracic spine will cause an extension movement. By aiming the force in a more cephalic direction, the movement created will be flexion. When the pressure is released, the spine, because of its natural elastic resilience, will 'spring' back or return to its resting position. Because of its short leverage, the joint movement will reach the end of range before any muscles that traverse more than one segment are at their full stretch, therefore springing has its effect principally on the passive structures of the joint rather than the muscles. However, if the joint is sensitive, then pressure will initiate muscle contraction which will be palpated by a rapidly increasing resistance under the applicator hand.

Manual traction

Traction can be applied to a body part in order to produce a longitudinal stretch, for example to the base of the head to stretch the neck, to the pelvis to traction the lumbar spine (Figure 4.5), or to the thigh to traction the hip joint. The rhythm may be fairly slow, ranging from perhaps 25 down to 2 times per minute. Sustained traction with quite large weights has been used in hospitals

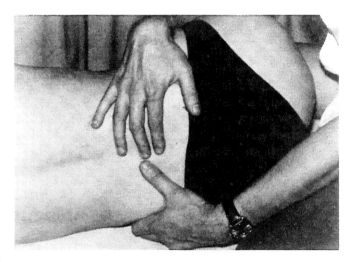

Figure 4.5 Manual traction is applied to the lumbar spine via a hand hold on the pelvic crests. The practitioner sits behind the patient and may apply the traction force by leaning backwards. The response of the local tissues is palpated and the technique modified accordingly.

by some therapists in the belief that this will reduce a disc bulge, though this remains a controversial hypothesis. Used more gently, the effect is probably to calm down the soft tissue reaction; the gentle traction force separates the joint surfaces and alters the tension in the joint capsule and this may cause an alteration of the mechanoreceptor stimulation of the dorsal horn of the spinal cord, with further reflex effects within the segment and beyond. This can be a particularly useful technique with acutely inflamed tissues. It is likely to be beneficial if it leads to a significant reduction of pain when traction is applied.

Rhythmic traction may also have an effect on the microcirculation by allowing venous stasis to be released by reduction of the tissue pressure. Even brief periods of intermittent traction may have a lasting effect.

High-velocity thrust

These techniques are the type that most patients remember after visiting an osteopath. The patient is positioned such that a joint is placed in a position of 'tension' (palpated by the osteopath in the local tissues, not merely the emotional state of the patient!), thus engaging a barrier (Figure 4.6). A high-velocity low-amplitude thrust is applied and frequently a click or crack is heard to emanate from the joint being stretched. This is believed to be the result of decompression of the joint synovial fluid (also known as cavitation) which temporarily becomes a gas bubble. This phenomenon has been observed using

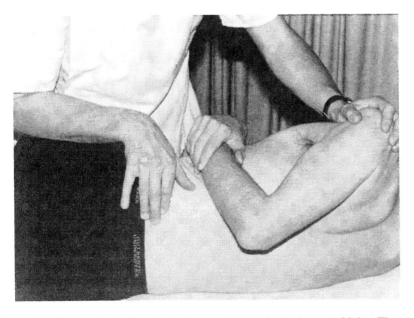

Figure 4.6 High-velocity thrust technique applied to the lumbo-sacral joint. The body position is modified until a point of tension is palpated at the level of the joint to be manipulated. A high-velocity thrust is then applied by the arm that is resting on the patient's pelvis.

X-ray techniques [46, 47]. However there is continuing debate as to the relationship of cavitation to any resulting improvement in joint range [48].

Following effective thrust manipulation there is an immediate increase in mobility of the individual joint. There have been various theories to account for this change. Lewit [49] argues that when a joint is restricted, this is because there is a synovial fold or villus trapped between the two surfaces of a facet joint, and manipulation releases this (Figure 2.6). Korr [50] suggests that the restriction is the consequence of aberrant muscle tone that has inappropriately limited the joint movement; the thrust promotes the resetting of the neurological tone. Stoddard [19] believes that there may be adhesions formed within the apophyseal joint which, when stretched by a thrust, are broken or stretched, thus allowing normal movement to be restored. Cyriax [51] held the view that the segmental restriction is due solely to alteration of position of the intervertebral disc and manipulation moves the misplaced fragment. Probably all these play a part in joint restriction, either individually or in conjunction with one another.

A thrust technique predominantly affects the local joint and its immediate surrounding and segmentally related structures. There may be changes in the autonomic nervous control of sweat glands and local circulation following manipulation. This suggests that altered neurological reflex activity is in some way involved in the dysfunction, although this in no way proves that the mechanism is solely the result of altered neurological activity. Specific joint manipulation does not stretch longer multisegmental muscles directly. Any alteration of tension in these muscles must therefore be a reflex effect rather than any influence on the passive connective tissue.

As seen in Table 4.1, there are a number of different ways of thrusting a joint depending on the leverage and application of the force, and personal tuition is probably the only effective way of learning them.

Low-velocity stress

In these techniques very small or even minimal force is applied. Careful positioning maximizes the body's relaxation, leading to a gentle release of tension in order to restore normal function. These types of techniques have been subdivided according to whether the low-velocity stress is applied with sustained leverage as in the case of 'muscle energy' technique, sustained traction, which is a variation on rhythmic traction discussed above, or sustained pressure, which is a variation of rhythmic soft tissue massage. These are types of direct techniques. Low-velocity stress may also be applied with sustained articulation, which includes 'functional' and 'strain and counter-strain' techniques. Cranio-sacral technique may also be included in this group. These last three are all indirect techniques.

Muscle energy [52, 53]

This is an active technique that involves the patient employing muscular effort. The aim is to place the patient in a position such that the joint or muscle group is in a position of tension, i.e. in a position where there is a sense of resistance to further movement, usually in three separate planes. The patient is then asked to push in a direction that is away from the direction of resistance – for up to 3–4 seconds is often enough. They are then asked to relax; if the technique is effective, as they relax it is found that the resistance has eased a little. The body is repositioned so that a new point of resistance is addressed, thus taking up the slack created after the muscular effort. It is wise only to take up this slack as far as the muscular resistance will allow and not to use excessive pressure. The process is then repeated three or four times. This appears to be the optimum number usually required but may be continued until the barrier cannot be moved further. This procedure is not a test of strength and the patient should be discouraged from attempting to overcome the practitioner's force. On the contrary, the aim is principally to contract the deep muscles that traverse only one or two spinal segments rather than the long superficial multisegmental muscles, since this enhances the specificity of the technique. This is most effective if localized to one spinal segment and may also be used on peripheral joints or muscles to enhance relaxation and stretch shortened tissues.

Variations on muscle energy technique are known by other terms among other groups of manipulative therapists, i.e. proprioceptive neuromuscular facilitation, or 'hold release'.

It is likely that the main effect of this technique is to reset the neurological tone to the muscles surrounding the joint, presumably by initially overstimulating it and then silencing the sensory input to the spinal cord during the relaxation phase. Joint cavitation sometimes occurs causing the sound of a crack or pop more commonly associated with a thrust technique. In the absence of this, the effect is less likely due to intracapsular effects and therefore probably neurological in nature. There will also be a mechanical effect of stretching the joint and surrounding tissues. This stretch may be maintained for a sustained period of more than 20 seconds.

Functional

In functional technique a joint is gently guided through a number of ranges of motion in order to find a position by palpation in which the surrounding tissues are maximally relaxed. This position is discovered by assessing all possible ranges of movement. It is the relative sense of ease or resistance (or 'bind') to the initiation of movement that is being assessed, rather than the range of movement, and requires very sensitive palpation. The soft tissue tension surrounding the joint is monitored by the 'listening' hand, while the other hand guides the patient's body through the various ranges of movement. As the joint is gently guided, for instance, into flexion, the tissue response as the movement is initiated is palpated in the surrounding tissues and then compared with extension. This is then repeated in side-bending, rotation, and also translation in an AP, lateral and vertical plane. The results are then summated and the body part is held in the position that combines all the directions of ease. The result of testing may have revealed ease in the directions of flexion, side-bending to the left, rotation right and lateral translation. The body is taken into a small degree of each of these movements and adjusted to find the position of maximum ease. If the technique is effective there will be a palpable relaxation of the tissues. On returning the joint to its normal neutral position it may be retested, and there should be a reduced resistance to movement, suggesting an alteration in the muscle reactivity.

Given the lack of force applied and the absence of stretch of tissues, any change resulting from this kind of indirect technique is almost certainly the result of altered neurological control of the local tissues.

Strain and counter-strain

Although this form of technique developed from different roots within the osteopathic profession, the underlying mechanism is probably similar to functional technique. Here there is an emphasis on tender points that develop in the body in association with particular dysfunctions. Thus as a result of a 'strain' the body's response results in a dysfunction surrounding a joint, whether it is an individual muscle that has been disturbed or the whole joint complex. Often a tender point may develop, not at the point of trauma or direct stress but in a related tissue, perhaps even in an antagonist muscle. Many tender points have been observed throughout the body. The tenderness of these points may be modified by holding the joint in a position that relaxes the tension around the tender point. This constitutes the 'counter-strain'. The gross positions to be used have been documented by Jones [54] but, as with functional technique, the position has to be 'fine tuned' based on palpation of the tissue texture surrounding the tender point. If the technique is effective when the joint is slowly returned to the 'normal' position, then there is a significant reduction if not a complete absence of tenderness. Practical details of this technique may be found in the text by Jones [54].

Cranio-sacral

This is also an indirect technique. The theory behind 'cranio-sacral' is complex and the practice requires considerable knowledge and individual tuition. In addition, the approach to assessment of problems in patients requires different techniques beyond those described in this text. The reader therefore is referred to specific texts for the full details [55, 56].

Visceral

Most of the above techniques have been discussed in relation to spinal or peripheral joints. In principle, osteopathy does not address only the tissues of the musculo-skeletal system but may be able to influence other tissues. Dysfunction (alone or in addition to structural abnormalities or pathologies) may occur in visceral structures. These may also be palpated and may respond to manual treatment. It is worth reflecting that the gastro-intestinal tract is a tube surrounded by smooth muscle which is clearly vulnerable to dysfunction, notably in the irritable bowel syndrome.

With accessible viscera, such as the gut, direct techniques may be used including abdominal massage. Because of the inaccessibility of some viscera (e.g. lungs) and the sensitivity of many visceral structures, indirect techniques may be more appropriate. These follow similar principles as functional techniques. Again readers are best referred to specialized texts [57, 58].

SELECTION OF TECHNIQUES

None of the techniques described above is exclusive and a variety might be used on the same patient at different times, even within the same treatment session. Patients with apparently similar mechanical problems may respond differently to the same technique, applied in the same way. This may be due to differences in physical, chemical or psychological factors.

The state of the tissues prior to as well as after the development of the dysfunction will have a bearing. For example, there may have been significant stress on the muscles around a joint due to postural fatigue. A sudden unexpected strain is then superimposed and dysfunction results. The tissues were already fatigued prior to the precipitating event and thus will not recover as quickly after the dysfunction has occurred.

It is obvious that some patients prefer one type of technique to another. Some welcome the use of high-velocity thrust techniques, even to the point of feeling that treatment is incomplete if they have not heard a 'crack', while others may request that they are not manipulated in this way even though they may have experienced relief from the use of such manipulation in the past. There may be times when it may be appropriate to persuade the patient to allow the use of forceful manipulation, but more often it is wiser to employ a different approach.

Different practitioners may prefer using particular techniques, because they find them most easy to perform and most effective; thus one may use thrust techniques frequently while others might never do so but use indirect techniques such as cranial or functional approaches. There is nothing inherently wrong in this so long as a successful outcome is achieved. However when a student or new graduate is developing technical skills it is wise not to ignore either thrust techniques or more gentle indirect techniques, since in the long term this will allow a wider range of approaches to a particular problem.

CONTRAINDICATIONS

With experience and sensitive application most osteopathic techniques can be applied to a wide variety of patients. Caution, however, must be employed particularly with patients in acute pain, since frequently the tissues will be very sensitive and therefore may react adversely after treatment. The possibility of a more serious pathological condition must be borne in mind even when the problem is apparently a benign musculo-skeletal one. Any suspicion of bone disease from the case history or examination calls for X-ray examination before proceeding with osteopathic treatment. This applies equally to the possibility of secondary bone cancer or infection, metabolic disorders such as osteoporosis, osteomalacia or Paget's disease, since all of them may cause weakening of bone and thus predispose to pathological fracture.

Severe degenerative changes in the spine also preclude the use of strong rotatory techniques, since in the neck this could compromise the vertebral artery flow. If there were significant encroachment into the intervertebral foramina, then strong rotation might cause aggravation of the symptoms by increasing or precipitating nerve root irritation or compression.

There have been reports in journals of vascular accidents occurring following cervical manipulation [59]. Although any accidents are to be regretted, when the number reported is compared to the number of manipulations performed world-wide it is found that there are only about two to three accidents per million manipulations. These are probably all related to high-velocity thrusts. In addition, from some reports it is probable that, with better management, at least some of these accidents could have been prevented [60]. It is therefore important to ask about symptoms and signs that might indicate brainstem ischaemia before and after manipulation and to cease treatment in the event of symptoms developing. The most important and common of these symptoms are dizziness, vertigo or light-headedness (Table 4.2). Although there are other causes of these symptoms, for example from abnormal proprioceptive inputs from upper cervical joints, it is safer to cease treatment and monitor the patient's progress. Then, at a later date, treatment may be continued with different techniques, if appropriate. It is interesting to note that the average age of patients affected is below 40, ranging from 23 to 60 years.

Table 4.2 Symptoms and signs of vertebro-basilar ischaemia

Dizziness (vertigo, light-headedness)
Drop attacks
Diplopia (or other visual problems)
Dysarthria
Dysphagia
Ataxia of gait
Nausea with possible vomiting
Nystagmus and/or numbness

Although the above conditions may contraindicate the use of some techniques, such as high-velocity thrusts and articulation at the extremes of joint range, other methods may be used which cause less distortion of the tissues; these may involve less amplitude or may be performed in the mid-range of joint movement. With older patients or those who are either not very fit or are unwell muscle energy may be used with much less risk and indirect techniques such as functional and counterstrain may also be used with minimal risk.

A more extensive review of contraindications to manipulative treatment may be found in other texts [61, 62].

WHERE TO TREAT – A CLINICAL JUDGEMENT

One of the philosophies of osteopathy is that the body is a unit (see Chapter 1) and thus what happens to one part of the body may influence any other. In principle therefore any dysfunction, whether in the musculo-skeletal system or the viscera, has an influence on the immediate cause of symptoms and so treatment could logically be applied to any and all areas of dysfunction. This is potentially laborious and in practice not appropriate or necessary. However, what is treated is a matter of clinical judgement. For instance, with a shoulder problem affecting the tendons of the periscapular muscles, treatment may be directed purely to this area to reduce any muscle hypertonia and enhance healing of the inflamed tendon(s). However, the presence of dysfunction in the neck or thoracic spine commonly affects the response to treatment. Disturbance of the function of the elbow or muscles surrounding it may also have a mechanical effect on the shoulder area. Disease within the thoracic cavity, such as a chronic infection or consolidation of part of the lung, might have either a reflex or mechanical effect on the shoulder girdle. Postural asymmetry may cause increased stress on the shoulder area. Clearly the indirect effects from within the body are virtually endless.

So should the thorough osteopath always treat all these areas? Is a problem in one area always going to have an impact upon the shoulder area? In practice this is not always the case. This is apparent from many practitioners' experience since without dealing with all observable factors (and there will always be unobserved problems) patients can still be helped. However when the problem is not fully resolved it may be that not all important factors have been dealt with and therefore there are residual problems which prevent resolution.

Thus there are a number of different approaches that are employed by osteopaths.

- Treat the local dysfunction.
- Treat anatomically related areas, particularly neurologically related spinal areas.
- Treat any musculo-skeletal dysfunction wherever present in the body.
- Attempt to restore normal postural balance or even normal postural symmetry.
- Treat any visceral dysfunction.
- Treat the whole body using cranio-sacral technique.

Two or more of these may be combined together, either in the same treatment session or at intervals. There are some who advocate only dealing with one area in a particular treatment and then dealing with a different area in the next. This has been described as specific adjustment technique. Conversely, there are others who assess all areas of the body in a regular sequence and deal with any and all dysfunction found. There are of course the majority of osteopaths who fall between these extremes and who will judge where and what they will treat according to a variety of criteria.

There have not been any comparative studies to establish which approach is more effective for any particular problem and therefore we are dependent on our own or other people's anecdotal experience. This has inevitably led to dogmatic opinions and to controversy among osteopaths. Further research is obviously required and, though this is strewn with difficulties, it will benefit the profession greatly.

5 Case history analysis

While taking a case history the osteopath has to integrate a variety of data, physical, psychological, cultural and spiritual (Table 5.1). The most obvious purpose of the interaction is for the practitioner to develop some understanding of the person before them and of their problem. As an osteopath it is not enough to establish what has happened in the symptomatic area. This local problem has not developed in a vacuum but within a complex living system. We therefore seek to explore whether there are particular factors that have made the body vulnerable, leading to the development of this problem now. For example, previous injury to or symptoms in another part of the body may have left residual stiffness or dysfunction. As discussed in Chapter 1, osteopaths place particular emphasis on the impact that diverse problems, both musculo-skeletal and otherwise, may have on each other.

Table 5.1 Aims of a case history

To develop a therapeutic relationship
To determine if there is acute or chronic breakdown
To determine any contributory factors
Differential diagnosis
Management considerations

While conversing with the patient, close observation is important. Often there are clinical signs to be observed in the face and hands of a patient and their body language may reflect the patient's state of mind.

As well as providing diagnostic information, the patient's words may give clues as to the management of the problem. A management plan needs to be tailored to an individual; thus the patient's general physical activity level, sports, hobbies, diet and stress level may all have to be considered and, if practical, modified.

DEVELOPING A THERAPEUTIC RELATIONSHIP

If any treatment, osteopathic or otherwise, is to be effective there must be a relationship of trust between patient and practitioner both during treatment and management. This is particularly important with a therapy such as osteopathy which involves very close, even intimate, contact and co-operation between the two parties. From the patient's viewpoint this will develop if they feel comfortable with and accepted by the practitioner. The practitioner needs to listen carefully not only because the patient's history will reveal much useful information but also because the patient needs to know they have been heard. There is more to history taking than just asking the right questions and interpreting the answers.

The practitioner must avoid imposing a set agenda while taking the history. This can be particularly difficult for students who may be insecure in their knowledge. Where possible the patient must be allowed to explain her own problem, prompted by appropriate questions to clarify particular clinical details. They are then much more likely to explain their real concerns and also reveal other related or apparently unrelated problems.

While listening to the patient, their natural sitting posture and other personal characteristics may be observed. These will include their general state of well-being both physically and mentally, as well as how they are dressed and how they present themselves. It is important not to jump to conclusions about the patient, since first impressions are often hard to overturn. It is helpful however to acknowledge consciously one's 'gut-feelings', since this may prevent them from unconsciously colouring one's view of the patient. Further discussion of communication skills is beyond the scope of this book but they are vitally important in any interaction with a patient.

BREAKDOWN IN COMPENSATION

The concept of compensation and its breakdown has been discussed in Chapter 1. Patients may often present with one problem that they are concerned about. Frequently, however, on further questioning it will be revealed that they have or have had other minor or significant problems. The initial aim is to differentiate how many problem areas there are. The osteopath needs to consider whether and how these may be related and also what other factors may have either predisposed or contributed to the problem. This requires the osteopath to make a value judgement about how significant any factor might be. Frequently this can only be based on experience rather than objective data. These contributory factors will be discussed below.

It is clearly important at this stage to be alert to any possible clues in the case history about the factors involved, as such clues will be pertinent to the management of the patient's problem.

Pain at one or more sites?

Pain at more than one site may have a number of implications:

- There may be two areas of pain, but one is actually referred from the other site. (Sites of referred pain are discussed later in this chapter.) Normally this can be recognized since the two pains will be aggravated by the same factors. For instance, pain referred to the arm from a cervical joint will usually be modified by neck movements. Also frequently with musculo-skeletal pain the referred site will act as a measure of the intensity of the pain [17]; if the stimulus increases when the patient attempts an activity that aggravates the underlying injured tissues, the pain may be referred more distally along the affected limb. Conversely, as the degree of irritation decreases the pain will reduce and disappear from the referred site before the local pain settles. There are exceptions to this where sometimes pain is felt only at the referral site or may last longer in this area than the local site.

- It may be an indication of two or more relatively separate mechanical problems, for instance a chronic rotator cuff and a recent acute low back problem. They are separate in the sense that treatment may need to be directed to both areas. They may however be mechanically related. For instance, sometimes a rotator cuff problem may be influenced by a problem in the low back area via neurological, postural or myofascial mechanisms.
- They may be two or more related mechanical problems, perhaps a cervical pain that is secondary to lumbar dysfunction or pelvic torsion which may have been predisposed by a disturbance of foot mechanics. Sometimes by resolving the primary problem the secondary dysfunction no longer needs treatment.
- There may be an inflammatory arthritic condition such as ankylosing spondylitis or rheumatoid arthritis causing polyarticular involvement. Details of these conditions can be found in rheumatology texts.

Acute or chronic 'mechanical' breakdown

The patient's story will often clarify whether the problem has just come to the surface, perhaps through a significant trauma, or whether it has been intermittent or even persistent over the recent or less recent past. The cause of the 'breakdown' may also be apparent; for example, the patient may have changed employment in the past few months, which has meant driving further during the week and the symptoms have gradually come on and are getting slowly worse. However, it may be that although the symptoms commenced quite suddenly, the problem has been developing over a period of time but eventually becomes symptomatic as a result of a minor trauma; for example, the patient has taken up a new sport recently which has demanded much more of her body.

The chronicity of the problem may also be assessed during the examination by the state of the soft tissues. If there has been a chronic breakdown then there will very likely be palpable changes in the muscles, demonstrating the attempt to cope with the altered demands; these may often include fibrosis or contracture. It is important to correlate the history to the examination. There are times when examination findings are inconsistent with the patient's history, and this prompts further questioning which reveals information that the patient did not consider significant.

Predisposing and contributing factors

There may have been other predisposing and contributing factors which a careful history may reveal. When discussing the mechanisms involved in dysfunction it was noted that the state of mind has a significant effect on the general level of muscle tone throughout the body and this can amplify any localized dysfunction. This applies to all forms of stress, whether physical, mental, emotional, social or even spiritual. So, when discussing the build up and development of the problem, it is usually worth probing any possible areas of stress, in work, home, family or other social contexts. It is also important to discuss sources of physical stress, either prolonged ongoing stresses imposed at work, both postural and dynamic, or changes in physical workloads. It may be as significant that the patient is now doing *less* physical work as it is if she is doing more. For example, Ron, a building worker, who had until 18 months ago done heavy manual work now runs his own business and is virtually office or car based. He has become significantly less fit and therefore does not cope so well with occasional manual work.

Sometimes the presenting symptoms may be a secondary result of a pre-existing problem. For example, the patient may have suffered a low back injury some months previously (the primary area). Although the symptoms from this subsided after a few weeks there may still be residual stiffness and dysfunction of the area. This may indirectly place altered mechanical stresses on other parts of the body, for instance the cervico-thoracic junction. If this area is able to adapt and tolerate the added stresses, then the patient is unaware of this. However, if there is a change in the patient's lifestyle or she experiences a minor trauma to the neck (the secondary area), the body can no longer adapt to the primary problem, and symptoms develop in the neck. History of previous dysfunction or disturbance, whether musculo-skeletal or visceral, needs to be considered as a potential contributing factor.

It can be seen, therefore, that although two patients may present with similar symptoms, perhaps of a lower lumbar joint injury, there may be quite different contributory factors which will alter the treatment and management of their varying problems.

DIFFERENTIAL DIAGNOSIS

When a patient consults an osteopath it is important to establish as far as possible the cause of her symptoms in each area, both the tissues that may be involved and their pathophysiological state. However, from an osteopathic viewpoint it is not just the tissue breakdown but the body's response to this (producing the total dysfunction) that is equally important. This will be assessed further on examination.

People are most commonly prompted to seek help because they are experiencing pain or alteration of some body function. There are a number of features of the patient's story that are particularly useful in establishing the underlying cause(s) of their symptoms. These include the location(s), character and severity of pain, behaviour of the pain including aggravating and relieving factors, the onset and development of the problem, previous history and related symptoms.

Pain location

Specific tissues tend to cause pain in characteristic areas. Many tissues of course cause pain in their local area, for example most joints will cause pain locally. (A common exception is the hip joint which frequently causes pain in the thigh or even the knee in the absence of pain in the hip or groin region.) Conversely, many visceral structures frequently cause pain at a distance from the source of pain. The heart commonly causes pain that is felt in the medial left arm; the gall-bladder causes pain that is experienced in the right shoulder (Table 5.2).

Table 5.2 Common causes and sites of referred pain

Visceral cause	Site
Heart	Anterior chest, left medial arm, anterior neck to mandible
Gallbladder	Right lower costal margin, point of right shoulder, right posterior mid-thorax
Stomach	Central upper abdomen, left posterior mid-thorax
Pancreas	Mid-thoracic spine
Kidney	Twelfth rib region unilateral
Uterus	Lower abdomen, anterior pelvis, sacrum

Referred pain may be defined simply as pain experienced at a site distant from its cause. As mentioned in Chapter 2, the phenomenon of referred pain appears to be the result of convergence of sensory nerves in the spinal cord. Because nociceptor axons from visceral and somatic structures synapse very close or even onto the same second order intermediary axons in the spinal cord, when information from the nociceptors is transmitted to higher centres, it is 'interpreted' as coming from other structures. So nociceptor fibre axons from the heart synapse in the left upper thoracic region of the spinal cord, where fibres also synapse from the medial left arm. The brain then 'experiences' pain caused by disturbance in the heart in the left arm. There is no disturbance of structure or function in the left arm.

Pain caused by irritation of different musculo-skeletal structures may cause a similar experience of pain in the same referral area. For instance, disc [63] and facet [64] structures may cause similar patterns of pain referral to the leg from the low back region.

As a starting point in diagnosis it is vital to know where particular tissues refer pain. The first stage of differential diagnosis is to consider the possible causes of pain in the area that the patient reports.

Although muscles and facet joints tend to cause pain locally they may also cause referred pain in related areas. There have now been many clinical studies using injection of an irritant into spinal tissues in order to reproduce referred pain and a number of pain maps have been produced [64–67] (Figures 5.1–5.3). From these studies it is clear that there is significant overlap of pain referral from adjacent spinal segments and pelvic joints and therefore the referral pattern is of little help in localizing which joint is causing the pain. For instance, groin pain has been elicited by irritant injections in and around facet joints from L1/2 to L5/S1. However, this is less problematical than it may seem, since if the symptoms suggest somatic dysfunction in a spinal region, then treatment will be directed to the segment or segments found on examination to be restricted rather than that which *ought to be* causing the pain referral pattern.

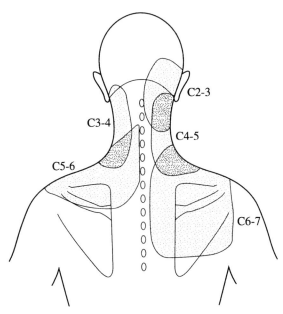

Figure 5.1 Distribution of referred pain from cervical apophyseal joints in asymptomatic subjects (taken from Dwyer *et al.* [65]).

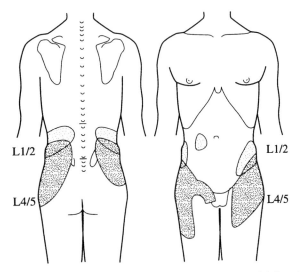

Figure 5.2 Distribution of referred pain from lumbar apophyseal joints (taken from McCall *et al.* [64]).

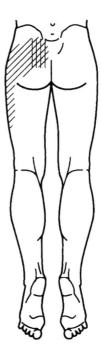

Figure 5.3 Distribution of referred pain from sacro-iliac joints (taken from Fortin *et al.* [67]).

These patterns of referred pain seen in asymptomatic subjects tend to be limited to the immediate trunk or proximal limb area. However, Mooney observed much more extensive referral patterns in symptomatic subjects; for instance, pain was sometimes referred down to the foot from a facet joint in the lower lumbar spine. He inferred from this that the extent of the referral was in some way proportional to the intensity of the stimulus in that particular individual. However, the extent of referral cannot be used to compare the relative intensity of pain in different subjects.

In the past, pain extending beyond the knee or elbow was inferred to be the result of nerve root irritation. Mooney demonstrated that pain may be referred to the end of the limb from other sources, such as the facet joint as well as the nerve root.

Intervertebral discs have been demonstrated to have a nerve supply [68] and are therefore a potential source of pain. Pain has been produced in subjects by irritant injection. Pain is mainly experienced centrally, with some bilateral spread. Referred pain may also be experienced into the limbs. These experiments, however, must be interpreted with care, since it is still conceivable that limb pain may be unilateral.

Nerve root pain

If a spinal nerve root is compressed, after a period of time the area of skin that is supplied by the nerve becomes numb because the nerve becomes ischaemic and ceases to conduct. The area of skin supplied by a spinal nerve root is known as a dermatome; these areas are fairly consistent between subjects, but frequently overlap adjacent dermatomes (Figure 5.4). They are not, however, reliable enough to distinguish which nerve root is being affected.

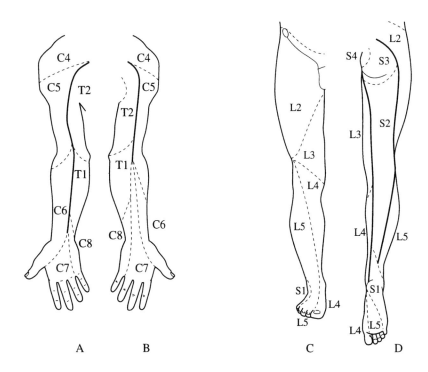

Figure 5.4 Distribution of dermatomes. A. The arrangement of dermatomes on the anterior aspect of the upper limb. There is minimal overlap across the heavy black line whereas there is considerable overlap across the interrupted lines. B. The arrangement of dermatomes on the posterior aspect of the upper limb. C. The arrangement of dermatomes on the anterior aspect of the lower limb. D. The arrangement of dermatomes on the anterior aspect of the lower limb.

If a spinal nerve is irritated, for example by a disc prolapse, pain is experienced typically in the related dermatome. By definition therefore all nerve root pain is a form of referred pain. *However, it is important to note that most referred pain does not involve nerve root irritation.*

There are certain characteristic differences between 'typical' nerve root pain and referred pain from other structures (Table 5.3). However, since nerve root pain is a form of referred pain, when the intensity of the stimulation is less marked, the differentiation becomes less obvious.

Nerve root pain is discussed in more detail in Chapter 11.

Table 5.3 Comparison of characteristics of nerve root and referred pain

	Nerve root	*Referred*
Proximal vs. distal	Worse in the limb	Worse in the back
Location	Usually linear within a dermatomal	Less well defined, not dermatomal
Character	May be intense, sharp, shooting	Vague
Effect of spinal movement	May be a few seconds delay before alteration of pain	Immediate change in symptoms depending on effect of spinal movement on structure causing referred pain

Character of the pain

It will be recognized that many different tissues may cause pain in similar areas of the body (Table 5.4). The character may sometimes help differentiate the type of tissue involved; for example pain from an inflamed nerve root may cause intense shooting pain in a dermatomal distribution. Likewise, if the pain from a viscera is colicky in character but referred to the spine, then it will be relatively straightforward to distinguish from pain of musculo-skeletal origin. However, both visceral and musculo-skeletal structures may cause a similar pain sensation, for instance the pain of an acute costo-vertebral joint strain may be very similar to that from a dry pleurisy. Due to convergence at the spinal cord level there may even be identical neurological pathways transmitting the pain sensation from the two structures to the higher centres. Also the character of the pain experienced from different musculo-skeletal tissues such as intervertebral discs, facet joints, spinal ligaments and muscles may be similar. Thus the character is not always of help in differentiating between pain from such structures.

Severity of the pain

This may give an indication of the type of tissue involved. For example, intense pain radiating down the leg in a dermatomal distribution may indicate a nerve root irritation rather than referred pain from a lumbar spine structure.

The severity will, to a degree, be related to the intensity of nociceptor stimulation, though this will be greatly modified by the limbic system under the influence of the patient's emotional and cultural background. However, the severity will not necessarily be related to the seriousness of the problem. For example, a patient may present with headache. A migraine headache may be debilitating intermittently, whereas a slowly growing intra-cranial space-occupying lesion is life-threatening. The latter may cause only a minor background headache for many months until it becomes more persistent and eventually more intense.

Table 5.4 Character of pain from various organs

Tissue	Character and site
Oesophagus	Retrosternal, radiating to midline of back at same level of lesion
Heart	Heavy, crushing sensation in chest, heavy ache in arm
Pleura	Localized ache in chest wall, sharp pain on deep or even shallow breath
Stomach	Indigestion pain upper abdomen occasionally radiating to left posterior thorax
Duodenum	Nagging pain in upper abdomen, rarely in midline of back or right scapula
Gallbladder	Nagging or colicky pain upper right abdomen, to right mid-thorax, to right point of shoulder
Kidney	Unilateral nagging ache at angle of twelfth rib, may radiate down loin to lower abdomen
Small intestine	Colicky pain in central abdomen
Colon (usually left half)	Colicky in left iliac fossa or hypogastrium
Uterus	Central lower abdominal aching and vague sacral aching

Behaviour of the pain including aggravating and relieving factors

Different tissues and different conditions are aggravated by particular stimuli. For instance pain caused by stimulation of nociceptors in heart muscle by ischaemia causes characteristic angina pain. This is typically aggravated by exercise, since this increases the demand on heart muscle and therefore increases the ischaemia. The gallbladder is stimulated to contract by a fatty meal; if the gallbladder is irritated by gallstones then the fatty meal will aggravate the organ and pain will be increased.

Likewise musculo-skeletal structures will be aggravated or relieved by different activities or postures and these should be discussed with the patient (Table 5.5). The majority of musculo-skeletal problems will be relieved when resting horizontally unless the involved structures are inflamed. Then chemical stimulation of local nociceptors may be persistent even though the mechanical stress of gravity has been removed.

Pain is much less likely to be musculo-skeletal in origin if it is not related to position or movement.

Differential diagnosis will be explored further in the survey of problems in each region. However, some general observations will be made here regarding the behaviour of pain in different tissues. This will, in some cases, depend on the pathophysiological state of the tissue or tissues involved. In addition, differentiation using active, active-resisted and passive movement testing is discussed in Chapter 6.

Table 5.5 Activities or postures that should be discussed

Neck and arm	Thoracic	Low back
Neck rotation	Twisting	Standing
Looking up	Bending	Walking
Sporting activities	Sitting	Sitting – home, office, car
Car driving	Lying	Lying
Sitting, reading, knitting, etc.	Sport	Bending
Work	Work	Straining
Sleep position and pattern	Coughing	Sport, etc.
Pillows	Deep inhalation	Work

Note that it is the predominant aggravating or relieving factor that is most important. For instance, with a tennis elbow, stretching the elbow in full extension may cause discomfort around the lateral side of the elbow, but this will be much less than when active gripping is attempted, whereas if there is a problem with the joint itself, stretching in full extension or flexion is more likely to aggravate the pain than active use of the hand. One should not assume, however, that there is necessarily only one tissue involved. For instance, the lateral ligament may be involved with a lateral epicondylitis.

Muscle injury will cause pain principally on active movement. Thus a tear of the gastrocnemius will be painful on attempting to take weight on the toes rather than the heels, for example when walking. Likewise, because a *tendon* acts 'in series' with a muscle, if the tendon has been damaged then pain will again be felt on activation of the muscle. This is experienced with a lateral epicondylitis of the elbow (tennis elbow), where gripping an object in the hand contracts the forearm extensor muscles and causes pain.

If postural fatigue occurs then muscles and ligaments will cause local aching which increases while the particular posture is maintained but is usually relieved by changing position. Postural fatigue rarely causes referred pain.

When *ligaments* are partially torn by injury, pain will be aggravated by stretching of the affected ligament, whether passively or actively. Thus with a lateral collateral ankle sprain, if the patient inadvertently inverts the ankle, particularly while weight-bearing on that side, pain will be experienced. A complete tear of a ligament may cause pain at the time of injury but will subside rapidly. Pain will not, therefore, be aggravated by stretching of the ruptured ligament.

If a joint *capsule* is acutely inflamed then there will be a constant dull ache with pain increased on any movement. As the swelling recedes pain is mainly felt at the end of range of movement. This is usually in a number of different ranges, though not necessarily all ranges. In comparison, when a ligament is strained there may be only one or two ranges affected. So for instance if the shoulder joint is affected, particularly if there are adhesions present (i.e. adhesive capsulitis/frozen shoulder), then there is pain as well as restriction of movement in all ranges, especially abduction and internal rotation. With early degeneration of the hip joint there is commonly loss of mobility and pain in flexion and internal rotation due to capsular shortening. As degeneration continues, the restriction is compounded by cartilage involvement. So in the early stage of hip osteoarthritis, pain may be experienced mainly when commencing walking; it then subsides, though it may return after a long walk. With a spinal apophyseal joint, unless it is acutely inflamed, pain is felt mainly on changing position, getting up from bed or from a chair, whereas the patient can be quite comfortable while remaining in one position.

It must be remembered that when one tissue is damaged and inflammation develops the resulting swelling does not remain confined to the immediate damaged tissue but spreads into adjacent tissues. For instance, a damaged apophyseal joint capsule may cause pericapsular swelling. Likewise, a lateral collateral ligament sprain of the ankle may cause swelling extending into superficial subdermal tissues. The significance is that the secondary swelling may well affect the behaviour of the pain.

The reported presence of swelling all around a superficial peripheral joint (e.g. knee, ankle, elbow, wrist) suggests that the problem is intra-capsular. In comparison, swelling on one side of a joint may suggest a more localized ligament injury. In most cases of intra-capsular swelling this is due to irritation of the joint capsule. This may be due to an autoimmune condition, such as rheumatoid arthritis, or due to trauma. In the case of the knee, and sometimes the temporo-mandibular joint, this may also be due to damage to an intracapsular *meniscus*. In the knee, one of the menisci (more commonly the medial) may become torn and cause locking or disturbance of the capsule, resulting in capsular irritation and pain. Pain tends to be worse on weight-bearing, particularly on movement, since this may 'trap' the cartilage meniscus between the two surfaces of the joint.

Another cause of joint locking in the older age group is a fragment of *cartilage* that breaks off from the joint surface and then disrupts the normal joint movement. This may also initiate joint effusion. If effusion is not marked, then crepitus may be felt.

Joint *cartilage* has no nerve supply and therefore cannot normally cause pain. Thus, even if the cartilage is damaged through trauma, the pain that is experienced is caused by underlying bone damage rather than the cartilage itself. When degeneration develops in the joint cartilage in osteoarthritis, or in the late stages of inflammatory arthritis, then the cartilage becomes thinner and eventually may be worn away completely. In the later stages of this process, as the cartilage becomes so weak that it becomes distorted by the stresses placed upon it, the underlying bone becomes distorted also. In addition, when the cartilage is destroyed, then the underlying bone that is less well adapted to allow minimal friction becomes eburnated and pain will occur from both the weight-bearing and the movement of the joint. Pain will be experienced therefore on weight-bearing and movement. With markedly degenerate joints pain is also experienced in the later hours of sleep. This results from reactive hyperaemia which develops while at rest, causing an increase of vascular pressure in the subchondral bone.

Another form of cartilage is found in the intervertebral *disc*. Until the 1970s, it was believed that the intervertebral disc had no nerve supply. It has, however, been demonstrated that at least the outer one-third of the disc does contain free nerve endings and thus is a potential source of pain. If there is injury to the disc, particularly in the younger age group up to about 45 years, pain tends to be worse when the patient is sitting due to the increase in intra-discal pressure. Characteristically the pain builds up while the person sits, sometimes to the point where they have to get up to relieve the pain. It may be painful then to get up also. Pain tends to be worse in the morning when first rising from bed and this may take an hour or two to ease. This is believed to be because during the night while vertical compression is removed by lying horizontal the disc imbibes fluid and thus swells. When the patient then sits up or stands the disc bulge is slightly greater. In the older age group disc injury may still occur but the pain is usually easier in the morning after rest, although there may be stiffness and pain on attempting to stretch.

If the *nerve root* is inflamed then the limb pain will be modified by vertebral movement. If the cause is a disc bulge encroaching on the foramen then frequently flexion movements or postures will aggravate the limb pain most and standing and walking may relieve it. With a large bulge all vertical positions may be painful and even walking may be painful. Where the root is compromised, predominantly by degenerative trespass of the foramen, and complicated by inflammation, then standing may be the more painful position, since relative extension narrows the foramen. Walking may become very painful also.

Usually the most obvious difference between pain from *viscera* and musculo-skeletal structures is that pain from the former is not related to movement or body posture but may be affected by stimulation of activity in the particular viscera. For instance, pain from an inflamed urethra will cause pain on urination, and pain from the gallbladder will be aggravated by a fatty meal once it reaches the duodenum since this causes contraction of the gallbladder. Pain from the gynaecological organs tends to be worse at the time of the menstrual flow. Visceral pain is commonly not relieved by lying down, unlike musculo-skeletal pain.

It is important to note that quite frequently disturbance of a viscera may not cause pain at all but may present only with other symptoms. For example, lung infection may cause a cough and sputum production and generalized malaise and fever, but there may be no marked pain from the lungs. It is only when the infection causes inflammation of the pleura that pain results from stimulation of receptors in the outer layer of the pleura.

Onset and development of the problem

It has already been mentioned that the onset and previous history can be important in identifying whether the current symptoms are part of a gradual breakdown or whether this is a sudden acute injury resulting from a particular trauma. The onset may also give us direct clues as to the nature of the immediate problem. If there has been substantial trauma, such as a car accident or an injury induced during lifting a heavy weight in an awkward position, there is the possibility of serious structural damage to bone, whereas if the patient merely twisted to reach a piece of paper and suddenly felt pain in the spine, the problem is more likely to be due to soft tissue or joint dysfunction than to a fracture. The patient's age has a bearing on this; a lady in her seventies (or even in her fifties) may have osteoporosis and a relatively trivial event, for instance tugging at a sheet caught under a bed, may be trauma enough to cause a vertebral collapse.

The problem is more complex if there is no trauma recalled. The symptoms may still have commenced quite quickly. The patient may report that they just woke up with the pain, or it gradually increased over a period of a few hours. In the absence of any initiating trauma the possibility of a non-musculo-skeletal cause has a much greater likelihood and we need to enquire specifically about other related symptoms (see below). However, a musculo-skeletal problem may also develop for no apparent reason, and may occur because:

- It results from a minor recurrent stress such as a habitual activity.
- The initial insult to the involved tissue is minor and does not initially cause significant nociceptor stimulation until local inflammation builds up over a few hours. This sometimes occurs with a disc injury, where initially the disc damage does not cause actual irritation of an intervertebral nerve, but the prolapsed nuclear material triggers off an inflammatory reaction which, after a few hours, causes pain.

The rate of development of symptoms may be of importance. With a traumatic injury, if swelling develops over a period of a few minutes, this probably indicates significant bleeding as the cause, whereas if swelling develops over a few hours inflammation is more likely.

Previous history

Previous bouts of pain in the same area may be an indication of a recurrent problem though this should not be assumed. It is essential to verify that the nature and behaviour of the pain is the same as with previous episodes. The patient may have previously had upper lumbar pain from a mechanical dysfunction, causing pain on movement and on taking a deep breath. At a later date a kidney infection might cause pain in the same area, but now pain would not be greatly altered by movement and would be present constantly, causing disturbed sleep and possibly urinary symptoms.

Though the problem may still be musculo-skeletal in origin, the nature of the tissue disturbance may alter over a period of time. A disc injury might occur at the age of 32. There may be further recurrence over the years, but by the age of 50, disc degeneration will have progressed and will lead to different tissue breakdown, a different pattern of symptoms and will require a different treatment and management approach.

Related symptoms

There are many non-musculo-skeletal tissues that refer pain to the spine which need to be considered in differential diagnosis. Many, though not all, will present with other symptoms (Table 5.6); pleural irritation will cause sharp thoracic pain which is aggravated by breathing; the problem may appear similar to costo-transverse dysfunction but the patient may also be feeling unwell and have had a cough recently. Gynaecological pain may well refer to the low back or pelvic area, but on specific questioning the patient may be aware of other gynaecological symptoms such as change in regularity, pain or bleeding or discharge between periods.

Table 5.6 Symptoms associated with various organs

Source of pain	Associated symptom/s
Oesophagus	Reflux into mouth of undigested food
Stomach	Reflux into mouth of partly digested food with unpleasant taste of stomach acid Vomiting especially of blood
Lower gastro-intestinal tract	Alteration of bowel habit Passing blood per rectum
Bladder, kidney	Dysuria, frequency, blood in urine
Gynaecological organs	Dysmenorrhea, bleeding or discharge mid-cycle, dyspareunia
Lung	Cough, sputum, dyspnoea

The absence of symptoms of visceral disturbance does not necessarily demonstrate that all is well within the abdominal or thoracic cavity. For example, a mass in the abdomen, for instance in the kidney or ovary, frequently causes no visceral symptoms until quite late in its development. The possibility of a serious visceral problem must be borne in mind constantly, particularly with a patient with apparently musculo-skeletal problems which do not conform to a common pattern or which do not respond as anticipated.

Conversely it should not be assumed that symptoms are necessarily causally related. For example, a lady might have painful periods which cause pain in the low back, but she might also develop a mechanical problem in her spine. The pain from this would be more obviously related to changes in position or to movement.

More specific differential diagnosis will be discussed in Part 2 of this book which looks at the different regions of the body.

MANAGEMENT CONSIDERATIONS

As well as providing important information about differential diagnosis, the history supplies clues to immediate and ongoing management.

Stage of condition: rest or activity?

Once initiated, inflammation tends to build up over a period of 2–3 days. During this time attempting to carry on regardless and ignore the pain aggravates the swelling induced and may make the inflammation more persistent. However, given sensible management in the early stage, controlled activity can be resumed and should be encouraged after this period unless the patient is still seriously disabled by muscle spasm. Sometimes a nervous patient needs some persuasion that activity will not put them back to square one and this is why emphasis on controlled activity is crucial. Usually, gentle walking around the house for short periods, avoiding household chores, will result in relief of pain and an increase in mobility. Being allowed to be vertical rather than horizontal is in itself psychologically therapeutic! There are very few exceptions to this principle of controlled exercise. However, the patient should not persist in activities that cause a gradual increase of pain. This is more likely, for example, with a large disc prolapse that is causing acute radicular pain.

Motivation

Often patient involvement in treatment is helpful, particularly by doing some form of exercise. If they are used to taking exercise, particularly if they are keen to return to their sport, then their motivation will be increased. Likewise if they need to get fit to return to work or have commitments or responsibilities, they are likely to be more disciplined and determined to help. This will affect the prognosis significantly, so it is wise to assess this early on.

It is also useful to discuss the patients' hopes, expectations and needs over the coming days and months. They may have unrealistic expectations about what they will be able to achieve. It is better to prepare them earlier rather than later that they may have to change their forthcoming plans. Not only is this pertinent to maximizing their progress but it will also demonstrate an interest in them as people rather than carriers of low back symptoms and will improve compliance generally. This is part of building the therapeutic relationship.

Results of previous treatment

When asking about past history it is useful to discover what previous treatment has been performed for the present or previous similar problem. This may give a guide to what may or may not be useful. As discussed in Chapter 4, different people respond better to different techniques, thus one person may improve rapidly with a forceful approach involving high-velocity techniques while another may react very badly to such treatment.

When a patient consults because they have not responded to another osteopath's treatment it is important to consider the possible reasons for this:

- The diagnosis may have been wrong and a more serious problem may be present.
- The local diagnosis was correct, but the osteopath did not take into account all the relevant mechanical or contributing factors. For instance this may be because only the symptomatic area was treated.
- There was poor compliance with the advice given by the osteopath, thus the tissues were not given the chance to settle down.
- The wrong types of techniques were used. It is therefore useful to discover what type of treatment was given. This is not necessarily very easy if only the patient's report has to be relied upon. Direct contact with

the other osteopath is ideal. It is logical that if the patient has not responded to another practitioner's use of high-velocity techniques or cranio-sacral methods, then it might be more appropriate, at least initially, to use a different approach.

Examination | 6

Osteopathic examination, with its emphasis on detailed palpation of the body framework, is a distinguishing feature of this form of manual medicine. It is vital that this is performed in the context of the information gained from the case history. The primary aim is to investigate the initial hypotheses developed from the case history to establish the cause of the symptoms. The area of the somatic dysfunction needs to be determined and, where possible, the nature of the tissue disturbance. Manipulative treatment is primarily directed at the abnormal function discovered on examination, whether through dysfunction or through other soft tissue changes which may have occurred through postural or dynamic adaptation (see Chapters 1–3). Manipulative treatment is contraindicated in some pathological conditions such as bone neoplasia, where the state of the bone may be weakened such that the more forceful techniques might cause damage. It is also important to consider whether the cause is in a non-musculo-skeletal structure. Often it is more difficult to be certain of the underlying pathological state with a visceral problem and therefore further tests may be necessary.

If we are confident that the cause is benign and that there is a mechanical component contributing to the problem, then any alteration of function that is present should be explored, including the specific range of restricted movements of joints and the nature of any abnormal soft tissue texture, since these may have specific implications for the type and application of treatment techniques.

As well as analysing the local area of dysfunction, this should be placed within the context of the rest of the body and also other aspects of the person, that may be affected by or contribute to the problem, should be taken into account. This may involve investigating the patient's musculo-skeletal system for any contributing mechanical factors in other areas of abnormal function. It may also involve examination of the patient's non-musculo-skeletal systems for any signs of disease or dysfunction, since this may cause reflex effects in the musculo-skeletal system as well as having a mechanical influence via fascial connections.

Limitations of differential diagnosis

Rarely can any particular problem be ruled out on the basis of the clinical information available. The probabilities of the various possible causes of the symptoms should be considered. For instance, in considering a patient with pain in the right elbow, the source of the pain may be local to the joint or soft tissues or may be referred from the shoulder, neck or upper back. The observation that the elbow pain is particularly aggravated by neck movements and not by elbow movements suggests that the cause is most likely to be in the cervical or thoracic spine, but it does not rule out a local cause as well.

Likewise the absence of symptoms related to the abdominal or thoracic contents does not rule out the presence of pathophysiology in these cavities. There may in fact be a retro-peritoneal mass that is causing referred pain to the spine without affecting the function of abdominal structures and that is why there are no symptoms of visceral disturbance. In theory such a pathology would not be altered significantly by the patient's posture or movement, but it is unwise to assume that this is always the case.

SELECTION OF EXAMINATIONS PERFORMED

It is not essential to perform a comprehensive examination of all body parts and all systems in all circumstances. These must be selected according to the information collected in the history. For instance, it is often appropriate to examine the related cavity when considering posterior spinal pain. Thus, with pain in the low back region, it is wise to examine the abdomen. Likewise if there is pain in a limb that may be referred from the spine, then neurological examination of that limb is advised to ensure there are no signs indicating root or cord damage. Features of a full examination, parts of which may be performed as clinically indicated, will be discussed below.

STATE OF GENERAL HEALTH

Visual features

When patients present to an osteopath, they may well be seeking help for a benign mechanical problem, but they may actually be suffering from symptoms caused by disturbance to a viscera and may have a disease which requires a different form of treatment. Thus differential diagnosis is important as a first step in the evaluative process.

In addition, as argued in Chapter 1, any disturbance of function in one part of the body may affect another part. Thus although the patient may present with an actual musculo-skeletal problem there may also be problems in another body system which interfere or aggravate the mechanical problem.

Therefore during the anamnesis, while listening to the patient, the patient's manner and mental state should be observed. There are also a number of features that may be observed in the face and hands relating to the patient's general health. The beginning of the examination is the examiner's first opportunity to observe the whole of the patient undressed. This may reveal more about their general health from the state of their skin which may be dry and flaky, or oily. A bluish colour of the skin may suggest poor circulation. The general distribution of body fat may indicate an hormonal imbalance (e.g.

central obesity in Cushing's syndrome) and the presence of oedema around the face and in the extremities may be a sign of myxoedema. Skin lesions may be indicative of an underlying autoimmune disorder that could have a direct bearing on apparent musculo-skeletal symptoms (e.g. psoriasis or systemic lupus erythematosus). Further details of these conditions may be found in medical texts.

Systems examination

The osteopath should be equipped to examine any body system for signs of disease or dysfunction. Examination of all systems is not necessarily carried out routinely but only where clinically indicated. This may include thoracic investigation of the heart and lungs as well as searching for peripheral signs of vascular or respiratory disturbance. Not only may signs of serious disease be observed, but also signs of abnormal function, such as shallow breathing, suggesting possible hyperventilation. Likewise abdominal examination may be performed for signs of both serious disease and for functional impairment – frequently there is tightness of gastro-intestinal muscle causing inefficient bowel function, which may be contributing to an irritable bowel problem. Thus osteopathic examination may use similar techniques to medical examination, as can be found in other texts [69], but in addition, gentle palpation may explore the more subtle functional aspects of visceral cavities. Information on visceral osteopathic techniques can be found in more specialist texts [70, 71].

Because of its close functional relationship to the musculo-skeletal system, relevant parts of the neurological examination will be included here.

Neurological

When there is limb pain or other neurological symptoms reported, neurological testing should be performed. With lower extremity symptoms, observe for muscle wasting or other deformity. Also test muscle power, reflexes and sensation. With upper extremity pain similar tests should be performed on both the lower as well as the upper extremity to explore the possibility of spinal cord as well as root compression. In addition, when performing neck movements the patient should be questioned carefully about the presence of any lower extremity symptoms, for example tingling or numbness in the feet caused by the neck movements. With thoracic pain, lower extremity neurological function should be tested.

Nerve stretch tests

The most commonly used are straight-leg raising (Lasegue's test) and femoral nerve stretch tests and neck flexion. In recent years upper extremity nerve stretch tests have been described by Butler [72] but these will not be included here.

Straight-leg raising Anatomical studies have demonstrated that straight-leg raising (SLR) moves the sciatic nerve roots within their intervertebral foraminae. If there is inflammation, tethering or compression by adjacent structures (e.g. disc) of nerve roots, the symptoms resulting tend to be aggravated by SLR, which is therefore limited by hamstring tension induced by the pain.

During SLR the following stages occur [73] (Figure 6.1):

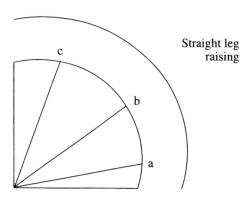

Figure 6.1 Picture SLR theory. Movement of the sciatic nerve in a normal subject: (a) nerve begins to move in sciatic notch; (b) nerve root begins to move in root foramen; (c) movement of nerve in foramen ceases.

a. Once the heel has been raised by 5 cm the sciatic nerve starts to move in the greater sciatic notch. As the leg is raised further the sciatic nerve gradually stretches.
b. At 30 degrees the nerve root begins to move in the root foramen. Between 30 and 70 degrees the normal nerve root is drawn down through the root foramen.
c. Beyond 70 degrees the root does not move; tension increases in the sciatic nerve and root.

SLR should be performed by slowly raising the affected leg and assessing the angle at which pain is experienced by the patient. It is important to ask where the pain is felt. Pain felt in the low back area cannot necessarily be attributed to nerve root involvement and is therefore non-specific. Pain of nerve root origin will be felt in the posterior leg and should reproduce the presenting pain to be significant. Confirmation of the nerve root as the cause can be achieved by lowering the leg a few degrees below the point when pain is initiated. If the foot is then dorsiflexed and pain is again reproduced, then the likely cause is nerve root irritation. Dorsiflexion will reintroduce the nerve tension released when the leg is lowered slightly. Only the nerve is therefore being stretched by this procedure.

SLR may cause pain when other structures are involved. Mooney and Robertson [17] reported that injecting an anaesthetic block into a facet joint not only resulted in pain relief but also improved a limited SLR to normal in 5 minutes. Mooney [74] further reported other patients with SLR of 45–60 degrees with positive EMG findings at the point of limitation who, after facet joint injection, had normal SLR. King [75] reported that treatment to trigger points in spinal muscles produced an increase in SLR and lasting reduction in pain.

Even marked SLR limitation does not inevitably indicate disc prolapse. Fahnri [76] reported three patients who presented typical symptoms and signs of disc prolapse including a positive myelogram. At operation no protrusion was found but the root was adhered to the disc. The nerve was released but the disc was left intact. Good results were reported in all three cases. This suggests that marked limitation of SLR indicates nerve root involvement rather than disc prolapse.

This was supported by work published by Thelander [77], who demonstrated that there is little correlation between size of disc bulge and SLR. He suggests that the limitation is more related to the degree of nerve root inflammation.

SLR also causes movement of the hip, pelvis and lumbar spine. Since all of these structures may cause not only low back pain but also posterior thigh pain, simply lifting the straight leg may reproduce symptoms from these sources. Therefore the addition of dorsiflexion is important to ensure clear differentiation.

In the younger age group (below 40) SLR is a very sensitive test, sometimes producing a false-positive result, particularly during the first week or two of an acute episode. It is therefore not highly specific even when dorsiflexion is included in the test.

Crossed SLR test In this test the pain-free leg is raised. SLR causes longitudinal stretch of the nerve root, but also draws the dural sac laterally. If there is irritation to the contralateral nerve root, then SLR of the pain-free limb may aggravate the symptoms in the painful leg.

A crossed SLR is positive if symptoms in the painful leg are reproduced when the pain-free leg is raised. It is not significant if pain is reproduced in the low back only.

Clinically, Hudgkins [78] demonstrated that the crossed SLR was a particularly specific test for nerve root irritation caused by disc prolapse. He reviewed a sample of 351 patients with diagnosed disc prolapse who all underwent operation. Of the 58 who had a positive crossed SLR, 97% had a proven disc prolapse whereas of the 293 who did not have a crossed SLR, only 64% had a proven disc prolapse. His conclusion was that when the crossed SLR is positive it is a very accurate indication of nerve root irritation by disc prolapse. But note that there were a further 187 with disc prolapse who had a negative crossed straight leg raising. Thus this test is much more specific as a test for disc prolapse than single straight leg raising, but it is less sensitive.

Femoral nerve stretch test Upper lumbar nerve lesions are much less common and therefore this test is used less frequently. For this reason much less research has been performed to assess its specificity. The nerve is stretched by flexing the knee of the painful leg while the patient is lying prone. This theoretically stretches the femoral nerve and reproduction of symptoms indicates irritation of the femoral nerve. However, the result must be interpreted with great care since prone knee bending will induce extension of the hip and secondary extension of the lumbar spine. Thus a number of musculo-skeletal structures will also be moved during this manoeuvre. Alternatively the procedure may be performed with the patient side-lying (Figure 6.2).

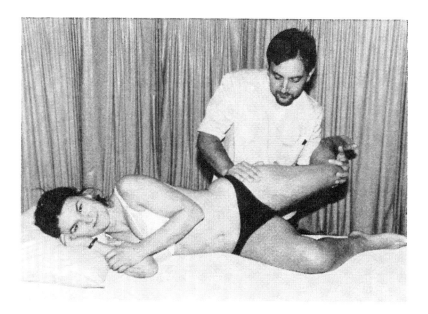

Figure 6.2 Femoral nerve test: the nerve is stretched by extending the hip. If this reproduces pain in the anterior thigh, particularly if it is accompanied by an increase in tingling or numbness, then femoral nerve irritation is the likely cause of the thigh pain.

Neck flexion while supine (Brudzinski's test) Neck flexion causes traction on the structures within the spinal canal. Movement may occur as far down as the lumbar region. Pain initiated in the thoracic or lumbar spine by neck flexion is likely to be caused by irritation of the spinal cord or its surrounding structures rather than by more superficial tissues. Neck flexion can also be used as an adjunct to SLR, since it may cause a greater stretch of the sciatic nerve.

STATE OF THE MUSCULO-SKELETAL SYSTEM

The main elements of the examination include:

- General observation of the patient's frame, including any obvious structural abnormalities.
- Dynamic postural balance.
- Assessment of the state of muscles when standing, sitting and lying.
- Active movements.
- Active resisted movements.
- Passive movements.

General features

Observations are made of any obvious abnormalities of the patient's normal structure; for example, do they have any gross deformity such as a scoliosis, increased antero-posterior curves or protective posture? Are they markedly overweight and how is the excess weight distributed? Is their muscle bulk and distribution consistent with their described activity level, i.e. have they reported playing squash regularly, yet have poor muscle bulk and tone throughout?

STATIC POSTURAL ASSESSMENT

Protection

With some musculo-skeletal and non-musculo-skeletal problems, the body may attempt to minimize further damage by taking up a protective posture (see Figure 7.1). This will usually be apparent, because any attempt to restore a more balanced posture will be met by resistance and pain. Conversely, if the patient naturally stands with their centre of gravity slightly shifted to one side (e.g. to the right), then when asked to actively bend to the left, the movement will be painless (see also Chapter 3).

State of mind

Before considering further the biomechanical assessment of posture, it must be emphasized again that a person's posture often reflects their state of mind. If a patient is anxious about the consultation, then this may be apparent; alternatively the patient may be feeling low as a result of their condition. In assessing a patient's posture this must be taken into account.

General

Now we start to assess the musculo-skeletal structure in more detail. The patient shall be viewed from all directions. It is a helpful discipline to take an overall view and then study the detail in a logical sequence. Remember though that the 'shape' and posture that is observed is not necessarily the patient's 'natural' posture. Much can be learned about the particular person's body from this initial assessment of their posture, but we must not read more into it than is reasonable. Observation of the patient's posture may reveal structural abnormalities which will reduce the adaptability of the body to different positions. They may also cause increased strain on other body parts when maintaining a particular posture. This is merely used as a starting point for the examination.

Posterior view (Figure 6.3)

Overall

Looking first from behind, observe for any gross abnormality in shape. Then consider the line of weight-bearing; is the weight distributed equally on both feet or is the trunk swayed to one side, so that the weight falls more on one leg?

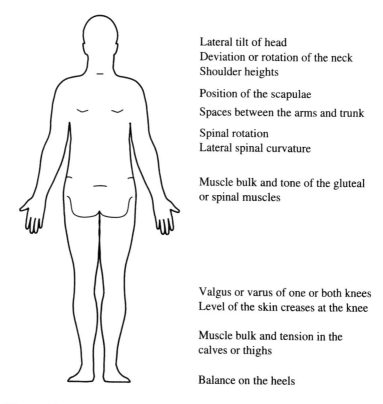

Lateral tilt of head
Deviation or rotation of the neck
Shoulder heights

Position of the scapulae
Spaces between the arms and trunk

Spinal rotation
Lateral spinal curvature

Muscle bulk and tone of the gluteal
or spinal muscles

Valgus or varus of one or both knees
Level of the skin creases at the knee

Muscle bulk and tension in the
calves or thighs

Balance on the heels

Figure 6.3 Postural examination: posterior view.

Detail
Consider:

- Tilt of the head in the lateral plane.
- Deviation of the neck in a lateral plane or any rotation. This may be as a compensation for asymmetry lower in the body or may be the result of problems with one of the special senses. A patient with a hearing problem in one ear may tend to hold their head rotated.
- Shoulder heights. Care must be used in assessing this since protraction or retraction of the shoulder may have an impact on the apparent heights.
- Level of the angles of the scapulae and the displacement of the scapulae from the midline. Any asymmetry may suggest spinal asymmetry or chronic shoulder dysfunction.
- Any apparent rotation in the spine suggested by an increase in the bulk on one side.
- Are the spaces between the arms and the trunk equal? Any difference between these spaces is commonly due to spinal asymmetry. Are the pelvic crests at the same height and is this consistent with the above?
- Any asymmetry of the line of spinous processes in the spine.
- Muscle bulk or tone of the gluteal or spinal muscles.
- Valgus or varus of one or both knees? Are the skin creases at the knee at the same height?

- Muscle bulk and tension in the calves or thighs. If there is any difference between the size of the two legs and is this consistent with any occupational or sporting history or the result of previous injury?
- Balance on the heels. Does one heel roll in or out more than the other?

Lateral view (Figure 6.4)

Overall

It is less easy to assess balance in this plane because of the lack of natural symmetry. Some have previously suggested a theoretical normal posture that has the line of weight-bearing passing through the mastoid process, point of the shoulder, just anterior to the hip joint, just posterior to the knee joint, and through the talus of the foot. Any deviation from this would then cause increasing stress on the muscles to maintain the posture. However, because soft tissues adapt to a degree to the person's natural posture, other postures may be reasonably efficient. It is the overall balance that has more significance. Therefore the line of weight-bearing of the body as a whole needs to be assessed. If the body has a tendency to lean forwards then there will be increased energy required by the posterior muscles to maintain the upright posture. Not only will this lead to postural fatigue but also to soft tissue changes, to adapt to the excessive demand.

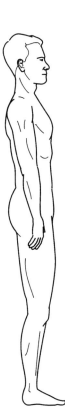

Cervical posture

Shoulder retraction / protraction
Increase or decrease in spinal curvature

Tone of abdominal muscles / anterior trunk contour

Angle of the pelvis on the femurs

Angle of the knees

Figure 6.4 Postural examination: lateral view.

Detail

Consider:

- Cervical posture. Does the head poke forward? This may be a psychologically trained posture, but it has implications for postural stress.
- Shoulder posture. Are the shoulders held in retraction/protraction?
- Spinal shape. Is there an increase or decrease in lumbar lordosis? Increased lordosis statistically increases the risk of low backache [79].
- Is there an alteration of thoracic kyphosis? Increased kyphosis (for instance caused by osteochondrosis) can lead to an increase in cervical lordosis, which may contribute to postural fatigue in the neck and shoulders.
- Tone of abdominal muscles/anterior trunk contour. A large abdomen has significant biomechanical as well as dietary implications for a patient.
- Angle of the pelvis on the femurs. Are the hips extended or in slight flexion. If flexed, is the pelvis relatively tilted forward? This may be due to a shortened capsule or ligaments of the hips, shortened ilio-psoas or to a relatively extended lower lumbar spine.

  If the knees are flexed is this because of the flexion of the hips and lumbar spine? If not, then the knee flexion is probably caused by restriction of the knee joint itself. Hamstring shortening will not be enough to prevent knee extension, since this would prohibit any hip flexion. Sometimes combined flexion of hips and knees is seen with a spondylolisthesis, as an attempt to reduce the shearing force on the lower lumbar spine.

  Note, however, that the increased pelvic obliquity may be the result of psychological rather than biomechanical factors. This will be apparent from passive assessment of the lumbar spine, hips and knees – if they can fully extend, then there is no biomechanical barrier to the posture.
- Angle of the knees. Are they held in full extension or in part flexion?

Anterior view (Figure 6.5)

Detail

Consider:

- Symmetry of the neck in relation to the head and face.
- Breathing pattern. Is it shallow, and is the movement greater in the upper or lower ribs or the abdomen?
- Symmetry of the thorax. Is this consistent with the posterior view?
- Contour of the waistline. This may be drawn in or bulge according to the abdominal muscle tone.
- Symmetry of the abdomen.
- Position of the patellae in relation to the knees and associated tension in quadriceps muscle. With poor vastus medialis tone the patella may be held more laterally.
- Rotation of limb as demonstrated by the position of the feet.
- Inversion/eversion of feet. Are the arches dropped?

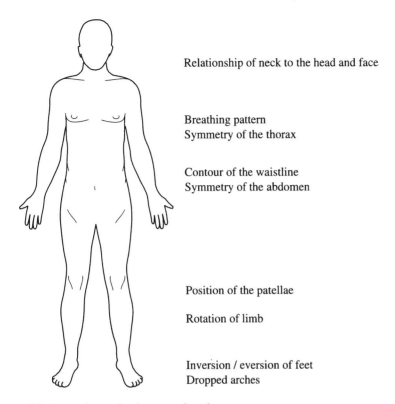

Relationship of neck to the head and face

Breathing pattern
Symmetry of the thorax

Contour of the waistline
Symmetry of the abdomen

Position of the patellae

Rotation of limb

Inversion / eversion of feet
Dropped arches

Figure 6.5 Postural examination: anterior view.

Palpation

Palpation is perhaps the osteopath's most important tool. Not only is it used for assessing both soft tissue and joint disturbance but it is also integral to effective osteopathic treatment, which must be continuously modified according to the response of the body's tissues. Having reached an osteopathic evaluation of the problem, we then work to release the body's reaction to the underlying tissue disturbance, to enhance normal healing and restoration of normal function. As the soft tissue state changes, so does the application of the treatment technique. Osteopaths do not apply a treatment by rote to a set of signs and symptoms. For the same diagnosis an osteopath may use a wide range of therapeutic techniques to achieve the same result, that of improving the patient's overall function. It is vital therefore to recognize that although the tissue state should be assessed as part of the initial patient assessment, it is an ongoing process whenever we are in physical contact with the patient.

Palpation is a skill that is better taught by practical tuition than by the written word, so some brief observations only will be made. The aim of the palpatory examination at this stage is to explore the superficial tissues and the underlying muscles, to identify signs of dysfunction and establish which muscles are posturally active.

First the superficial tissues are palpated. By gently passing the back of the hand over the skin any variation in skin temperature is evident (the back of the hand is more sensitive to temperature than the palm). Skin drag is assessed by gently stroking the surface of the skin. Drag may be increased by a slight increase of moisture in a local area as a result of alteration of sympathetic tone secondary to acute somatic dysfunction. More prolonged dysfunction may cause a decrease of drag, because of mild atrophy.

Erythema may be assessed by rubbing the skin on both sides of the spine and watching the resulting skin response. There may be blanching or reddening. Normally this will be symmetrical in its colour and the length of time that it lasts. Acute dysfunction of an area tends to prolong the red response.

Superficial oedema may be palpated with gentle pressure. This may result from underlying tissue damage or congestion. Tenderness may be reported by the patient, but this is a variable sign and highly subjective. More weight should be given to objective palpable findings.

Next the resistance of deeper tissues to pressure is sensed. Does the tissue feel taut, 'rope-like', nodular, soft and springy? Does the muscle tighten rapidly as we increase the pressure, suggesting that it is very reactive (often when protecting an underlying structure or in dysfunction), and is it tender?

Deeper palpation may also reveal whether there is scar tissue or thickening of tendons, ligaments or capsule around a peripheral joint. This requires an accurate knowledge of the underlying anatomy of the area under examination.

Palpation of muscle states

When a patient is standing, there are certain muscles that are active, at least intermittently, to maintain the posture. As discussed in Chapter 3, these will vary according to how the body shape relates to the line of weight-bearing. At this stage of our assessment we can palpate those muscles which are posturally active. If there is spasm (i.e. excessive tension resulting from protection of a damaged area), then the tension will be greater than that needed to maintain balance and will tend to prevent movement in one or more directions. However if, on palpating muscles, tension is found in non-painful areas, it is not always easy to judge what state the muscle is in (for instance, whether there is hypertonia or fibrosis). This can be clarified by assessment with the patient lying down, when the postural muscles relax (see below).

DYNAMIC STANDING POSTURAL ASSESSMENT

Observation of a patient's posture gives a static impression of the balance of the patient; we are effectively comparing with a theoretical 'normal'. However, a different impression of the patient's balance may be obtained by palpating her response to being swayed gently.

Balance testing

Lateral sway (Figure 6.6)

The practitioner stands behind the patient and places his hands laterally on the patient's shoulders. He gently imparts a force to one shoulder towards the midline and at the same time monitors the patient's response to this movement. The intention is to sway the patient gently from side to side within the stable range. If the patient is swayed too far, then she will feel unstable and resist any further movement. It is important to explain in advance what you are trying to achieve. The patient should be instructed to allow you to gently sway her, but *not* just to go limp as if you will take her weight!

There are two aspects to assess:

- Initial response to movement.
- Centre of weight-bearing.

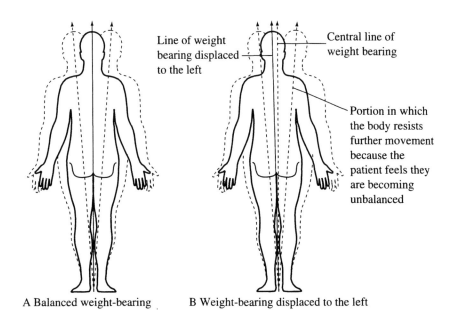

Line of weight bearing displaced to the left

Central line of weight bearing

Portion in which the body resists further movement because the patient feels they are becoming unbalanced

A Balanced weight-bearing

B Weight-bearing displaced to the left

Figure 6.6 Sway testing for postural balance: the patient is gently swayed, first to the left and then to the right. The practitioner senses the point at which the patient starts to resist further movement to avoid becoming unbalanced. A. The range of movement is equal in both directions, thus the patient has reasonably central weight-bearing. B. The range of movement is greater to the right than the left, therefore the patient normally leans to the left.

Initial response to movement

As the practitioner initiates the movement in either direction, he should palpate the resistance to movement, especially comparing the two opposite directions. If the spine is relatively symmetrical in its structure, then the neurophysiological posturing mechanism should allow fairly free movement in both directions. However, if there is dysfunction, particularly in the spinal column, then the posturing mechanism may be altered (see Chapter 3) and there may be unequal resistance when tested. The resistance is due to inappropriate exaggerated muscle reaction to the movement.

However, if there is structural asymmetry due to spinal curvature, there may be a difference in passive connective tissue tension which will alter the palpated resistance to movement.

This kind of sway test may be applied elsewhere on the body, for instance at the level of the pelvis; this is known as the hip shift test and was discussed in Chapter 3. Notice that hip shift may be altered even by dysfunction in the cervical region, though it is most commonly affected by problems in the lumbar spine.

By testing before and after treatment this may be used as a gross test to assess the outcome of treatment. If effective, the overall resistance to swaying should be more equally balanced.

Centre of weight-bearing

If the patient is swayed through a greater range, a point will be reached where we can sense that the position is feeling slightly unstable. This will be at the point where the centre of gravity is close to the edge of the stable base, i.e. the feet. Beyond this point, unless the patient takes avoiding action by putting a hand out or moving a foot to broaden the base, she will fall over. This is not the intention! We are trying to assess the stable range from the position of the patient's normal comfortable posture, i.e. her starting point. Is the range equal in both directions? If it is, then her weight-bearing is central. If she reaches the point of instability more quickly to the left than to the right, then it infers that she is already leaning slightly to her left in the normal posture.

Weight-bearing that is off-centre might be visually obvious if the patient has a fairly straight spine, but with a lateral curvature this is not necessarily so apparent.

Antero-posterior sway

This can be tested by placing one hand on the upper thoracic region posteriorly and another on the upper thorax anteriorly, and the patient gently swayed. In this plane there is of course no anatomical symmetry, therefore assessing the resistance to initiation of movement and the point of weight-bearing is more difficult. As with all palpatory testing, it is a skill that only develops by routine conscious use. Assessment becomes more useful as a library of palpatory memories is built up. In effect we learn to compare the balance of one patient with another.

So what is the importance of weight-bearing? If the body is not evenly balanced then the muscles use more energy to maintain the vertical posture. This is therefore less efficient and puts increased stress on certain postural muscles which then may adapt by hypertrophy, shortening or fibrosis. This in turn interferes with the mobility of affected areas, predisposing them to strain.

Assessing other postures

Assessing a patient's structure when standing will reveal much, but very few of us spend very much time standing in this one position. Many people spend much more time sitting at a desk or workbench, which may alter their weight-bearing and the consequent stresses on their body. To understand these stresses better it may be appropriate to ask the patient to take up the particular posture in which they work. First, there may be features of their workstation that may be contributing to their problem which may come to light through such an exercise. Addressing such features may do more good than any treatment. Second, viewing these postures may reveal areas where the patient's body may not effectively adapt to the demands of their workstation and which may need to be addressed in treatment or management.

GAIT

Gait involves a smooth co-ordinated movement of the arms, spine, hips, knees and ankles. It can therefore be affected by biomechanical or neurological disturbance. The altered gait may be gross, as in the case of hemiparesis, and will be apparent as the patient enters the room. It may be much less evident and may require careful observation, with the patient undressed, though when the patient is aware of being observed she often unconsciously walks more carefully and disguises the abnormal gait. Wherever possible it is wise to watch the patient as she enters the consultation room. It is when the patient is walking that abnormalities of the lower extremity joints are most likely to be observed.

Normal gait involves taking even steps, with the weight equally distributed on each limb in turn. During the weight-bearing phase (stance phase), weight is transferred from the heel to the lateral foot and then to the medial forefoot. The pelvis remains approximately horizontal, but sways from side to side. The spine curves slightly to accommodate the pelvis, moving mostly in the mid-lumbar region. The head should move very little and the arms should swing symmetrically.

Abnormal features of a patient's gait to observe may include:

- Shortened stride length.
- Increased pronation of the foot or leg in the early stance phase.
- Alteration in the weight-bearing sequence of the foot during the stance phase.
- Restriction of flexion or extension in one or both legs.
- Increased pelvic movement, involving more sway or raising of one or both hips in turn.
- Increased sway of the whole body.

When gait is painful the most obvious feature is the alteration of rhythm. The duration as well as the length of the stride is reduced, particularly when the patient tries to walk quickly. This may be *heard* as easily as seen. Pain may be related to dysfunction in the lower extremity, pelvis or spine.

Abnormal gait may be painless; it is then the contour of the gait that is altered. There are a number of causes of abnormal gait.

Neurological damage

Gait depends on intact proprioception and higher centre function including the cerebellum and the extra-pyramidal system. Therefore disturbance in the neurological system commonly causes more obvious characteristic gait patterns. Hemiparesis causes a markedly altered gait; the affected leg is stiff and swings forward in a circular manner rather than being lifted from the ground. In the early stages of Parkinson's disease the sufferer tends not to swing the arms and shuffles along with short steps.

More localized damage to a nerve root by disc prolapse or to a peripheral nerve, such as the common peroneal nerve at the head of the fibula, can cause 'foot drop' because of weakness of ankle dorsiflexion. This may be recognized by the sound of the foot slapping the floor because of the poor muscle control. It may be seen bilaterally in polyneuropathy and in tabes dorsalis, causing a 'high stepping' gait.

Spinal stenosis may cause neurogenic claudication (see Chapter 11). Because of ischaemia of nerve roots within the spinal canal the patient experiences pain on walking. The patient tends to stoop when walking, since this enlarges the cross-section of the canal, thus improving blood flow marginally.

Bone shortening or deformity

This causes asymmetry of the stride pattern. This should be apparent with the patient undressed.

Joint instability

With congenital dislocation of the hip the gluteal muscles are unable to hold up the pelvis, therefore the patient seems to 'waddle'.

Myopathy

In muscular dystrophy the gluteal muscles are weak, also causing a waddling gait.

Joint stiffness, laxity or deformity

An ankylosed or stiff hip will be apparent at the end of the stance phase, as the lack of hip extension will shorten the stride length and the gluteal muscles will be unusually prominent.

A stiff knee joint is more obvious, since the leg seems to move as a whole. Walking up stairs is achieved by stepping up with the good leg and then bringing the affected leg up to the step, thus always leading with the good leg.

A stiff ankle joint is less obvious, causing a slight alteration in the length of stride. It may only be noticed that the heel of the affected foot is raised more quickly during the stance phase.

Dysfunction in the spine, pelvis or lower extremity

Apparent joint stiffness or subtle gait changes may actually be caused by muscle imbalance, shortening or dysfunction. Restriction of extension of either pelvic or lower lumbar joints will shorten the stride length.

ASSESSMENT OF ACTIVE MOVEMENTS

Gross regional movements are performed. Some practical points are relevant when assessing any active movements.

It is important to tell the patient to stop if the movement hurts. The patient should not be allowed to force the movement, unless the osteopath has good reason to request it.

The selection of the first movement is sometimes important. For example, if, from the history or from initial observation, a particular movement is anticipated to be painful, then this movement should be performed last, since this may cause a prolonged reaction in the muscles, thus reducing the potential movement in other ranges.

When observing active movements there are a number of features to consider, which are mentioned below.

Willingness to move

This gives a general indication of the patient's level of discomfort and disability. However, it may also reflect the patient's level of anxiety regarding their pain. Sometimes a patient who has been in acute pain, but is now somewhat improved, may still move with excessive caution, to avoid any risk of reproducing the pain.

Pain behaviour

A number of questions need to be considered here. Because of this it is often helpful to ask the patient to repeat the movement. Communication is particularly important, since it is not enough to know whether it hurts to move but where the pain is being felt on each particular movement. How quickly does the pain increase during the movement? When does it occur – throughout the range, at the end of range or is there a painful arc? How intense is the pain? Although this is a subjective judgement it may give some indication as to how irritable the problem is. This will have implications for the type of treatment and techniques to be used in treatment. Is the character of the pain similar to the presenting symptoms, i.e. are some or all of the symptoms reproduced?

Overall quality of movement

Is the movement free and flowing throughout the range or is it jerky? Is there any deviation or adventitious movement? For example, if there is instability in a lumbar segment, sometimes a momentary pause is seen when returning from a flexed position. This flexion 'catch' is characteristic and may or may not be painful. Alternatively, a disc injury may cause slight deviation during flexion; part of the way through the range the trunk side-bends slightly and then returns to the midline for the rest of the range. This deviation may be associated with pain (i.e. a painful arc of movement).

Is the normal range reduced?

If the range is reduced, the cause of the limit needs to be considered. As mentioned above, the patient may be fearful to move because of previous sharp pain, but the movement may actually be limited by pain. If asked to move further through the range of movement the patient may be able to go further. Pain will be accompanied by a degree of muscle tension or spasm, which eventually will prevent further movement. In the absence of pain, movement is either prevented by the elastic limit of tissues that are stretched by the movement or by tissue compression. The effects of various tissue states on ranges of movement are discussed later in this chapter.

What movement should be assessed?

In the thoraco-lumbar spine, flexion, extension, side-bending and rotation are performed. With lumbar pain, rotation is least helpful. However, it is a significant movement in the thoracic spine. Commonly, with ankylosing spondylitis, spinal rotation is lost early, as is spinal side-bending, and this is more obvious than flexion restriction.

When viewing flexion and extension the movement of the hips must be carefully noted, since this will greatly affect the overall range of spinal flexion. Some people may be able to touch the floor yet have a quite restricted lumbar spine, while others with shortened hamstrings may only be able to reach halfway down their tibias, yet have good lumbar range. A normal lumbo-pelvic rhythm involves initial flexion of the lumbar spine to about 60 degrees and then the hips begin to move allowing a further 80–90 degrees (Figure 6.7).

It is important to look at the shape of the spinal contour from the side of the patient, looking for areas either of curvature or flattening, to identify a section of the spine that is not moving. Note that one is unlikely to identify a *single* restricted spinal joint on active movements.

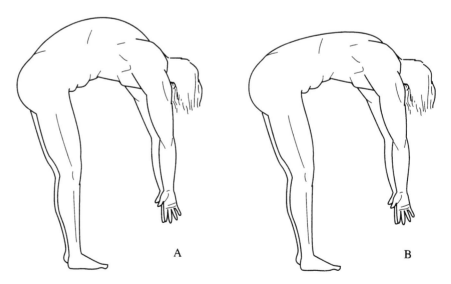

A   B

Figure 6.7 Limitation of flexion: notice the difference in the contour of the lumbar spine. A. Short hamstrings limiting hip flexion – curved lumbar spine. B. Restricted lumbar spine – flattened lumbar spine with hips flexed to 90 degrees. The lumbar spine is therefore approximately horizontal.

Deviation on flexion to one side away from the midline is often, though not invariably, a sign of disc injury. This may be associated with a painful arc of movement in flexion. As the patient bends, she reaches a point that is painful; if she then carries on through the range, the pain eases and she can pass on to a less painful position in flexion.

In the neck flexion, extension, side-bending and rotation are performed. Most commonly affected are rotation and side-bending; restriction of these is usually associated with joint dysfunction.

The shoulder girdle includes a complex of joints. Active movements performed are flexion, abduction, extension and reaching behind and up the back (this involves internal rotation in extension).

Lower extremity joints may be assessed in a similar way, by specific active movements, but an overall view may be useful during observation of gait, which may well reveal functional abnormality.

Tissue differentiation by pain behaviour

Pain reproduction on movement will help, first of all, to identify the area that contains the local source of pain. For instance, pain in the left arm and forearm may be caused by disturbance in the neck, shoulder, elbow, forearm soft tissues or heart. By considering what factors aggravate the arm pain, the area involved can be localized (Table 6.1).

Table 6.1 Activities that aggravate arm pain from different areas

	Neck movement	Shoulder movement	Elbow movement	Gripping hand	Walking upstairs
Neck	Pain				
Shoulder		Pain			
Elbow			Pain		
Forearm muscle				Pain	
Heart angina					Pain

Then the tissues that may be involved need to be established. Different tissues when injured will cause pain under different conditions of loading or use (Table 6.2). Their behaviour can be compared when actively moved, when active movement is resisted by the practitioner or when moved passively. Passive movement assessment will be discussed in more detail later, but pain behaviour will be discussed here.

Active resisted movements are used mainly to differentiate muscle and tendon injury. Thus if damage to a hamstring muscle is suspected, then the patient is asked to contract the muscle against resistance. Pain will be felt on initiation of movement at the site of damage in the muscle. With pain in the extremities, it should not be difficult to differentiate the cause using these principles. However, when considering spinal tissues, the problem is more complex. When active movement is resisted, not only is the muscle contracted but also the muscle tension generated may compress an underlying joint or intervertebral disc. Injury to either of these structures may therefore cause pain on active, resisted movement testing, which may be in the same region as any muscle damage.

Table 6.2 Pain behaviour of various tissues when damaged

Tissue	Active	Active, resisted	Passive
Ligament	End of range of ligament stretch	No pain	End of range of ligament stretch
Capsule	End of many ranges when capsule stretched	No pain unless capsule swollen, then pain when muscle contracted	End of many ranges when capsule stretched
Muscle	On initiation of movement involving muscle contraction	On initiation of movement involving muscle contraction	On passive stretch of muscle
Tendon	On initiation of movement involving muscle contraction	On initiation of movement involving muscle contraction	On passive stretch of muscle
Tendon sheath	During movement	No pain	Sensation of tissue crepitus on movement
Bursa	When overlying muscle is contracted, particularly during movement	When overlying muscle is contracted	No pain
Meniscus	May occur during range	Pain if joint compression traps meniscus	May occur during range

The theoretical behaviour of various tissues is now reviewed. In practice it is unlikely that only one tissue is involved, particularly in the spine, but in the extremities the problem is more often related to predominantly one tissue. The following observations are made, based on a knowledge of anatomy and biomechanics rather than research data.

Ligament

If a ligament is injured and sensitive, then pain will be felt as soon as it is stretched, whether actively or passively. If the joint is moved, the pain tends to occur at the end of range of movement. Depending on the anatomy of the joint and ligament, the pain will be reproduced mainly by only one or two movements.

Capsule

Pain will be maximal when the capsule is stretched actively or passively, but unlike a ligament this will occur usually in a number of ranges of movement rather than only one or two. Commonly a particular joint will be painful and restricted in a characteristic group of movements. For example, with a hip capsule problem the most restricted and painful movements are usually flexion, abduction and internal rotation. Other ranges may also be affected.

When a capsule is highly inflamed, then there may be pain on all movements, even on initiation of movement. This is more obvious when some form of inflammatory arthritis is the cause, for example, gout or rheumatoid arthritis.

Muscle

An injured muscle will cause pain if it is activated during a particular active movement, for example with a torn gastrocnemius, pain will be reproduced by active plantarflexion of the ankle. The pain will be initiated as soon as the muscle is activated. If the movement is possible at all, pain will continue through the range of movement.

In addition, discomfort will also be caused by passive stretching of the damaged muscle, especially in the early stage of the injury. Conversely, if there is no pain caused by active or active resisted movement involving the suspected muscle, then it is very unlikely that a *muscle tear* is the cause of the problem. In this case it is likely that the pain is referred from elsewhere.

Tendon

Because a tendon acts in series with a muscle, if there is damage to a tendon, then pain will be reproduced by similar testing as muscle. Differentiation is made on the basis of the site of pain. For instance in the calf, if the pain is just above the calcaneum, the cause is the Achilles tendon but, if it is 8–12 cm above the ankle, the cause is more likely the musculo-tendinous junction. If it is higher, then the damage is in the muscle itself.

Tendons can also be irritated by compression. For example, if the supraspinatus tendon is swollen then compression may occur between the head of the humerus and the acromial process. Pain is then caused mainly and quite often only on active shoulder abduction at between 70 and 120 degrees. Pain will also be caused by active resisted movement, not necessarily just in the painful range of the joint but even in the neutral position.

Tendon sheath

When inflamed, a tendon sheath will be aggravated particularly as the tendon moves during active *movement*, more than by active resisted movement. On passive movement, if the tendon sheath is highly inflamed, then there may be a crackling sensation palpated over the tendon. This is most commonly encountered with tenosynovitis of the extensor tendons of the wrist and fingers.

Bursa

A bursa reduces friction between muscles or muscles and bone. If a bursa is inflamed, then movement of the area involved will reproduce pain, which will be worse on active than passive movement. Active resisted movement may cause compression and therefore pain, but this tends to be less so than on passive movement.

Meniscus

A cartilage meniscus is found in some joints. The knee is the most important of these, containing one in both the medial and lateral compartment. Active movement of the joint compresses the joint surfaces together and the cartilage between them. If the meniscus is torn, or there is a loose fragment, then this may cause painful locking or blocking of the movement through part of the range. It is therefore frequently painful on walking.

Effects of tissue swelling

Inflammation of one tissue may spread to adjacent tissues and therefore, although a ligament tear may be the initial injury, swelling may extend into surrounding tissues. With an inversion strain of the ankle, swelling may extend down the lateral side of the foot and even to the whole foot. Pain will then be initiated by static weight-bearing, an activity that does not necessarily put stress on the ligament. This effect of inflammation must be borne in mind when considering the hypothetical behaviour of specific tissues, particularly when analysing the spine, which is a more complex system to assess.

It must be emphasized that, although diagnosis of specific tissue damage is important, it will not lead to a consequent treatment plan, since treatment will be directed at the overall dysfunction as a consequence of the body's response to the injury.

PASSIVE EXAMINATION

Watching the patient carefully during the process of lying down sometimes reveals that the symptoms are not as severe as reported. For an acute patient the action of lying down is a difficult movement and usually fairly painful. Absence of this may indicate either malingering or at least exaggeration. Once the patient has managed to lie down, observe whether the body will now relax and allow all joints to stretch or whether there is residual muscle tension and joint restriction. Some low back sufferers, for instance, may not be comfortable lying supine, because extension is painful. In this case it may be wise to examine them in another position, since they may then relax more, and the underlying tissue state may be palpated more easily. If there is a visceral problem, for example a kidney infection, it is more likely that they will not be comfortable in any position but will tend to be restless.

With the patient lying down the effect of gravity is eliminated. Any residual muscle tone is the result of excessive and inappropriate neurological input, due to dysfunction or connective shortening. This may be palpated directly in the muscles or indirectly by passively moving a joint. However there are other influences on joint function which will be discussed later.

Muscle states

When assessing muscle states it is always important to compare one side of the body with the other where possible and one region with another. With experience, and with a knowledge of the underlying anatomy, the texture of the various layers of myofascial tissues can also be palpated.

The variety of muscle states that may be encountered are considered below (Figure 6.8).

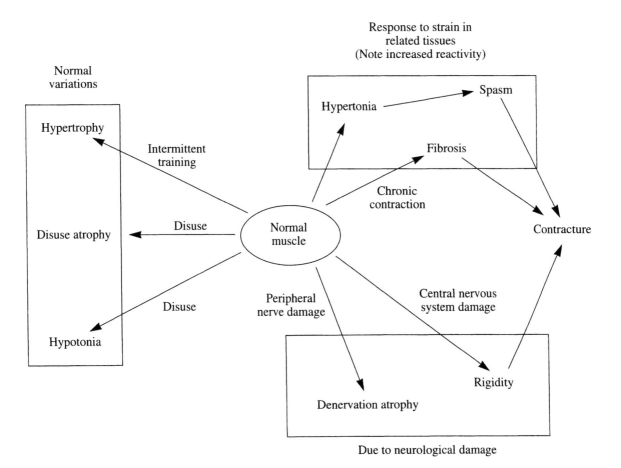

Figure 6.8 Summary of various muscle states.

Normal muscle

'Normal' muscle will relax when there is no stress placed upon it and it is not tender to touch. Normal, of course, is a relative term and is only recognized by comparing to abnormal states. It is only by building up a palpatory 'library' that useful differentiation can be made.

Hypertrophy

If a muscle is intermittently and repeatedly contracted by muscle training exercise, then the muscle will be stimulated to hypertrophy. There is a thickening of muscle fibres because of an increase in the number of individual muscle fibrils within each fibre. To achieve hypertrophy, forceful muscular activity is required or at least repetitive activity at moderate levels. When examined, there is increased bulk of the muscle. If stretching exercises are not performed along with the muscle training, then shortening of the muscles may also occur. On palpation the muscle is enlarged, but is unreactive to touch, similar to the 'normal' muscle state.

Fibrosis

Ischaemia may occur if a muscle is held in a state of persistent tension; for example, because of postural stress. This results because when the muscle contracts it is harder for blood to flow through it. In response to this the muscle develops more fibrous tissue and fibrosis results. This is an adaptation to reduce fatigue, since the fibrotic tissue acts more like a ligament, thus saving the muscle from contracting continuously. However, on palpation, fibrotic muscle is frequently tender and may feel as if there are rope-like bands through the muscle. It is important to note that a muscle is unlikely to become completely fibrosed and therefore there will still be some contractile elements within it. Fibrotic tissue may therefore be hypertonic also.

Hypertonia

Due to increased neurological stimulation there is increased tone of the muscle. Initially this is a reversible state, but within a short time congestion may develop within the muscle. When the patient lies down the muscle may become neurologically inactive, but there will still be increased passive tone (and therefore greater resistance to stretch). This results from both the congestion and also connective tissue shortening that occurs when a muscle is held in a sustained state of contraction (see also Chapter 2). When observed, the muscle will be visibly more tense than normal and on palpation it may be tender and more reactive to gentle pressure. If the muscle is congested then it may feel 'boggy'.

The neurological stimulation is a result of a reflex response. This may be initiated at:

- A brainstem or higher level. This will lead to widespread increase in muscle tone. This is commonly seen when a person is anxious. Activity in the limbic system causes stimulation and a large area of hypertonia results, usually most obvious in the neck, but it may involve the rest of the spine and even the whole body. This appears to be part of our 'protection' response. The person is 'keyed-up', ready to cope with any stresses that await them.

- A segmental level in the spinal cord, causing quite localized hypertonia in response to injury within the related segment (i.e. this is a normal component of dysfunction). The degree of extra-segmental spread of the muscle hypertonia will depend on the intensity of the noxious stimulus and on the more general state of arousal as above.

The two stimuli may co-exist. If there is a joint disturbance that triggers local hypertonia, for instance in the neck, this will add to any existing level of muscle tension. This probably helps to explain why some are prone to 'tension' headaches and others are not. If there is pre-existing local joint dysfunction, then if further muscle tension is added, caused by anxiety or being keyed-up due to pressure or volume of work (the result is the same), then the accumulative tension generated is enough to cause symptoms to be felt.

Spasm

Spasm is a higher level of hypertonia. It is a more intense form of local protection to damage in one or more tissues and is therefore a local reflex effect. It tends to cause marked limitation of movement, at least in one or two ranges of movement, and all ranges may be affected, depending on the tissues damaged. Spasm is characterized by an intense contraction which may become even more obvious on attempting a movement that is painful. On palpation, when standing or even when lying, the muscle is very reactive; even gentle pressure may cause an involuntary flinching reaction.

Contracture

Contracture occurs when a muscle is allowed to maintain a shortened state. This happens:

- When a muscle is held in a state of persistent hypertonia.
- Due to postural stress leading to fatigue or due to lack of stretching following an injury to the muscle. In the case of injury the muscle may well become shortened as a result of scar tissue, as well as connective tissue shortening due to lack of stretching.

Muscle contracture can be recognized, because there is multisegmental restriction of movement in the ranges that stretch the muscle, and it is not reactive to touch, unlike a muscle that is protecting underlying tissue damage.

Hypotonia

Poor muscle tone may develop in a person with a relatively inactive lifestyle. In this case the poor tone will be generalized and on palpation there will less resistance to pressure than normal. It may be more marked in cases of atrophy.

Atrophy

This refers to a state of wasting away of the muscles. Individual muscle fibres decrease in size due to a progressive loss of myofibrils. This is the result of a reduction of the flow of nervous impulses.

Disuse atrophy

This may develop in a group of muscles that are little used, for example in the bedridden or those who have a cast after a fracture. It may also occur in muscles surrounding an arthritic joint. There is visible loss of bulk and poor tone.

Denervation atrophy

If the nerve supply to a muscle is cut, then the muscle will waste and in about 6–24 months the muscle will be one-quarter of its size and the muscle fibres will be replaced by fibrous tissue. When the change to fibrous tissue is complete it is irreversible. Flaccidity is another term used to describe this form of muscle state. A common example of this is the classic 'foot drop' associated with S1 nerve root damage caused by a lumbo-sacral disc injury. As the patient walks, the affected foot 'drops' on to the floor since there is no strength in the foot dorsiflexors.

Rigidity

Rigidity results from central nervous system damage, most commonly associated with a cerebral infarct. The brainstem and the pons usually act as a 'brake', by inhibiting local spinal reflex pathways, so when these areas are damaged the motor output of the anterior horn cells is exaggerated; the muscle is held in a much greater degree of tension and when it is passively stretched the muscle is much more resistant.

Trigger points

Travell [80] discovered that certain points in muscle may become extremely sensitive and act as a source of pain with a characteristic distribution. These trigger points are also reactive when palpated, causing an exaggerated increase in tension. Using injection or spray and stretch techniques these could be eliminated and the pain relieved. They also respond to soft tissue techniques. These may commonly occur alongside or as part of joint dysfunction and may respond to treatment to the joint dysfunction. With persistent or refractive dysfunction, attention to altered muscle states, including trigger points, can be very important.

Assessment of passive joint movement

The assessment of passive joint movement is fundamental to osteopathic practice, because in the first instance most osteopathic treatment techniques are designed to alter passive function, and thereby reduce or eliminate dysfunction in order to relieve symptoms. Without the ability to palpate joint dysfunction we can therefore neither identify it nor treat it.

Whether peripheral or spinal joints are being assessed, there are various aspects of joint movement that need be to considered:

- *Total range of movement.*
- *Ease of movement.* Consider ease of initiation and ease of movement through the range (Figure 4.2). Does the resistance increase very quickly, suggesting increased muscle reactivity, or does the joint move freely to the end of range? The resistance will be related to both the passive and active state of the soft tissues around the joint, including the muscles and fascia. The joint viscosity may also contribute. If there is significant degenerative change in the surface of the joint, this may be palpated as crepitus. This is easier to feel in peripheral joints, but can sometimes be elicited from spinal facet joints.
- *'End feel'.* At the end of range, what appears to prevent further movement? If there is a gradual increase in resistance which reaches a springy end point, this suggests that muscles are the main limiting factor. If there is hypertonia then the resistance will build up quickly within the range and limit it short of the expected range, e.g. a gastrocnemius tear; dorsiflexion would be limited because pain would be initiated by passive stretching early in the range and reflex contraction would restrict further movement. In comparison, a non-traumatized joint would reach the end point without such an increase in resistance. Only in the last fraction of the range would the ligaments resist the movement, causing a firm end feel but with a small degree of elasticity.

Note: The findings on active and passive movements of various other tissue states will be discussed later in the chapter.

Assessment of passive movement is most easily performed with the patient lying down, although some areas may be examined passively in the sitting position. Generally the patient is more able to relax when lying and thereby the tendency to resist or help the practitioner is minimized. The aim is always to move the body in a careful but firm manner, so that the patient feels supported but not uncomfortable (unless, of course, one needs to stretch a painful part). Heavy-handedness will cause the patient to resist. The examiner cannot then gain accurate information and the examination could even become a painful struggle between patient and practitioner. It goes without saying that this puts at risk the patient's confidence – and her co-operation.

Observation of active movements and gait may have already indicated specific areas which will need more detailed assessment. At this stage we are looking for evidence of abnormal function in particular areas of the body; this may be more subtle than that which is seen on active examination. For instance, although gait may be normal, there may be restriction of rotation of the hip which may have implications for pelvic and consequently spinal function. Likewise, gross spinal movements may be normal, but there is specific restriction of passive movement in a thoracic spinal segment contributing to a neck problem.

General screening examination

In each position, first the muscles that are accessible in this position are assessed and then particular joint movements are assessed as described below.

Supine

Muscles (starting from the feet and working up the body)

Anterior leg muscles, quadriceps, adductors, tensor fascia latae, abdominals, pectorals, anterior, lateral and posterior cervical spinal muscles (these are more easily palpated with the patient supine rather than prone – it is not so easy to relax the neck when face down), biceps, forearm flexors and extensors.

When palpating spinal muscles it is important to be aware of the depth of different layers of muscles. A detailed knowledge of the anatomy of the musculo-skeletal system is crucial. Generally, superficial muscles will be larger and longer and therefore, if there is a disturbance in these, the tightness is more widespread. However there may be discreet localized tender points or trigger points. In the deeper layers, especially close to the spinal joints (i.e. multifidus), there may be localized tender hypertonic muscles, usually indicative of dysfunction around the joint beneath.

Movement testing

Ankle dorsiflexion Limitation is commonly due to muscle or ligament shortening due to previous or present damage.

Knee extension This is lost if there is any mild swelling in the joint or commonly with mild to moderate degenerative changes. Limitation may also be due to poor leg posture, with hips and knees held in flexion, leading to chronic shortening of soft tissues.

Hip internal and external rotation Limitation may indicate early degenerative changes, muscle imbalance, pelvic joint dysfunction.

Lateral lower rib springing Gently spring with both hands in a medial direction. This gives a general overall impression of the mechanical compliance of the rib cage, with its impact on the spine and torso and on the effort of breathing. This has a particular bearing on patients with intra-thoracic problems.

Circumduction of the shoulder The *elbow* is taken passively through the maximum range of movement, starting with flexion with adduction and internal rotation. The arm is raised past the ear and, when the shoulder joint reaches full flexion, the arm is then returned to its starting position through an abduction-adduction range and returned to the side of the body (Figure 6.9).

Any limitation of this full arc of movement indicates dysfunction in the gleno-humeral, acromio-clavicular or scapulo-thoracic joint. Occasionally acute pain in the upper back may lead to painful limitation of the shoulder, but the pain is then felt predominantly in the upper thoracic or scapula region, rather than in the gleno-humeral or lateral arm area, as is usual with shoulder girdle problems.

Neck rotation and/or side-bending In the neck an area of dysfunction is most easily palpated with one of these movements.

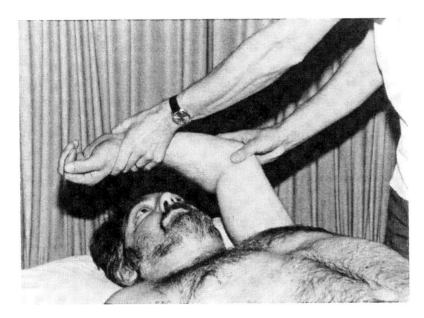

Figure 6.9 Testing the shoulder for full range of movement: with the elbow bent at 90 degrees and the gleno-humeral joint in 90 degrees of internal rotation, the shoulder is taken through a flexion range (as shown). When the shoulder reaches full flexion then the arm is returned to its neutral position at the side of the body through an abduction-adduction range.

Limitation in any of these tests indicates abnormal function and therefore more thorough examination of that area is required. This is discussed further in the specific chapters on various regions of the body.

Prone

The patient lies prone with arms over the side of the examination table, with the head either facing down if the table has a 'nose hole' or with the head turned to one side (as preferred by the patient).

Muscles
Calf, hamstrings, gluteals, spinal extensors, periscapular muscles.

Movement testing
Spinal springing This is performed by placing the heel of one hand over each spinal joint in turn and gently leaning in a postero-anterior direction. The line

of force can be varied from this vertical direction to a more cephalic or caudal direction (Figure 6.10). Alternatively, pressure may be applied bimanually to the transverse processes, using the hypothenar eminence of one hand and the thenar eminence of the other. The aim is to sense the resistance of a region or a specific segment. Abnormal muscle reaction to mild pressure indicates dysfunction. Excessive reaction may indicate serious pathology of bone (fracture, metastasis, infection) or a serious disc injury.

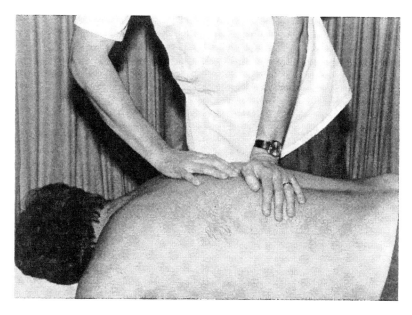

Figure 6.10 Springing the thoracic spine: this may be used as an examination technique to assess the general mobility of an individual spinal joint or region. By modifying the direction of the force flexion, extension or side-bending can be palpated. This may also be used in treatment either as an articulation technique or, by applying the force to the transverse processes, as a high-velocity thrust.

Sacral springing There is considerable controversy not just about where any line of axis of movement occurs through a pelvic joint but even whether there is any movement at all. However, most manipulating therapists of a wide range of persuasions do now agree that there is palpable movement. Assuming an approximate axis through the body of S2, we attempt to 'spring' or 'hinge' the sacrum about this axis between the two relatively stable ilia. Pressure is applied by the heel of one hand, while movement is monitored by a finger or thumb of the other hand palpating the sacro-iliac joint. There is only a very small movement available even in a normal pelvic joint. It is therefore very easy to push too hard or too far and 'jam' the joint before the movement has been perceived. It is often easier to feel the movement as the pressure is released than as it is applied (Figure 6.11).

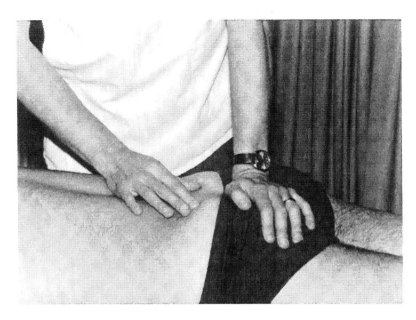

Figure 6.11 Springing the sacrum: pressure is applied by one hand to the sacrum with the intention of causing a rotation movement about a theoretical axis through S2. Movement is palpated by the fingers of the other hand at the upper pole of the sacro-iliac joints.

Hip extension The hip may be hyper-extended by lifting the leg with a hand under the thigh. Extension is commonly reduced early with osteoarthritis. Psoas shortening will also limit hip extension. This may be a secondary feature of a lumbar disc injury due to prolonged muscle spasm.

Side-lying examination of the spine

Although muscles may be palpated in a side-lying examination, it is easier to compare opposite sides when lying prone or supine so it is mainly movement testing that is performed in this position. With the patient lying on their side with their knees and hips at 90 degrees, small movements of the lumbar spine may be performed by moving the legs in a rhythmic flexion-extension range (see Figure 4.3). If a patient, however, has stiff hips, then the lumbar movement may begin before 90 degrees of hip flexion and passive assessment of the spine must be performed with the appropriate degree of hip flexion. The actual range of movement may be palpated by feeling the movement of the spinous processes as they move apart in flexion and approximate in extension. Also the adjacent muscles may be palpated as the spine is moved. The reactivity can be palpated; if there is dysfunction for any reason the muscles tend to tense actively during the movement and the increase in tone is palpable.

Similarly lumbar and thoracic rotation may be performed in this position, although not through their full range. By initiating small movements the response of the local soft tissues may be palpated. Any excessive reactivity in the soft tissues indicates dysfunction.

Causes of limitation of movement

Although osteopaths are concerned with altered function, it will be recalled from Chapter 1 that function may be changed not only by dysfunction, a reversible state involving inappropriate physiological activity, but also through structural changes, which are usually less amenable to change (Table 6.3). Therefore, the behaviour of various tissue states found on active and passive movement will be considered.

Table 6.3 Causes of movement restriction

Tissue state	Examples
Congenital	Facet anomalies Abnormal segmentation Spondylolysis, olisthesis
Developmental	Osteochondrosis Organic scoliosis Stenosis
Degenerative	Disc – spondylosis Facet arthrosis Stenosis
Inflammatory	Ankylosing spondylitis
Neurological	Ischaemic damage, e.g. cardio-vascular accident
Myofascial adaptation	Postural strain causing myofascial shortening Fibrosis
Somatic dysfunction	Response to tissue injury or strain
Psychological (altered muscle tone)	Anxiety Depression

Congenital

Congenital anomalies are not uncommon in the lower lumbar and, to a lesser extent, in the thoraco-lumbar region. Failures of segmentation occur around the lumbo-sacral area. There may be fusion of this joint with the disc calcified (sacralized lumbar segment) or fusion of one or, less commonly, both facet joints. Occasionally the L5 transverse process is fused to the iliac crest or the ala of the sacrum.

The planes of the facet joints may be anomalous. These are usually in a sagittal plane in the lumbar spine, but, at the lumbo-sacral level, they may be virtually coronal, allowing much greater rotation and thus increasing the torsional strain on the soft tissues at this level. Asymmetry of the facet planes (tropism) is common, affecting up to a quarter of the population. The facet planes have been observed to be angled, with the inferior joint surface facing medially and inferiorly.

The clinical significance of these anomalies has received much debate, with no statistically definitive results. Logically there is likely to be some mechanical impact on the adjacent tissues, but it is important to note that such anomalies have been observed on X-rays of non-symptomatic people – symptoms are not inevitable. Most anomalies described above will cause markedly reduced mobility of the segment, except where facet planes are coronal rather than sagittal; rotation then is more easily palpated. Anomalies are frequently not evident on active movements since usually only one joint is involved. On passive examination the segment is limited, although the muscle response may be normal in the absence of dysfunction.

Total or partial sacralization will cause complete immobility. Sometimes this causes confusion about the level of the lumbo-sacral joint. A guide to the level of the spine is that the lumbo-sacral joint is approximately at the same level of the posterior superior iliac spines.

Spondylolysis is a defect of the pars interarticulares where the posterior arch does not fuse to the anterior portion. The two are joined by cartilage which is less strong. Depending on the forces imposed and the strength of the surrounding soft tissues, the cartilage defect may become weakened, allowing anterior slippage of the body of the vertebra, while the posterior arch is held back by the superior articular processes of the vertebra below. This is known as spondylolisthesis. It is not inevitably a symptomatic condition, even when slippage is present; patients have been seen with the defect observed on X-ray, but no low back pain reported. The variety of possible clinical presentations will be discussed in Chapter 11.

Developmental

Spinal osteochondrosis (Scheuermann's disease) is caused by a defect in development in puberty. There is softening of the cartilage end-plates of the vertebrae, usually the lower border of the vertebral body, leading to narrowing and anterior wedging of the disc space. The commonest area involved is the thoraco-lumbar junction area (T10–L3), followed by the middle and occasionally the upper thoracic spine. It is very rarely seen in the lower lumbar or cervical area. There is, as yet, no adequate explanation for this distribution.

Sometimes symptoms are experienced in teenage, more commonly in males, causing low-grade aching, but frequently there are no symptoms and the kyphosis is blamed on the teenage psyche. The presence of osteochondrosis predisposes to degenerative changes, but not to a serious extent. However, Stoddard [19] considers that it also predisposes to mechanical back pain in adjacent areas of the spine by the fourth or fifth decade, due to increased dynamic or postural strain. This will depend on the lifestyle of the person; physical fitness will reduce the likelihood of symptoms.

Muscles overlying areas of osteochondrosis are typically fibrotic and tender on palpation, but not reactive on passive movement. Posturally there is increased flexion of an area, in the thoracic area seen as an increased kyphosis and in the thoraco-lumbar region as a flattening of the normal lumbar lordosis (see Figure 11.2). This is accompanied by chronic restriction of movement in all ranges, felt on thoracic springing as an almost rigid block.

Since a group of segments are affected together, the limitation is obvious on active as well as passive movements.

As discussed in Chapter 7, there are structural changes in the bones and joints that occur in an organic scoliosis which cause palpable rigidity of the area.

Degenerative changes

These occur predominantly in the lower cervical and lower lumbar areas, and to a lesser extent in the upper cervical region. However, if there has been trauma to other parts of the spine, the resulting damage and scar tissue may accelerate degeneration in these areas also. The clinical significance of degenerative changes is discussed in Chapter 2.

Disc degeneration may lead to hypermobility in the early stages, with accompanying instability. This can sometimes be palpated in the lumbar spine on passive flexion by an increased degree of AP shift; in flexion the upper vertebra seems to move more anteriorly than is usual.

Early changes in the facet joints occur in the capsules and ligaments due to previous damage and scarring. Shortening of these tissues may lead to a loss of flexion and, to a lesser degree, side-bending. As facet joint arthrosis advances and the joint cartilage surfaces deteriorate, osteophytes form around the joint margins and this leads to further reduction in movement, particularly of extension. Extension may be lost entirely and the lumbar spine loses its lordosis completely and may even become flexed. This effect is probably a combination of the facet and disc thinning changes.

In the absence of somatic dysfunction, loss of movement may commonly be observed in all ranges and passive movement will characteristically be limited with a relatively sudden end feel, having lost some of the surrounding soft tissue elasticity.

If there has been previous trauma to an area with or without actual bony damage, then this often leads to scar tissue and immobility. On passive movement there is again a rigid feel. The history gives the pointer as to the reason for this finding.

Inflammatory arthritis

Ankylosing spondylitis is discussed in Chapter 11 in more detail. It is an inflammatory arthritis that most commonly starts in the sacro-iliac joints or around the thoraco-lumbar region. In the early stages there may be no X-ray changes that will identify it and there are some cases where the ESR may not be raised, which makes recognition of the condition difficult. However, even before the appearance of the X-ray features, there will probably be significant stiffening of the spine. Since it usually begins in younger people (20–40 years at presentation) it should be suspected in a patient with recurrent or persistent stiffness, with or without pain. In these patients there will be loss of movement in all ranges, often most noticeable in side-bending or rotation.

In the later stages when ankylosis has occurred the problem is obvious because there is complete loss of active and passive movement in all ranges as one or more regions of the spine become like a single bony rod rather than a series of segments.

Neurological

Structural damage may occur in the nervous system resulting in altered movement of a body part. A stroke may cause damage to part of the brain leading to abnormal motor control, seriously impairing mobility as well as the control of the affected joints. Usually the cause is apparent from the history but neurological examination will generally clarify the underlying problem. With a lesion within the pyramidal system, muscle tone is increased in the affected area, which is commonly a complete body region (e.g. a whole extremity). When the patient lies down, initially the tone is maintained. If soft tissue techniques are applied the muscles may relax, but any attempt then to move the area causes immediate contraction again and movement is resisted. Unlike acute muscle spasm secondary to mechanical dysfunction, the muscle reaction is not accompanied by an increase in pain or discomfort.

Myofascial adaptation

Chronic postural strain may lead to persistent muscle contraction (Figure 6.12). This may then cause fibrosis within a muscle. This involves an increase in connective tissue which is non-contractile and less elastic. In addition, there may be connective tissue shortening both in muscle and fascia due to cross-bridging of collagen. Fibrotic muscle is usually tender on palpation and feels 'ropy' under the fingers. The fibrosis is relatively irreversible but the sensitivity may well be due to accompanying hypertonia caused by the original muscle fatigue.

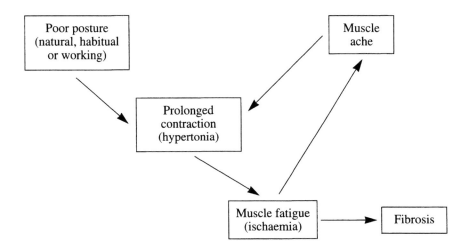

Figure 6.12 Muscle changes that may result from postural strain.

The muscles most affected are the larger postural muscles – in the neck the trapezius, in the thoracic and lumbar spine the more superficial erector spinae muscles that traverse many segments. The result of these muscular changes is to reduce the flexibility of the underlying spinal region.

This may also occur with extremity joints. For example, hip extension may be restricted by a shortened hip capsule, shortened psoas or rectus femoris. To differentiate between the two muscles hip extension can be tested, first with the knee straight, then with it flexed. If the rectus femoris is limiting the hip extension, then hip extension will be greater with the knee extended. Knee flexion will have no effect on psoas. Since the psoas muscle is attached to the spine and acts as a weak side-flexor of the spine, then if the psoas muscle is shortened, side-bending the spine towards the restricted hip should allow slightly more hip extension. Take care not to abduct the hip since this might allow more extension.

If a broad muscle like the trapezius is shortened, as is the case with many typists and keyboard operators, then side-bending in the neck is often reduced. It is possible to palpate the joint movement individually, using the side-shifting technique discussed above. However, the trapezius muscle is often shortened as well as there being joint restriction. If the trapezius is the main cause of restriction when full side-bending is tested, then the upper border of the muscle will form a tight band from the upper cervical down towards the shoulder area. If the restriction is mainly in the cervical joints, then the trapezius is less taut.

In a similar way if there is restriction in the lower lumbar spine it may be from shortening of the superficial erector spinae muscles or from soft tissue shortening at a segmental level. Since the superficial muscles traverse a number of segments, we may compare the range of flexion of the lower lumbar spine with the upper lumbar joints flexed or extended. If the lower lumbar joints themselves are restricted, then the relative position of the upper lumbar spine will have no effect. If the limitation of movement is due to the superficial muscles, extending the upper lumbar spine will allow more flexion movement in the lower lumbar area.

Somatic dysfunction

If the patient is complaining of pain, then almost inevitably there will be some degree of dysfunction in the area that has been disturbed (whether the cause is somatic or visceral and the effects of dysfunction may be in both). Note that because of the effect of the phenomenon of referred pain the pain may not be in the area of the disturbed function. There is likely to be some degree of muscle reaction. However this may not be apparent on active movement. In its most subtle degree there may only be some *palpable* increase in muscle reaction on initiation of passive movement and restriction of range. The other extreme is when there is an acutely inflamed area due to tissue damage. There is then acute spasm with severe loss of range of active movement. In addition, there is frequently no palpable movement in a number of segments due to the spasm which is maintained, even when lying down.

With *somatic* dysfunction in the absence of serious structural damage (e.g. fracture) usually some, rather than all movements are restricted to some degree. Marked restriction of movement in all ranges is more often a sign of serious underlying damage such as fracture or a large disc prolapse.

Visceral dysfunction may also cause restriction of movement in the musculo-skeletal system as part of a protective reaction. Acute peritonitis causes complete bracing of the abdomen and spine. However, the patient's overall state of health and abdominal symptoms and signs usually are a guide in differential diagnosis. On the other hand, less intense visceral dysfunction may cause palpable reflex changes in the musculo-skeletal system, particularly in related spinal segments. There may be reflex muscle contraction and restriction of passive movement which may be erroneously interpreted as due purely to somatic dysfunction. This must always be borne in mind, even in the absence of visceral symptoms, and, if in doubt, appropriate examinations and tests should be performed to clarify the diagnosis.

When an area of dysfunction is palpated the muscle will be more reactive to touch. On passive movement there will be a greater response in the muscle on initiation of movement. This 'twitch response' is used particularly in functional technique, where the ease or restriction of initiation of movement is crucial to finding a position of greatest ease of an area of dysfunction (see Chapter 4). In addition, there will also be limitation of the range of movement in one or more directions on passive testing. However it is the increasing muscle resistance, both on initiation of movement and throughout the range, that is characteristic of dysfunction rather than reduced range of movement, since as discussed above there are many other tissue states that may reduce the overall range of movement. This is probably the most important finding that an osteopath can observe to confirm the presence of dysfunction.

Dysfunction may persist for months and even years without full resolution, but it is rarely persistently painful. Thus even in an asymptomatic area there may be signs of somatic dysfunction. These may include joint restriction, increased muscle tone, and exaggerated muscle contraction on movement. With chronic dysfunction the skin may become dry rather than the increased sweat response seen in acute dysfunction and skin rubbing may result in a very brief skin weal only (this tends to be more persistent in acute dysfunction). Clearly, therefore, the body's neurological response has changed over a period of time, yet is still abnormal compared with other parts of the musculo-skeletal system.

Psychological factors

A further cause of altered muscle tension that will affect joint mobility is the patient's state of mind (see Chapter 1). Anxiety and other stress states may cause an increase in muscle tension, which may add to muscle reaction of dysfunction. Generally this will be widespread and not localized to one or two specific joints and therefore may be differentiated from joint dysfunction. At times this may be the overwhelming influence on the musculo-skeletal system. It is important to recognize this and refer to some form of psychological therapy if necessary. Sometimes it may be the worry of the symptoms, caused by their dysfunction, that may be the major cause of anxiety, which may account for some remarkable improvements after initial treatment!

Multiple causes of restriction

It cannot be overemphasized that dysfunction may occur in addition to all the other causes of restriction. It may be superimposed onto a spine that is already degenerate (and frequently is), it may be found complicating a neurological deficit caused by a stroke, it may occur in a patient who has currently or has previously had inflammatory arthritis. In these cases it is entirely appropriate for an osteopath to treat, but it is important to acknowledge that there are various components to the mobility restriction, since this will affect the response expected from treatment.

Hypermobility

Emphasis in the above sections has been on hypomobility of both joints and soft tissues. This is because hypomobility occurs when there is tissue disturbance and clinically we are most frequently called upon in such circumstances. However, either localized or generalized hypermobility can also occur; when localized it is frequently a secondary effect to hypomobility in an adjacent area of chronic somatic dysfunction. Generalized pathological hypermobility may result from a congenital abnormality, such as Marfan's syndrome, or from a neurological disorder. Others are constitutionally hypermobile. This can be recognized by assessing elbow and knee extension, where there is usually at least 10 degrees of extension beyond the normal.

If hypermobility is generalized, then, although the flexibility this provides may be helpful in certain sports or occupations, it may be a problem for more static activities. The ligamentous laxity that accompanies the hypermobility also reduces the stability that the ligamentous structures usually provide, and thus the person is more vulnerable to postural fatigue. If, therefore, the postural fatigue is principally the result of the generalized hypermobile state, then manual treatment is less likely to be helpful. Attention must be given to the maintenance of good posture and the strengthening of postural muscles.

Hypermobility may be found adjacent to areas of joint restriction which may result from a variety of causes (see Chapter 1), including congenital abnormalities, degeneration and dysfunction. If dysfunction is present in adjacent areas, then treatment of this may well improve any tissue disturbance and reduce strain on the hypermobile segment. The hypermobile joint may or may not be the site of the cause of the symptoms. If it has been strained, then reason suggests that there will be consequent somatic dysfunction and reduction in range of movement and this does indeed happen. Thus what appears to be a restricted joint prior to treatment may turn out to be hypermobile (though not purely as a result of treatment). With a lesser degree of restriction, the joint may actually seem to be hypermobile and yet is still restricted compared to its normal range; this can of course only be assessed retrospectively, after treatment (Figure 6.13).

Extension   Flexion

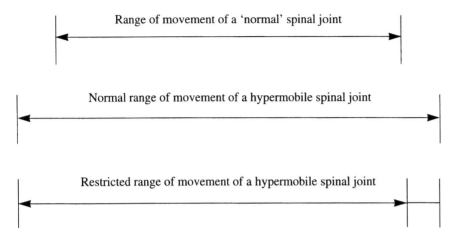

Figure 6.13 Restriction of movement of a hypermobile joint.

Should a hypermobile joint be manipulated? It is probably inappropriate to use forceful techniques such as high-velocity thrust techniques in the area of hypermobility, if they are performed at the end of range. However, minimal leverage thrusts which are performed in the mid-range may be used, since these may help improve the quality of movement and alter reflex behaviour of the surrounding tissues, without stretching the already lax ligamentous structures.

OTHER TESTS

Further tests including blood tests and X-rays may be necessary to clarify the local diagnosis. These are no less a part of the osteopathic diagnostic process than the manual examination already described, since they will give important information about the state of the patient's health and the nature of her problem.

X-rays are not requested routinely for all musculo-skeletal problems. Their use is important when serious pathological disease is suspected, including infection, neoplasm and metabolic pathology. Observation of degenerative changes needs to be interpreted with great care since, as discussed in Chapter 2, there is no correlation between degenerative changes and clinical symptoms [34]. Thus the presence of degeneration should not be assumed to be the cause of pain. Only when there is gross signs of degeneration is this of importance.

Currently access to more specialized scanning techniques, such as computerized tomography and magnetic resonance imaging, is only available through a medical specialist and then only used prior to possible surgery. It is important that osteopaths understand both the value and the limitations of these techniques.

SUMMARY

There are three main aims of the examination:

1. To differentiate between possible hypothesized causes of symptoms generated from the case history. This may involve differentiation of the various tissues by attempting to reproduce the symptoms. The objective is to determine what has happened to the various tissues involved rather than purely label the patient with a particular 'syndrome'.
2. To discover how the body has responded at a local, regional and whole body level to the cause of the dysfunction. This emphasizes the fact that though somatic dysfunction may have localized effects, it may be much broader and thus treatment and management may be required at each level of the person.
3. To discover any predisposing factors that may have contributed to the development of the presenting problem by exploring the body's mechanical function, principally the musculo-skeletal system but also muscle and fascial tension surrounding the viscera.

Clinical Aspects

PART

2

Spinal curves | 7

The adult human form will always show a certain degree of curvature in the antero-posterior (AP) plane when in the standing posture. The amount will often reduce when in the lying position. However, this seldom disappears completely. The rare exceptions are seen in the very supple, for example, ballet-trained individuals. The reason for the retention of a slight curve is usually due to the changes which occur in the spinal ligaments.

In childhood, however, these curves are often more apparent in the standing position, and can disappear completely when lying. The changes are able to take place because the ligaments are very flexible and can accommodate change.

Curvature of the spine was first described in the fourth century BC by Hippocrates. With him originated the term scoliosis, which is taken from a Greek word meaning to twist or bend. The term denotes lateral curvature of the spine. The deformity can be permanent; this situation arises as a result of permanent changes in the bones or soft tissues. Alternatively, it may be no more than a temporary disturbance, produced by reflex or postural activity of the spinal muscles.

SPINAL CURVES IN PRACTICE

It must be emphasized that most spinal curves do not give rise to symptoms. Clinically, an osteopath may be faced with any of the following situations:

- A case of previously diagnosed scoliosis, i.e. a patient presents with a set of symptoms which have a defined history. The patient also volunteers that they have been previously told they have a scoliosis, which was confirmed on X-ray.
- A patient seeks a consultation about their 'twisted' spine, not necessarily with symptoms, only an anxiety about the appearance of the spine. Quite commonly the consultation is with the parents who are uncertain about the nature and prognosis of the deformity of their child's spine.
- A defined set of symptoms and history, which has resulted in a visible side shift of the spine. The patient will make reference to the appearance of a 'bulge' at the base of the spine; or that their 'bottom' has moved to one side.
- A clinical presentation of symptoms which can be attributed to the presence of the scoliosis. This may arise in cases where the patient has no prior knowledge of the curve.

For convenience, four main types of scoliosis can be identified:

1. Sciatic scoliosis.
2. Compensatory scoliosis.
3. Idiopathic or primary scoliosis.
4. Secondary structural scoliosis.

Sciatic scoliosis

This is the most temporary of the deformities. It is produced by protective action of the muscles in certain conditions of the spine. The underlying pathology can be any sudden acute cause of pain in the lower back. The predominant clinical feature is severe back pain with or without sciatica, aggravated by any spinal movement (Figure 7.1).

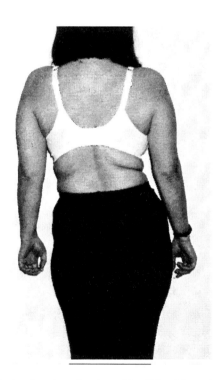

Figure 7.1 Sciatic scoliosis: showing clearly a side shift of the spine.

Compensatory scoliosis

This is seen when present in order to compensate for an underlying deformity of the pelvis or lower limbs. It is commonly seen with a hip pathology or prosthesis. The curve which arises in the lumbar spine is temporary and disappears when the patient is recumbent or the pelvic tilt is corrected. (However, in cases of many years' duration, the lumbar scoliosis may become fixed by adaptive shortening of the tissues in the concave side.)

The above two categories can be broadly described as being *'functional curves'*. This group can be defined as curvatures in the lateral plane which have *not* undergone any pathological or physiological changes.

Categories 3 and 4 are part of a general group which can be termed *'structural curves'*. This group includes spinal curvature, in any plane, which has undergone irreversible and hence permanent changes of the bones and soft tissues (Figure 7.2).

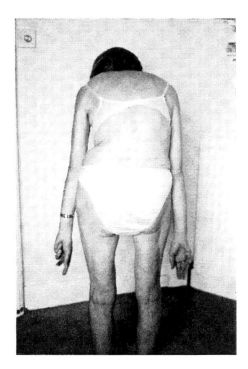

Figure 7.2 Structural scoliosis.

In childhood, a well-defined group of curves of unknown cause is known as idiopathic or primary scoliosis.

Idiopathic or primary scoliosis
This is the most important type of structural scoliosis which must be identified and monitored. It starts in childhood or early adulthood and tends to increase progressively until cessation of skeletal growth. Left unattended, it can result in severe and prominent deformity. This is especially so if marked in the thoracic area. Any part of the thoraco-lumbar spine may be affected.

Secondary structural scoliosis
In this group the spinal curvature is secondary to a demonstrable underlying deformity. The commonest underlying causes are congenital abnormalities, especially hemivertebra. Other causes include neurological conditions which result in a residual weakness of the spinal muscles, for example poliomyelitis.

In its mildest state, a *functional curve* will only be noted by the trained eye. A *structural curve* can usually be seen clearly when the subject is in a state of suitable undress. The higher the distortion, the more marked the presentation. The individual may suffer from local pain caused by the musculo-skeletal tissues. In some cases, the gross distortion of the rib cage will cause changes in function of the contained organs. These changes will be experienced as symptoms of the respiratory or cardio-vascular systems.

THE 'SPECTRUM' OF SPINAL CURVES

Understanding the biomechanics of how and why curves occur demonstrates that if, in cases where the line of the spine is initially straight, and is then, for whatever underlying reason, made to deviate from the 'normal', we can observe the spine going through a '*transitional*' phase.

Pathogenesis

There are several known, and some still disputed causes for the development of spinal curves.

Muscle paralysis

'The literature implies that damage to the neuromuscular unit may be responsible for some types of scoliosis, but existing evidence does not support this contention' [81].

Heredity

Many authors have found a significantly increased incidence of idiopathic scoliosis in close relatives, indicating a dominant form of inheritance. According to the literature, similar curves have been noted in identical twins [82].

Vertebrae

Vertebral shape variations can be responsible for the development of idiopathic scoliosis (Figure 7.3). Heuter–von Vokmann's law [83] reports that the effect of pressure and traction on growth plates, producing asymmetrical expansion is a basis for changes that develop in scoliosis. These variations can be due to either unilateral epiphyseal injuries, resulting in uneven growth and development of the vertebrae, or to abnormal pressures on a developing spine leading to uneven loading. Ultimately, a wedge-shaped vertebrae develops, with compensatory spinal changes, the resultant effect being a lateral curve.

Biomechanics

The body is a segmented structure; it must be able constantly to adjust the segments one to another in order to maintain equilibrium. This action is instinctive. However, it is dependent on the presence of an intact nervous system as well as a normal musculo-skeletal system.

The normal spine is capable of three movements:

1. Flexion.
2. Extension.
3. Combined rotation/side-bending or side-bending/rotation.

Flexion occurs by bending the body forward; approximating the torso and the thighs. It is accomplished in the spinal joint by gliding upward and slightly forward of the inferior facets upon the superior surfaces of the vertebra below. At the same time there is an anterior compression of the intervertebral disc and a stretch of the posterior ligaments.

Extension is a backward bending of the spinal column and is a restricted movement due to the facet apposition and limitation of the anterior longitudinal ligament.

Rotation is always one part of the compound movement, the other being *side-bending*. The physiological reasons are complex and outside the scope of this book. It is sufficient to acknowledge that the spine acts as a series of wedges, bony and cartilaginous, held together by strong bands. These act together as a flexible rod, which being naturally bent in one plane, cannot be turned in another without twisting. The human spine *in vivo* responds to rotation differently in different areas depending upon the plane of the articulating surfaces and upon the initial position of the spine, whether flexed, extended or erect.

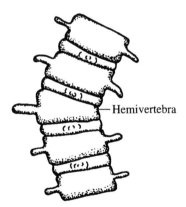

Figure 7.3 A hemivertebra: in this anomaly a vertebra is formed in one lateral half only. The defect may occur at any level. The body of the half-vertebra is wedge shaped, and the spine is angled laterally at the site of the defect.

ASSESSING SPINAL CURVES IN THE LATERAL PLANE (FIGURE 7.4)

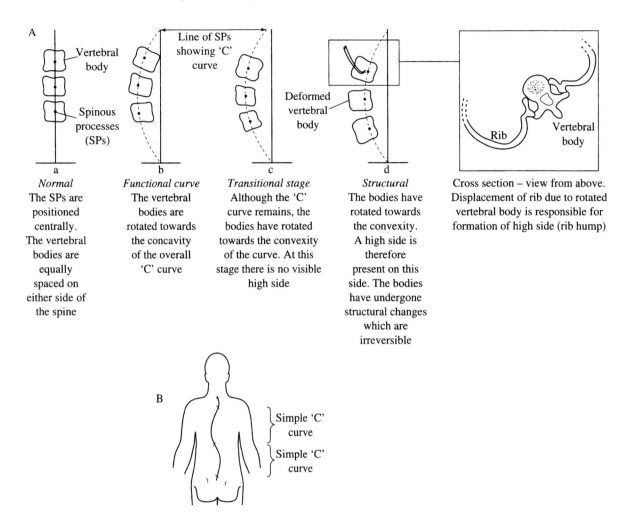

Figure 7.4 A. Schematic representation of a line joining the spinous processes in a spinal curvature: (a) a 'normal' spine; (b)–(d) progression from a functional to a structural curve. This diagram represents a simple 'C' curve throughout the spine. This conceptual interpretation can be used to work out what is happening at different levels of the spine by reducing all curves to simple 'C' curves. B. Diagram showing how once a complex curve can be split into simple 'C' curves the various stages of development of that curve can be identified.

In assessing the standing posture, we concern ourselves with the presence of an efficient posture and not a particular 'normal' shape. An efficient posture is achieved when there is minimal energy consumption. The balanced state occurs when the line of weight-bearing falls vertically from the inion of the occiput to between the feet. In the absence of any anatomical, physiological, neurological and psychological deviations from normal, this line will follow the line which links the spinous processes (SPs) in the erect position. The line of the SPs can only be linear in the absence of any vertebral rotation. As a point of practical reference, an imaginary line is drawn to link the tips of the SPs. The so called 'normal' can therefore be seen as a straight line from the occiput to the midpoint of the base of the sacrum.

Lateral curves are present as soon as this line assumes a bend in the lateral flexion (side-bending) plane. We have already seen that side-bending is always part of a compound movement, the other being rotation. Therefore, vertebral rotation will occur, giving rise to displacement of overlying tissue. Classically, the ribs are clearly seen in this displacement in the thoracic spine, giving rise to a rib hump or high side. It is the precise location of that rib hump within any curve that indicates at what stage that curve is along the hypothetical spectrum.

A mild functional curve is seen when the side-bending and rotation of the vertebral bodies have occurred to the same side and only to a minor extent. In a structural scoliosis the rotation of the vertebral bodies has occurred to the contralateral side of the side-bending.

Hypothetically, a midway stage exists along the spectrum where the vertebrae have initially rotated toward the concavity of the side-bending curve, and then start to rotate in the reverse direction. Once the vertebral bodies are positioned directly in front of the SPs (the side-bending curve still existing), the curvature can be defined as being in the 'transitional' stage. In other words, the spine may have started off as being balanced and in the midline.

As discussed earlier in this chapter, there are several possible causes for the development of a curve. The example in Case study 7.1 is used to illustrate how an injury eventually resulted in a structural scoliosis. Here we see how the spine initially compensated by developing a 'functional' curve; went through the 'transitional' stage, and eventually resulted in a 'structural' stage, this end stage being the most stable compensation achievable.

Case study 7.1

Following a road traffic accident, a patient was left with a lower limb length difference of 2 cm which remained uncorrected. The initial adaptation was in the form of a 'functional' curve. (This can easily be demonstrated practically by standing with one leg on a small platform.) This is not an efficient way to maintain the static, standing posture. Over a period of time, the vertebral bodies will rotate away from the high load position. They will move toward the line of least resistance, which is toward the contralateral side of the side-bending curve. A stage will then be reached when the vertebral bodies will be aligned directly in front of the SPs – the 'transitional' stage. This can be viewed as the midpoint of the spectrum. The time which elapses during this process is variable and dictated by several factors. The most important is age. The younger the individual, the faster the progress. Weight is another variable. The heavier the individual, the faster the process. The bones are able to do this owing to their 'plastic' property. Once re-moulding has taken place, the process becomes irreversible; the spine is at this stage entering the structural stage of the spectrum. This stage eventually reaches a stable and permanent phase. It is responsible for the final shape that the scoliotic spine will assume.

Clinical assessment

Having briefly explored the physiology of vertebral movement, this knowledge can be used in clinical detection. For ease, two anatomical pointers are chosen (Figure 7.5):

1. The line of the SPs.
2. The position of the high side or hump.

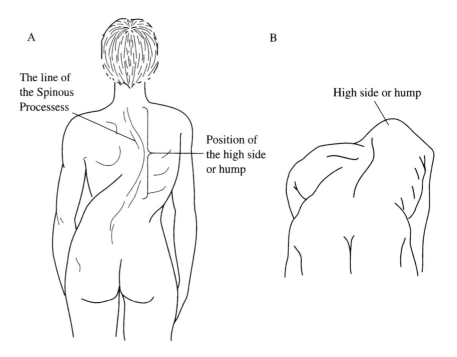

A

The line of
the Spinous
Processsess

Position of
the high side
or hump

B

High side or hump

Figure 7.5 A. Structural scoliosis: the rotation of the vertebral bodies has occurred to the convexity of the curve. B. High side or hump: posterior view of patient flexing forwards to accentuate the rotation of the thoracic vertebra, thus making the high side more visible.

In some cases these two points are not clearly seen. This may be because the changes are not very marked, or because the patient has a deep layer of underlying adipose tissue or may be heavily covered with hair. In order to accentuate the amount of vertebral rotation, forward flexion can be introduced.

This is easily achieved by asking the patient to bend forwards. As the patient bends, any underlying rotation becomes more visible and the high side becomes more obvious. The curves that are easily seen are the structural curves. These are easily identified by the high side being on the contralateral (or convex) side of the side-bending curve. The greater the degree of thoracic rotation, the greater the rib displacement and consequently the more marked the curve. It is the curves that occur at the milder end of the spectrum that are more difficult to identify and thus need more clinical scrutiny.

Case study 7.2 provides an example of clinical assessment and treatment of a patient with a structural curve.

Case study 7.2

Yvonne was first seen as a young 12-year-old when she noticed that her dress was not hanging properly at the shoulders. When she expressed her disappointment with the evening dress, her mother noted the 'lump' in Yvonne's back. The standing assessment revealed an obvious scoliosis both in the lumbar spine as well as the thoracic spine. On forward flexion the 'high side' was evident on the convex side of the curve, thus confirming a structural curve. The local orthopaedic department fitted Yvonne with a plastic brace and she was initially advised to wear it for 23 hours each day. Unable to tolerate this in the heat of the summer, Yvonne was allowed by her parents not to wear it. Corrective surgery was then suggested but subsequently refused by the family. She was treated osteopathically regularly and vigorously throughout her growing period and was given a regime of exercises to follow under parental supervision. Figure 7.6 shows a 'respectable' curve at the age of 20.

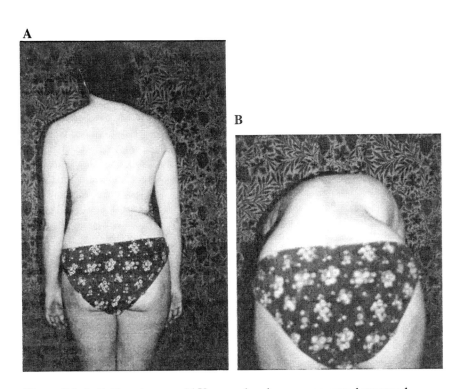

Figure 7.6 A, B. Twenty-year-old Yvonne showing an uncorrected structural scoliosis.

The most common complaint heard from people with 'structural' curves is usually of unsightly appearance. Functional disability includes reduction in spinal movement ranging from minimal to extensive inability to use the spine to any degree. The ligaments will shorten in time and the bones will fuse. Some of the paraspinal muscles will waste and others will become fibrotic. The thorax shows the most dramatic changes. The rib attachments will distort. The ribs themselves will alter in shape and the intercostal musculature will also waste. The rotation of the ribs will have the net effect of a decrease in the overall volume of the rib cage. The curvature shortens the length of the thorax, resulting in further decrease in total volume. These changes are reflected in a decrease in vital capacity. In a study of patients with scoliosis of many years' duration, Nachemson found that after 40 years of age pulmonary disability becomes evident, and patients with severe curvature have significantly increased disability and shortened life expectancy [84].

Although diminished vital capacity is the rule, it is not until the thoracic scoliosis exceeds 50 degrees that altered blood gases are anticipated. The oxygen tension is generally reduced, carbon dioxide tension increased and oxygen saturation diminished [81].

CURVATURES IN THE ANTERO-POSTERIOR PLANE

Increased curvature in the AP plane of the spine will result in a clinical condition known as lordosis in the lumbar spine, kyphosis in the thoracic spine.

Kyphosis

As a clinical state, in a kyphosis there is usually an underlying condition such as a vertebral fracture. The wedging of the vertebral body will result in an overall change in thoracic shape. Other causes are numerous. The following are the most important:

- Tuberculosis of the spinal column.
- Scheuermann's osteochondritis (Figure 7.7).
- Ankylosing spondylitis.
- Senile osteoporosis (Figure 7.8).
- Tumour of the spinal column (especially metastatic carcinoma).

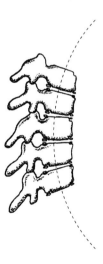

Figure 7.7 Scheuermann's vertebral osteochondritis. Diagrammatic representation of the active stage. The upper and lower margins of the vertebral bodies are irregularly indented in front, and the corresponding parts of the ring epiphyses appear isolated from the main mass of the vertebral body (taken from Crawford Adams [85], copyright © 1983 Churchill Livingstone, reproduced with permission).

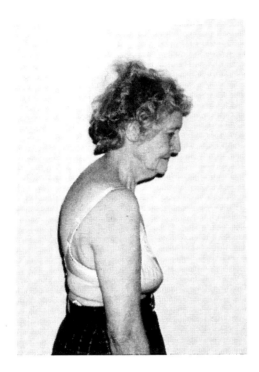

Figure 7.8 Senile osteoporosis. Showing accentuated thoracic kyphosis, particularly at the upper thoracic vertebra.

A mild version of a kyphotic spine, which is not associated with an underlying clinical condition, is more likely to be a postural deformity. This is classically seen in the rounded shoulders of a student.

Lordosis

Lordosis is the opposite deformity to kyphosis. The term denotes excessive anterior curvature of the spinal column. In practice, lordosis is seen only in the lumbar region where a slight anterior curve is normal. Strictly, the term lordosis should be used only when this normal curve is exaggerated.

Spinal disorders tend to cause kyphosis or scoliosis, rather than lordosis. In many cases lordosis is simply a postural deformity, predisposed by lax muscles and a heavy abdomen. Sometimes it is compensatory, balancing a kyphotic deformity above or below, or a fixed flexion deformity of a hip.

CLINICAL SIGNIFICANCE OF SPINAL CURVES

The descriptions so far relate to the main categories of spinal curves when they occur in isolation. More often, in practice, changes occur in both the AP plane as well as in the lateral plane, as seen in a kyphoscoliosis. They can occur partly in the thorax and partly in the lumbar spine. The components of the spectrum can often be seen to occur together, one part of the spine being at the functional stage, whilst other parts of the same spine have undergone complete fusion and hence become organic.

Clinical Assessment

As a rule of thumb, the primary aim is to assess along which stage of the spectrum the presenting curve can be placed. Having established the degree of changes which have occurred within the spine, assess the degree of lifestyle changes that the patient has noted.

These lifestyle changes can be simple alterations in driving position to give support to a different part of the spine. The change may have been necessary because of a recent breakdown in the compensation of the curve. At the other extreme, we find that the patient with a severe structural curve, who has been happily playing tennis for many years, is beginning to find that her stamina is decreasing. This has been gradual over a 2–3-year period. This deterioration in stamina is attributed to the overall decrease in the lung capacity, which is in turn related to the lessening volume of the thorax, as seen earlier in this chapter.

Having established a more general picture, we must try to relate any presenting symptoms to mechanical areas of dysfunction. Commonly seen is nerve root impingement at sites where curves change direction and plane. The local symptom may be muscular from local reflexes or distant from root entrapment. Soft tissues undergoing changes can also be responsible for symptoms; for example, ligaments under stretch, tendons under load, discs under compressive forces or ribs being simply squashed.

APPLICATION OF 'OSTEOPATHIC PHILOSOPHIES'

Many of the 'osteopathic philosophies' discussed in Chapter 1 can be observed in a person with a spinal curve. This is particularly so in cases where the curve is intricate and complex, as seen in patients with a kyphoscoliosis.

Philosophy 1

'The body is a unit' can be seen in the example in Case study 7.1 with the difference in length of the lower limbs following a traffic accident, where, at a physical level, the pelvis and spine undergo changes to compensate for the difference by introducing areas of flexion and side-bending to the spine in the form of a functional curve. At a physiological level, this same patient may eventually develop signs and symptoms related to poor respiratory physiology, as a direct effect of altered ventilatory mechanics, if the shape of the thorax becomes markedly deformed and ultimately inefficient. Psychologically, the patient may suffer anxiety from the resultant change in the shape of his spine and thorax.

Philosophy 2

'Structure and function are reciprocally interrelated.' As mentioned above when discussing pathogenesis, interruption of the growth plates of the vertebrae may result in a wedging effect. Altered vertebral shape will significantly change spinal mobility because of the direct mechanical effect.

Philosophy 5

'When normal adaptability is disrupted, or when environmental changes overcome the body's capacity for self-maintenance, disease may ensue.' Perhaps the most surprising feature of spinal curves is how in many instances, the patient with even the most striking curves does not suffer any symptoms. However, in adult life, a new external factor such as a change in occupational posture (e.g. a shop assistant who was used to standing and moving around all day, is promoted to an administrative role, sitting all day using a computer) may be suddenly plagued by episodes of pains in the chest and the thoracic spine in general. The pains may become so unbearable that she is forced to give up her regular sport. Over a period of time her thoracic movement can become more and more inefficient; her tolerance to chest infections can decrease as a result of greater stasis in the chest and her general lifestyle quality diminishes!

TREATMENT AND MANAGEMENT CONSIDERATIONS

A convenient approach to dealing with complex curves is to separate the spinal column into 'component curves'. That is to say, one person may present with a double scoliosis or a triple scoliosis. The same person can have part of that curve still in the functional stage. Therefore, for simplicity, identify the areas that form simple 'C' shaped curves. Assess the type of curve that each 'C' curve is and deal with the various components accordingly (Figure 7.4B).

The treatment and management of a patient will vary according to the following factors:

- Patient expectations.
- Stage within the spectrum.

Patient expectations

The patient needs to decide whether they prefer a treatment approach solely to calm the symptoms down or a more overall approach. That is to say, if there is a general 'breakdown' in the patient's adaptation to that curve, which has led to a specific area of dysfunction, the patient can choose to have the symptoms treated without any management of the overall curve. This can usually be done by taking the specific area of dysfunction and treating it in exclusion from any other area. The aim is to quickly, and with minimal disruption, rectify the local dysfunction. This can however be a very short-term solution because there may be physical or physiological underlying causes, which will once again create the dysfunction. This approach is in total opposition to the osteopathic philosophies; but, the patient's wishes, which may be shaped by finances or other personal factors, have to be respected.

Alternatively, the complete curve, as part of the whole physical, physiological and psychological make-up of that person, is assessed and analysed with the aim of identifying, as accurately as possible, why one or several levels of dysfunction have developed. This wider, analytical approach may ultimately require a 'maintenance programme' which is not what the patient wishes to undertake. Some osteopaths are strongly opposed to the approach of treating only the symptoms as they arise. They have a right to such feelings and the patients will be advised accordingly.

Stage within the spectrum

Before entering into any short- or long-term considerations or treatment programmes, it is essential to try and identify where in the 'spectrum' (described above) the curve is at the time of consultation. It must be remembered that the main limiting factor to the success of any treatment is the tissues' ability to respond to treatment. Therefore, it is futile, for example, to try and improve the mobility of a curve that has undergone large areas of organic changes. It is however extremely important to maintain/improve the mobility of parts of the curve that are still resilient enough to cope with change. Therefore, strong direct treatment can be applied to the whole curve when it can be identified as being still in the non-structural stage. In addition, the nearer it is to the normal (Figure 7.4A(a)) end of the diagrammatic spectrum, the more emphasis should be placed on mobility and activity. This will hopefully discourage the progression toward the structural end.

Occasions will arise when the post-operative progress of a patient may have to be followed with appropriate advice and treatment administered. Case study 7.3 is a good example of a case which was followed from initial recognition of a double scoliosis, which was referred to surgery, to post-operative treatment and management.

Case study 7.3

Elenor was initially seen as a young 11-year-old, who was very aware of a 'lump' in her spine. Whilst accompanying her mother for osteopathic treatment, she was asked to expose her spine for an opinion. It was immediately obvious that she had an adolescent idiopathic scoliosis right thoracic, left lumbar double curve pattern. On questioning, she admitted to pain in the left leg on exercise as well as unexplained breathlessness. The examination showed at least 75 degrees of lateral deformity in both curves. Her trunk was shortened by the concertina effect of the spinal shape. She was referred to a consultant orthopaedic surgeon, who carried out the following procedures when she was 13 years old:

1. *Anterior correction T12 to L4*
Through a left thoraco-abdominal incision dividing the diaphragm, Webb–Morley instrumentation was used following discectomies at the levels T12/L1 to L3/4.

2. *Posterior AO instrumentation*
Through a midline posterior incision the spine was exposed from T3 to L4. Continuous spinal cord monitoring

was used throughout and showed normal traces. A steady progressive correction of the curvature was performed, using a de-rotation technique on the concavity and a flattening rod to reduce the rib hump on the convexity of the thoracic curve.

Her initial post-operative progress was very good and she was allowed home 8 days after the operation. She was then referred back for osteopathic treatment 2 weeks later. Her main complaint, once the initial soreness had calmed down, was pain in all ranges of shoulder movement. This was found to be of muscular origin; the infra-scapular muscles were under considerable stretch following the re-alignment of the spine. Gradually, the paraspinal muscles were also stretched to accommodate the straight spine. Her abdominal muscles were found to be poorly toned, mainly because, prior to surgery, they were constantly slack as a result of the torso flexion. Progress in their tone made a noticeable difference to her stamina and general level of fitness. Two months after the operation she is being monitored every 2 weeks. General spinal movements are checked; abdominal tone tested and the exercise regime stepped up accordingly.

Elenor's case (Case study 7.3) illustrated how an apparently innocent remark made by this young girl to her mother about the lump on her spine, triggered a response which eventually resulted in surgery. This example of what at first appears to be merely a comment about the odd appearance of the spine is not an unusual presentation for spinal curvatures. It must be remembered that even the most complex and 'tangled' spine may not be initially obvious to the untrained eye. In some cases, most of the vertebral rotation that occurs is not very visible and hence does not actually present externally until the subject is asked to bend forwards which, in turn, exaggerates the rotation. Therefore, each and every case of suspected spinal curvature, particularly in the lateral plane, must be asked to bend as far forward as possible and the appearance of the rib hump must be identified.

8 The head and neck

Head movement is a complex motor task. It can seldom be achieved by the action of a single set of muscles or by changing the position of a single joint, but usually by combined movements of several sets of muscles and as a result of movements across several cervical and thoracic vertebrae. Head movements are controlled by the activities of muscles that link the skull, spinal column and shoulder girdle in a variety of configurations. The limiting factors to these actions are the physical properties of the vertebral column, whose articulations differ in their ranges and directions of mobility. A synchronous set of movements is then co-ordinated by the nervous system.

Neck problems appear in practice with, perhaps, the most dramatic presentations. An acute episode of neck pain is seen as very obvious distress and pain in the face of the sufferer. Movements will be minimal so as to avoid any jarring of the neck. Eye movements are exaggerated to make full use of the visual field without needing to turn the head or neck.

STRUCTURE

The human cervical column has seven vertebrae. As a point of interest, this number of vertebrae is even common to a giraffe and a whale, but not a tree sloth, which has nine! The upper cervical spine is composed of the atlas and axis, respectively; this area is looked at in some detail later in this chapter. The lower cervical spine includes the remaining five cervical vertebrae, which have structural features more typical of vertebrae at other spinal levels. They are linked anteriorly by the intervertebral discs and have gliding synovial joints on each side. Differences in bone and joint structure between the mammals introduce a degree of variability into the biomechanics of head movement from one species to another. Vidal *et al.* [86] have shown that a cat, rabbit and a guinea pig all hold their cervical column in a 'human-like' vertical orientation when they are sitting or standing quietly (Figure 8.1).

This posture appears to be advantageous in reducing the energy required to support the head against gravitational forces.

ANALYSES OF JOINT MOVEMENT

The maximum range of motion permitted at different cervical levels has been studied in some detail, because it provides an important base of information for clinical assessment of the musculoskeletal dysfunction.

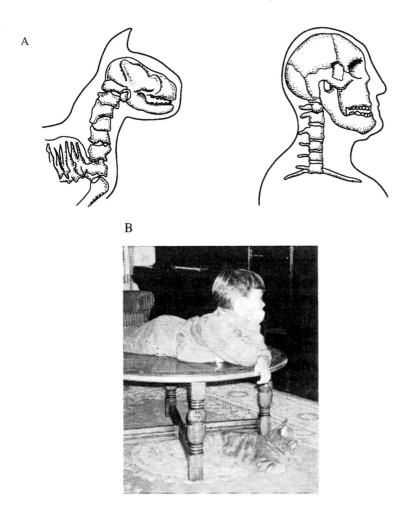

Figure 8.1 A, B. Comparative morphology and spinal orientation in the human and cat.

The variability in the reported values is shown in Table 8.1. The differences shown in the results stem in part from the use of different techniques, such as examinations of cadavers and radiographic analysis, as well as indirect estimates derived from information about head and neck posture. This data highlights certain important features of vertebral organization that must be considered when trying to analyse movements of the head and neck. First, head and neck movements in any direction can involve most joints of the cervical column. Second, and more important, the co-operation between certain joints may be essential if certain types of movements are made. For example, pure rotation of the head and neck can only occur if the upper two vertebrae compensate for the side-bending that always occurs during rotation at the lower cervical levels. The need for interrelated movements along the whole cervical column illustrates the complex relationship between long muscles that span several joints and short muscles that cross only one or two.

Table 8.1 suggests that most of the lateral flexion (side-bending) occurs at the lower cervical vertebrae in the human neck. Graf *et al.* [88] successfully showed, using preliminary fluoroscopic investigations, that the cervico-thoracic region may be even more flexible in the quadruped than in the human.

Table 8.1 Range of mobility at different cervical joints, measured in degrees

Comparative results from

	Flexion-extension		*Lateral bending (from midline)*		*Axial rotation (from midline)*	
	(A)	(B)	(A)	(B)	(A)	(B)
Skull/C1	13	15	8	3–8	0	12
C1/C2	10	5+	0	0	47	12
C3/C4	8	100+	10	37	9	56
C3/C7	58	100+	27	37	42	56

(A) and (B) are results from two different studies [87].

MUSCLE STRUCTURE

For detailed information on the organization of specific neck muscles, the reader is directed to detailed anatomical texts [89, 90]. To understand the complexity of human mechanical function, including spinal movements, we must first identify the muscles that link the different parts together, and then study the functional behaviour of these groups. This chapter is used to illustrate the depth of detail needed in order to fully appreciate how and why anatomical links are used during the diagnostic thought process.

Muscles that link the shoulder girdle with the skull

There are two large and clinically significant muscles which run between the shoulder girdle and the skull in humans. *Trapezius* is a large shawl-like muscle which is attached cranially at the medial part of the occiput and nuchal midline. It wraps itself to insert onto the clavicle. More distal parts of the trapezius originate from the spinous processes of the seventh cervical vertebrae and all the thoracic vertebrae. These fibres run laterally to insert on the scapula. *Sternocleidomastoids* originate as two separate heads from the clavicle and the sternum, respectively. The two heads mesh to form a single wide strap that runs obliquely to insert on to the mastoid process and the lateral half of the occiput.

Muscles that link the vertebral column with the skull

Learning the different muscle names can be made easier in this section by remembering that the muscles that link these two vital areas are distinguished by the noun '*capitis*' in their names. There are three distinct sets: a superficial set of muscles that crosses several vertebral joints, an intermediate set of suboccipital muscles that links the skull with the atlas and axis, and a very deep set that links the skull with the anterior surface of the vertebral column.

The superficial set

There are three long muscles which run in differing directions between the skull and the vertebral column. *Splenius capitis* originates from the lower half of the nuchal ligament, spinous processes of seventh cervical and upper thoracic vertebrae and inserts in the mastoid part of the temporal bone. It extends and rotates the head. *Longissimus capitis* originates from the transverse processes of four or five upper thoracic vertebrae, articular processes of three or four lower cervical vertebrae and inserts onto the mastoid process of the temporal bone. It draws the head backward and rotates the head. *Semispinalis capitis* has a complex origin from the transverse processes of the upper thoracic and lower cervical vertebrae, and is attached to the medial part of the occiput. It extends the head.

The intermediate set

These are primarily the *suboccipital muscles*. These lie deep to the long thoracic muscles described above.

    Rectus capitis posterior major originates from the spinous process of the axis and inserts along the inferior nuchal line of the skull. *Rectus capitis posterior minor* has a shorter and more medially directed course, from the posterior arch of the atlas to the medial part of the occiput along the inferior nuchal line. *Obliquus capitis superior* is located laterally to the paired recti muscles. It runs between the transverse process of the atlas and the lateral part of the occiput. *Obliquus capitis inferior*, although conventionally included in the suboccipital grouping, differs from the others in that it has no attachment to the skull. Instead it runs from the lateral aspect of the spinous process of the axis to insert onto the transverse process of the atlas.

The deepest set

Only three deep ventral muscles run between the skull and vertebral column. *Longus capitis* originates from the transverse processes of the third to sixth cervical vertebrae and attaches onto the basilar portion of the occipital bone. It flexes the head. *Rectus capitis anterior minor* is more laterally placed and connects the lateral part of the atlas to the base of the occiput. *Rectus capitis lateralis* is found more deeply and laterally. It originates from the transverse process of the atlas and inserts onto the occiput.

Muscles that interlink vertebrae

The long muscles that insert onto the skull appear to be specialized elements of a more extensive muscle system that runs the length of the vertebral column. Thus it is not surprising that the 'capitis' muscles are often matched by corresponding 'cervicis' muscles that have similar fibre orientations but insert on cervical vertebrae rather than the skull. In humans, three large intervertebral muscles correspond with splenius capitis, longissimus capitis and semispinalis capitis, respectively. Splenius cervicis is located caudolaterally to splenius capitis. Longissimus cervicis runs along the lateral margin of the vertebral column and semispinalis cervicis runs obliquely between the transverse processes of T1–T6.

Beneath the longer intervertebral muscles, a deeply placed network of shorter muscles connects adjacent vertebrae. In addition to muscles interlinking vertebrae, there are scalenus muscles that link the vertebral column with the rib cage.

Other 'neck' muscles

Head movement depends not only on motion at upper cervical joints but also on the posture of the neck determined by the relative positions of lower cervical and upper thoracic vertebrae. As a consequence, additional muscles that act exclusively across the cervico-thoracic column have to be recognized as part of the effector apparatus for head movement. Not only may these muscles actively contribute to head-neck movement, but their various activities may also establish the posture that will define the axes of motion of other muscle groups. Particular attention must be paid both to muscles that span the cervico-thoracic junction and to muscles that run between the scapula and the cervical vertebral column. The main groups are the rhomboid muscle complex (including rhomboideus major and minor) and levator scapulae.

Functional behaviour of neck muscles

Descriptions of muscle anatomy are typically used to support theories about the physiological capabilities of individual muscles. A knowledge of muscle shape, attachment and fibre architecture has often been used to predict the mechanical actions of an individual muscle, and this prediction is usually placed as a postscript to the anatomical descriptions that appear in most textbooks of anatomy. A detailed knowledge of muscle structure can bring us closer to understanding the physical adaptations and constraints that will affect the physiological behaviour of muscles. However, this information is often insufficient to identify the functional role of a muscle, because patterns of muscle recruitment will depend on a number of other factors, such as the concurrent operation of other muscles or the positions and degrees of freedom of movement of the joints across which the muscle must act. In the neck, most muscles are attached at both ends to bones that move, so their action will depend on the stability of the muscle origin and insertion at any given time. A further complication is that because many neck muscles cross several vertebral joints, the movement produced by these multi-articular muscles will depend on the initial position of each joint and the degree to which the joints are free to move in each of one or more planes. Thus, patterns of muscle synergy during normal head movements are complex.

In summary, head movements are made by changing the alignments of the cervical vertebrae that link the skull with the body. The bones composing the cervical vertebrae have specialized structures and articular arrangements. Thus individual joints differ in their abilities to move and these specializations have a significant affect on the way that head movements can be executed in any particular plane. The particular role played by a single muscle cannot be predicted simply from its pulling direction; it also depends on its biomechanical properties, its fibre-type composition, and its relationships with different cervical joints.

Having briefly explored the biomechanics of head and neck movements, the other structures of the anterior aspect of the neck will be studied. A working knowledge of this area is necessary for the practitioner to be able to carry out a complete examination.

THE FRONT OF THE NECK

To aid learning, the front of the neck will be divided into the following regions:

- Anterior triangle and median line of the neck.
- Carotid triangle.
- Submandibular triangle.

The most superficial structure to be found in the neck is the subcutaneous sheet of muscle which extends from the face to the level of the second rib, the platysma. It is continuous above with the facial muscles, but the most anterior fibres are attached to the lower border of the mandible and others merge with the opposite platysma for 2–3 cm behind the chin. Its anterior border slopes from this point to the sternoclavicular joint. Hence the platysma leaves the midline of the neck and the lowest part of the anterior triangle uncovered, whereas it covers the lowest part of the posterior triangle. There is a deep fascia which envelops the neck, forming a snug collar (Figure 8.2).

Anterior triangle and median line of the neck

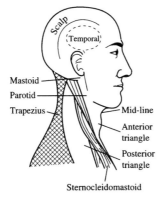

Figure 8.2 Superficial regions of the head and neck showing the anterior triangle and the posterior triangle.

The anterior triangle of the neck is bounded by the anterior border of the sternomastoid, stretching from chin to manubrium, and by the lower border of the jaw together with the hinder part of the posterior belly of the digastric. The median line is a broad strip, bounded above by anterior bellies of the digastrics, below by the sternothyroids, and between these the sternohyoids. The mylohyoids form the floor of the *submental triangle* which is bounded by the two digastrics (Figure 8.3).

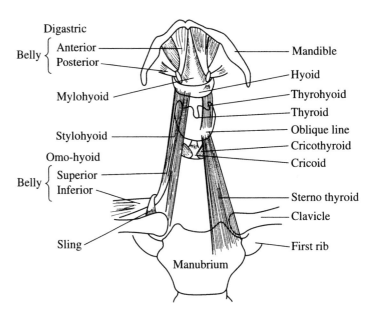

Figure 8.3 Anterior view showing the muscles bounding the midline of the neck.

There are four visceral tubes and the thyroid gland which can be found in the front of the neck. They can be collectively termed the 'cervical viscera'. The visceral tubes are the pharynx and oesophagus, with their offshoots, the larynx and trachea. The pharynx descends on the vertebrae from the base of the skull to the level of the sixth cervical vertebra; it is continuous with the oesophagus. At this level the larynx becomes the trachea. The back of the trachea is applied throughout to the front of the oesophagus.

The common and internal carotid arteries, the internal jugular vein, and the vagus nerve extend from the cranial cavity to the thorax. These structures are enveloped by the carotid sheath. This sheath is applied to the side of the cervical viscera, and is partly under the cover of the sternomastoid.

The thyroid gland is wrapped around the front of the four cervical 'visceral tubes' (Figure 8.4).

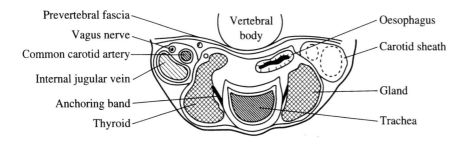

Figure 8.4 Cross-section of the neck at the level of the thyroid gland and the carotid sheath.

Carotid triangle

The carotid triangle is bounded by the anterior border of the sternomastoid, the superior belly of omohyoid and the posterior belly of the digastric. It is an area which houses very important structures – nerves, arteries and veins. The nerves contained within the triangle are the accessory nerve, the hypoglossal nerve, the ansa cervicalis and the vagus nerve. The arteries in this triangle are parts of the common, internal, and external carotid arteries, and the stems of most of the six collateral branches of the external carotid artery. Veins of the anterior triangle are the superior thyroid, lingual and facial veins, as well as a middle thyroid vein which crosses superficial to the carotid arteries and joins the internal jugular vein. The facial vein unites with the anterior branch of the retromandibular vein to form the common facial vein. The pharyngeal plexus is drained by several veins into the internal jugular vein.

Submandibular triangle

The boundaries of the submandibular triangle are the two bellies of the digastric and the lower border of the jaw. A broad band of fascia, stretching from the styloid process to the posterior border of the ramus of the mandible, and hence called the stylomandibular ligament, separates it from the parotid region behind. The triangle contains the submandibular gland and the lymph nodes, hypoglossal and mylohyoid nerves, lingual and facial arteries, and facial vein.

EXAMINATION OF THE NECK

Once the major landmarks of the neck are known to us and we can confidently recognize 'normal' from 'abnormal', we can begin to assess a neck problem. It is not enough to predict that an apparent trauma to the neck has resulted in what seems to be a mechanical injury of the neck, without palpating for any related or unrelated problems of the 'cervical viscera'.

Case study 8.1

Linda is a 54-year-old mother of two active teenagers. Six weeks prior to her first consultation she was involved in a car accident. She was driving slowly in a traffic jam when she was hit from behind. She was not aware of any problems immediately after the accident but gradually noted that she was developing aches in the front and left side of the neck. The aches became constant and irritating. Her neck movements were all reduced. She was advised to take paracetamol regularly to help with what had been diagnosed as a mild whiplash. Over the weeks she noted increasing tiredness which she attributed to looking after her children and her constant pain.

The main feature of the initial consultation was her overwhelming tiredness – slowing of mental activity and physical activity as well as generalized pains. She noted that the pains were spreading down her spine and gradually extending to her other joints. Her face looked pale and her eyelids were puffy. Her skin was generally dry and her hair was distinctly brittle. All neck movements were slow and deliberate to avoid deep aches; however, this seemed to be the general pattern of all of her movements. During the passive assessment of the neck a firm diffuse enlargement of the thyroid gland was noted. This was particularly obvious when the neck was slightly extended in the supine position. Subsequent blood tests showed that she was suffering from spontaneous primary hypothyroidism with an associated goitre.

Linda's case (Case study 8.1) highlights how symptoms can merge into each other without the patient necessarily realizing that an underlying condition had already been established. Here we see how it was the anxiety of an unresolved whiplash that prompted further help. It seems that although Linda was previously able to cope with her underactive thyroid, her tolerance level was tipped over a threshold which she could not tolerate. She simply could not cope with the additional pains and tiredness that the accident caused. The resulting knock-on effect made her condition of hypothyroidism state more obvious.

The active examination

Close inspection and observation of the neck must be carried out with the patient sitting in front of the osteopath, undressed down to the waist. The neck should be free of any jewellery. Glasses and earrings must also be removed. With the patient sitting, any visual or hearing impairment can be taken into consideration. For example, hearing loss on one side will result in the patient turning slightly to allow the good ear to face the operator. In the same way, visual loss on one side will also result in a slight turn of the head.

The acute neck

Severe neck pain will prevent the patient from turning the head in any direction. This is clearly seen as a totally rigid neck. The patient will use the extremes of her visual field by moving the eyes much more than normal. Exaggerated shoulder movements are seen to compensate for the lack of neck movement. Look out for any areas of high muscular tone, particularly of the anterior neck muscles. Note any imbalance from one side to the other, keeping a close eye on the trachea as the main anterior plumb line.

In order to establish the exact amount of movement possible in the neck the patient is instructed to follow closely the movements carried out by the practitioner, who is standing in front of her. This is easily done by asking the patient to keep the shoulders fixed and follow simple movements that the operator performs. Small ranges of slow nodding movement, gradually increasing the amplitude, is often the simplest way to start. The next movement should be dictated by the actual protective position. For example, the patient may present with the head firmly held in slight flexion with an element of lateral flexion to one side or the other. In such cases, attempt to side-bend the neck further, whilst maintaining the same amount of forward flexion, always returning to the exact starting position of ease. The last ranges to be assessed are lateral flexion away from the protection, i.e. toward the shoulder that is furthest away from the head and, finally, extension. It must be continually emphasized that these movements must be carried out slowly and stopped if the pain increases suddenly or radiates down the arms.

The 'subacute' neck

Where the patient can comfortably move the neck, without too much discomfort, start by asking the patient to nod and carry the movement through to cover as much of the flexion range as possible. Again stand facing the patient. Next ask the patient to turn the head slowly, first one way and then the other. This is followed by lateral flexion to each side and then finally extension of the neck. Once these pure movements are completed, introduce selective combined movements.

The above sequence describes a standard routine. A tailored sequence of movements should be worked out for individuals. As a rule of thumb, from the history work out which ranges are particularly difficult for the patient or the ones that cause the most pain – for example, extension with rotation right, when shaving under the left side of the chin. Perform the *opposite* movements first, working toward the most painful. In this case flexion; rotation left; lateral flexion left; lateral flexion right; rotation right; extension; extension with rotation left and, finally, very carefully extension with rotation right.

Often it is a combination of two or three ranges that is particularly painful. Bending the head down whilst slightly turning to one side and side-bending to the opposite side to take out a contact lens is a common example. Therefore look for ease of movement in all the normal ranges first, follow this by combining the ranges in the opposite direction to the ones complained of and, finally, work toward the range that gives the most discomfort.

Careful observation is an essential part of familiarizing oneself with the 'potential' for movement, the 'potential' being the maximum range that the patient feels that they can carry out. This observed potential is then compared with the 'actual' movement possible during the passive examination. The main question to be answered at this stage is whether the patient is unable to carry out a set of movements because of the muscles, or because of 'physical' obstruction. This simplistic interpretation aims to differentiate, on the one hand, between the muscular resistance to movement, in cases where the muscles are contracting because of muscular injury or reflex protective action, and, on the other hand, the inability to move because of structural changes in the vertebra, for example, an enlarged facet joint or degenerate disc. In the above examples, in a protective condition, the patient will find it difficult to move the neck actively, but will allow some movement when this is carried out passively. In contrast, however, the degenerate joint will show a decreased range of active movement, which will be similar to the reduction in range seen during the passive exam.

The aim of the active examination is to assess the patient's ability to perform movements of the neck. This will establish the 'normal' range for the non-acute case. In an acute case, it will indicate the degree of movement remaining in the neck, which will begin the differential diagnostic process. Secondly, it is a useful indicator as to the type of therapeutic techniques which may be used in treatment. On a more general point, it begins to build up the overall 'mobility' picture of the patient.

The passive examination

Sitting

It is important to allow the patient to choose the most comfortable position for this examination. It can easily be carried out in either the sitting or the supine position.

If the patient prefers to sit, use a stool, preferably one which allows the top of the head to reach operator chest level. Stand behind the patient while supporting the head. Allow the head to fall slightly forwards whilst supporting the forehead, thus allowing flexion to be tested (Figure 8.5). The palpating hand should feel for the following:

- The tension/tone of the superficial tissues such as the skin and fascia.
- The resting tone of the muscles.
- The separation of the spinous processes whilst flexion is occurring.
- The quality and end feel of the joint movements.

Repeat the procedure, testing rotation, lateral flexion and extension. Once again combined ranges of movement are then carried out.

Supine

Making the patient comfortable at the onset of this examination can make all the difference in establishing the exact nature of the problem. Use a pillow to support the head, but allow room for the examining hand to pass under the neck. Always allow the head to rest in the position where it feels comfortable. This may be slightly rotated round to one side or in any combination of positions. One of two hand holds can be used – either one hand on each side of the head, ensuring that the ears are not squashed (Figure 8.6), or one hand under the head and neck, while the other supports the forehead (Figure 8.7). In either hold, the palms support the head, while the fingertips move up and down the neck to palpate.

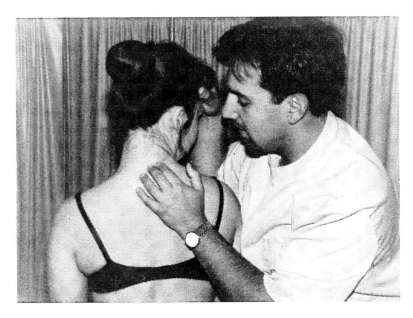

Figure 8.5 Passive examination of the neck in the sitting position. The osteopath is supporting the patient's head with one hand whilst palpating the neck posteriorly.

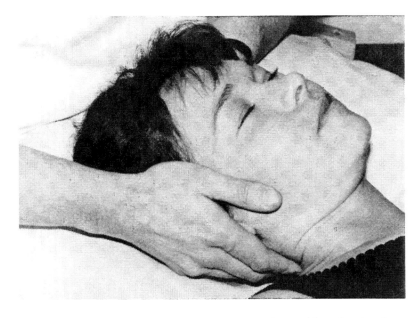

Figure 8.6 Passive examination of the neck in the supine position, showing the handhold where the osteopath has one hand on each side of the head.

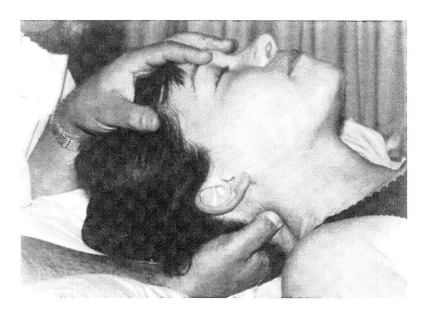

Figure 8.7 Passive examination of the neck in the supine position, showing the handhold where the osteopath has one hand under the patient's head and neck whilst the other supports the forehead.

Initially the examining hands should play a passive role, simply allowing the patient to get used to the feel of the operator's touch. The hold should gradually increase in firmness to assess the feel of the superficial tissues. At first this is done at rest, then some gentle oscillating movement is introduced. At this stage the aim is to feel for any increasing resistance to movement. Sudden mounting resistance indicates a protective, muscular spasm mechanism which is guarding an underlying 'acute' problem. (This will be explored later in the chapter.) Asking the patient which range of movement she feels most comfortable in performing is a good way to choose the sequence of examination movements. Once again, all the ranges must be examined, including any combined movements which are indicated as aggravating in the history.

Assess the following for each range:

- Degree of mounting resistance of the soft tissues. Is it gradual and then comes to an 'elastic' end point? Or is it sudden, and comes to a solid stop? The former is the normal presentation, as seen in healthy individuals with no signs of degenerate disease. The latter is seen in cases of protective spasm, which is seen in painful conditions such as disc prolapses or whiplashes.
- Character of end feel to movement. The normal end point feels like trying to stretch a bicycle tyre. One can almost project a little more 'give' with a little more effort! For example, marked degenerative changes in the neck will show a limited range of movement in all directions; the movement often comes to a sudden end stop and is accompanied by a grating sound known as crepitus.

- Relative ranges of travel in rotation and lateral flexion of the two sides are compared and contrasted.

Once the overall range is tested, the different segmental levels are examined individually. This is done by holding the head firmly between the two hands and using the fingertips as points of fulcrum whilst the joint lines are tested for movement. When applying the momentum force, test for the amount of give in the ligaments and the amount of separation of joint space at the facet joints.

When examining the different segment levels:

- Look out for any 'binding' of joint movement. This implies a local joint dysfunction.
- Feel for any localized mounting resistance from the small intervertebral spinal muscles.
- Constantly compare the relative movements of one side of the joint with the other.
- Try to incorporate all of the ranges of joint movements available, including any particular combined ranges which may be relevant to the case being examined.

Passive versus active movements

Active movements are motivated by muscular activity. Thus the movement will be limited by any pain caused by the active muscles, by the resistance created from the protective muscular spasm and by any preconceived anxiety that the patient may have in anticipating pain. Active movements are therefore merely a general indication of the person's perception of movement possible. That is to say, the passive range of movement will often show a greater overall range. This is particularly the case when the practitioner carries out the movements with a firm and confident hold.

During the passive examination, the direction of movement can be altered marginally to allow further travel. The slight alteration in direction of force may be sufficient to take off partial tension on certain ligaments and then continue the movement unhindered. This requires sensitive palpatory skill in order to be guided by the slight changes in resistance which build up during the examination.

It is important to be alert to any unusual movements carried out during the active movements. These should then be explored passively to try and assess the reason for the deviation. For example, during active lateral flexion, the patient may deviate toward the flexion range. This may be due to a sharp pain felt as a direct result of compressing the emerging nerve root. The sudden move towards flexion will increase the size of the intervertebral foramen, thus reducing the pressure. This simple hypothesis can be confirmed during the passive phase by carrying out lateral flexion, whilst holding the head in some flexion from the onset, then repeating with a slight degree of extension from the onset. The extended position is likely to cause local neck pain and even some arm pain. The advantage of the passive examination is that the influence of the muscles on both range and pain production can be minimized right from the start.

Both the passive and active examinations must be carried out whenever possible. In some cases, where it appears obvious from the start that the patient is in too much pain to be able to carry out the active range, then the passive movements will suffice to gain a general idea of the situation.

Experience in practice will allow the osteopath to introduce certain techniques which, although strictly speaking are therapeutic, can be used to improve the accuracy of the passive examination. For example, when testing a passive range of movement, an end stop to the movement is felt, which is identified as being caused by muscular spasm. At this precise stage, the patient is asked to resist actively by gently pushing against the practitioner's hand, for just 3–4 seconds; this will result in a small reduction in the protective spasm, which will, in turn, allow slight advancement to the range tested. This combination of examination/treatment procedure is a very useful way to achieve an easing of the symptoms in the very early stages. That is not only greatly appreciated by the patient, but also allows the practitioner to assess an area more accurately.

DISORDERS OF THE NECK

The neck is richly supplied with spinal nerves innervation as well as copious vertebral joint receptors. This richness contributes to extensive reflex effects upon the cervical muscles resulting in exaggerated protective spasm to any injury. Perhaps the clearest example of this is seen in the condition known as wry-neck or acute torticollis. Here the patient presents with an unprovoked episode of severe neck pain, which is 'stuck' in a fixed position. The episodes can last from just a few hours to several days. Clinically, the absence of any known injury and normal findings in all aspects of neurological testing, is indicative of the cause as being one of these alternatives:

1. Neuromuscular dysfunction resulting in an over-reactive muscle spasm.
2. Underlying joint dysfunction with an accompanying protective spasm.

Early attention to these cases provides rapid relief for the sufferer. Often the diagnostic/therapeutic use of localized active-resisted movements described earlier in the chapter can be sufficiently helpful in returning most of the neck movements.

Other neuromuscular/musculo-skeltal presentations in the neck include cervical joint dysfunction or somatic dysfunction. These tend to be more specific in presentation, with the patient identifying a particular direction or movement which is solely responsible for the sudden onset of a 'sharp', 'stabbing' pain. Usually the patient learns to keep the neck perfectly still and will allow it to relax only when support is provided. The support can be in the form of a pillow or the safe cradle provided by the osteopath's hands when assessing.

Other acute conditions seen in the neck are caused by injury of the intervertebral disc. This is examined in detail below.

At the other end of the clinical spectrum, one finds the chronic aching neck with a distinct 'grating' on movement, which is found in osteoarthritic states.

Practitioners must be aware of some of the more typical conditions seen in practice which are associated with certain age groups. The infantile and juvenile groups are considered below.

Infantile disorders

Infantile torticollis and congenital short neck

Sometimes children as young as 3 months are brought to an osteopath with a contracted sternomastoid on one side, which is felt as a tight cord. The ear on the affected side is approximated to the corresponding shoulder. The characteristic diagnostic feature is the cord-like contracted sternomastoid muscle, with some facial asymmetry. In the absence of other forms of wry-neck which may include structural deformities of the cervical spine or local inflammation from an infected gland, these cases respond well to repeated stretching of the affected muscle. In more established cases the contracted muscle is divided at its lower attachment surgically. A less commonly seen congenital disorder is Klippel–Feil syndrome. The degree of abnormality varies widely. The bony deformity consists of fusion of two or more of the cervical vertebrae. Clinically the neck appears short or absent, and the hairline is low. Movements of the head and neck are restricted. This condition is more commonly seen in adults as the reduced localized movements can cause a mechanical strain on the rest of the neck. Radiographs show the underlying bony abnormality.

Juvenile disorders

Torticollis and 'facet locking'

A wry-neck is commonly seen in young adults and older children. Cavaziel [91] reported that a segment between C2 and C7, more usually C2–3, is the site of a usually transient but acutely painful unilateral joint condition, often manifest on rising in the morning, which is seen as a typical posture of the head held in slight flexion and side-flexion away from the painful side. Often the arm movements of the painful side are also painful and limited in range. All attempted movements are suddenly interrupted by a sharp stabbing pain. Characteristically, the patient wakes with pain, which can be localized to the concave side of the deformity and often restricted to the top of the neck. As the day wears on, a generalized ache is superimposed upon the local pain and sudden movements will elicit jabs of pain spreading to the upper trapezius and shoulder area. The patient is then less able to localize the pain. This condition can be extremely distressing when the subject retires normally and then wakes with this severely painful condition. It is established that some people can be very active during sleep, showing activities such as powerful tooth grinding (bruxism) or fist clenching and back scratching or powerfully twisting the neck during sleep. This powerful stretching of the neck, which is probably held in a fixed position for a period of time, induces slight oedema which congests and thickens a meniscoid synovial villus, inducing it to remain as an impacted synovial inclusion on subsequent change of neck posture during the night [15]. Other schools of thought have proposed a slight shift of cervical disc substance during this strained posture at night. Some cases have suggested that the irritation may be caused by cold. The physiological response of the cervical muscles to cold can result in sudden spasm. 'I slept in a draught' and 'I had the window open all night' are common underlying statements in the history. Another type of common onset for this condition is the sudden one which is associated with a particular movement, commonly termed 'facet lock'. The abnormal neck posture is immediately assumed and the pain comes on from that instant. The onset may be at night, on waking or at any time during the day. Grieve speculates that, in this type of onset, the underlying mechanism is probably impaction of a meniscoid structure between the surfaces of a cervical facet joint. Associated with these conditions there may or may not be associated impingement upon the neighbouring nerve roots. In this handful of cases there will be associated neurological signs. The history is essential in distinguishing the possible mechanism involved, as it will dictate the therapeutic approach. The sudden traumatic type will frequently respond well to the appropriate high-velocity thrust technique. Results of a study which reviewed the efficacy and mobilization for the management of neck pain and headache showed that spinal manipulation and mobilization probably provide at least short-term benefits for some patients with neck pain and headache [92], whereas, probably due to the disturbed disc material, the gradually induced onset is more likely to respond favourably to traction with some degree of flexion. This is then followed by support and warmth applications for the following 3 days.

Prolapsed cervical disc

Displacement of disc material in the neck is less common than in the lumbar spine. However, when it occurs, it is an extremely painful condition which is commonly associated with neurological signs and symptoms in the upper limb and occasionally with signs of spinal cord compression.

Injury may be a predisposing factor, though often a history of injury cannot be obtained. Probably an intrinsic change in the substance of the disc predisposes to rupture and displacement. This occurs most frequently in the lower cervical spine; discs between C5 and C6 and between C6 and C7 are the most frequently affected. Part of the nucleus pulposus protrudes through a tear in the annulus fibrosus or there may be a partial displacement or bulging of the annulus itself. The weakest part of the disc tends to be the postero-lateral aspect.

For ease of diagnostic classification, three degrees of protrusion/prolapse can be identified:

1. If slight, the protrusion bulges the pain-sensitive posterior longitudinal ligament, causing local pain in the neck.
2. If large, the protrusion bulges the ligament and may impinge upon the nerve leaving the spinal canal at that level. This is a postero-lateral prolapse.
3. Less frequently, the protrusion bulges through the ligament and may impinge upon the spinal cord itself. This is a central prolapse.

Healing is more likely to be by fibrosis and shrinkage. Reposition within the disc is unlikely to occur. The concept of the old osteopaths 'putting the disc back in' has survived among grateful patients who received the magic 'click' in instances of severe neck pain. It must be appreciated that is only a working model and the audible 'click' is more likely due to joint cavitation or separation of facet surfaces than the 'bone going back in'! Disc prolapses predispose the acceleration of degenerative development of osteoarthritis in later years.

Clinical features

Although a characteristic picture outlining a classical sequence of events can often be recognized, variations are common. A typical picture of a postero-lateral disc protrusion often presents with a history of a jarring or a twisting strain which may seem slight at the time and may cause no immediate effects. Several hours or even days later, the pain may begin to radiate over the shoulder and throughout the length of the upper limb; it is felt along the course of the cervical nerve. Paraesthesiae are felt in the digits. The clinical examination shows limitation of certain neck movements by pain, but often movement in at least one direction is pain free. This is commonly lateral flexion away from the affected side. Examination of the upper limb shows full range of joint movements. Varying degrees of muscle wasting will be present, along with slight sensory impairment in the distribution of a cervical nerve. The corresponding tendon reflex is depressed or absent.

Some cases will present without a history of injury. The symptoms may be confined entirely to the upper limb. Motor changes (wasting or weakness) may be marked, sometimes amounting to almost complete paralysis of a muscle or a group of muscles; or, on the other hand, they may be absent. Similarly, wide variations in the degree of sensory impairment are noted. Radiographs are characteristically normal. Narrowing of one of the disc spaces, however, is often demonstrable – usually C5–6 or C6–7. Such narrowing denotes previous disc degeneration; it cannot be explained simply by extrusion of disc substance because the extruded matter forms only a small proportion of the total volume of the disc.

Case study 8.2

Lucy is a fit 32-year-old mother of two young children. Six months prior to seeking treatment she felt a gradual tightening of the neck, with a mild degree of limitation when bending her neck to the right. The pain and stiffness fluctuated in severity and mounting tension in the build up to Christmas seemed to make matters worse. She decided to seek help when it became increasingly painful to change gear while driving. Over a period of about 2 months she noticed that her left hand was feeling 'numb' occasionally, for no apparent reason. On examination her only limited range of movement was lateral flexion to the right actively and lateral flexion to the left passively. Her arm movements were full and pain free. The left triceps jerk was depressed slightly. All sensory tests of the upper and lower limbs were normal.

Her neck symptoms did not respond to two treatments of gentle neck traction and stretching of the soft tissues of the neck. X-rays were requested at this stage and they did not show any abnormal findings. She was then sent to the Orthopaedic department on the suspicion of a disc protrusion. Scans confirmed the presence of a large postero-lateral bulge at C6–7.

Lucy's case (Case study 8.2) is a good example of one of the many diverse presentations of a disc picture. Although seemingly atypical, it underlines the need for constant vigilance.

Cervical disc derangements vary from a minor internal derangement, with minimal distortion of the annulus, to a frank herniation where the nuclear material has escaped the confines of the anulus fibrosus [93].

In the study conducted by Stevens and McKenzie [93], it was found that patients exhibiting a derangement syndrome of the cervical disc were typically between the ages of 25 and 55 years. In 1990 McKenzie extended this age range to 12–55 years. He considered that the incidence of cervical derangement in teenagers was high in comparison to similar problems encountered in the lumbar region. He also posited that in patients under approximately 55 years of age internal derangement of the intervertebral disc may result from excessive flow or displacement of the fluid nucleus pulposus. In patients over 55 years derangement may result from displacement of a sequestrum from the degenerated annulus or now fibrosed nucleus pulposus or both [94].

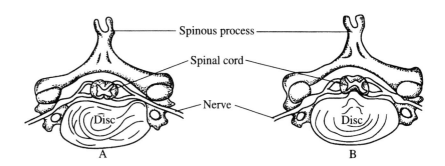

Figure 8.8 Prolapsed cervical intervertebral disc. A. Compression of the issuing nerve root from a posterolateral prolapse. B. A central prolapse with impingement upon the spinal cord.

Sometimes the protrusion is in a more central position, which will lead to manifestations of spinal cord compression (Figure 8.8). This must be differentiated from a space-occupying lesion in the cord. If there is any doubt, the patient must be immediately referred to a neurosurgeon for further assessment. Typically, the effects are seen as root pains at the level of the lesion, which are followed by lower motor neurone changes at the same level and progressive upper motor neurone paralysis and visceral dysfunction below the lesion.

Osteoarthritis of the cervical spine

Several terms are used to describe this condition – cervical spondylarthritis, cervical spondylarthrosis, cervical spondylosis. They all describe this commonly occurring condition, which afflicts the cervical spine and causes pain and stiffness of the neck. Osteoarthritis in the neck begins in the intervertebral discs and then affects the intervertebral joints posteriorly. This condition is often simply a manifestation of the widespread degenerative changes that occur with increasing age, however the primary degenerative changes are often initiated by injury.

Among the most commonly heard statements of desperation by patients is that they have been told that they have to 'live with it'. This means that once the arthritis is present the symptoms will always be there. It must be emphasized, however, that it is often the superimposed joint dysfunction that is responsible for the symptom picture. Osteopathic treatment to the area can therefore improve joint function and hence alleviate the pain.

Degenerative arthritis occurs most commonly in the lowest three cervical joints. The initial narrowing of the cervical disc causes a bone reaction at the joint margins, leading to the formation of osteophytes. Wearing away of the articular cartilage, together with the formation of osteophytes, reduces the space in the foramen. The reduction in the space encroaches on the cervical nerves. If the restricted space in a foramen is still further reduced by oedema, clinical manifestations of nerve pressure are likely to occur. Rarely, the spinal cord itself may suffer damage from encroachment of osteophytes within the spinal canal.

Clinical features

Commonly the symptoms are at first in the neck and subsequently in the arm/s. Sometimes they can occur in both the neck and the arms at the same time. Symptoms consist chiefly of aching pain in the back of the neck or in the trapezius area. Often stiffness and a 'grating' is felt and heard in the neck. Occipital headache may also be a feature. In the upper limb there may be a vague, ill-defined, localized, 'referred' pain over the shoulder region. However, in cases where there is more widespread narrowing of the foraminae, signs and symptoms from interference with one or more nerve roots may be experienced. The main feature in these cases is radiating pain along the course of the affected nerve or nerves, often reaching the fingers. There may also be paraesthesiae in the hand, commonly described as 'pins and needles'. Noticeable muscle weakness is uncommon.

On examination the neck may be slightly kyphotic. The posterior cervical muscles are usually tender, but not in spasm. The operator will identify a 'flaccid' response to pressure. Often fibrotic tissue will be felt interspersed in the main muscle bundles. Marked soreness will be experienced from palpatory pressure, particularly at the attachments to bony points, commonly at the skull attachments. Active movements are not necessarily markedly reduced except during acute attacks. The passive examination, however, shows a definite reduction in the movement of the affected level. In many cases audible crepitation can be heard during even slight passive movement. The passive examination is best carried out in the supine, recumbent position. Support the head using a pillow and gently straighten the kyphosis out before testing any of the movements. This makes identifying the level you are palpating easier. Splint the neck using both hands and then apply a rotatory force to encourage turning of the neck. Use the tips of the index fingers and next two fingers to gain the feedback. Repeat the procedure for lateral flexion and again for forward flexion. Leave extension as the last movement; this is usually the most painful and more likely to cause nerve root pressure if the foraminal space is reduced. Although palpatory pressure should be firm, ensure that a gentle hand is used. Tenderness is the main feature of this condition and it can easily be aggravated by too much palpatory pressure.

In the upper limb, objective signs are usually absent or slight. This is because nerve pressure is seldom great enough to produce neurological signs. Although demonstrable motor weakness or sensory impairment is exceptional, depression of one or more of the tendon reflexes is fairly common.

Radiographs will show narrowing of the intervertebral disc space, with formation of osteophytes at the vertebral margins, especially anteriorly.

A serious, although uncommon, complication of osteoarthritis of the neck is a marked narrowing by osteophytes of the spinal cord. This may lead to progressive upper motor neurone disturbance, affecting all four limbs and possibly the bladder.

'Whiplash'

'Whiplash' is primarily a legal term. It is used to describe what happens when a person riding in a car is suddenly and unexpectedly struck from behind. It is therefore more simply described as an extension strain of the neck. As a result of inertia, the head tends to stay in the same position while the body is rammed forward. This tends to whip the neck. When this happens the spinous processes tend to 'kiss' each other posteriorly; anteriorly the anterior longitudinal ligament may be sprained or strained. Fractures can occur, although these are rare. The nerve roots involved are usually C5, C6, C7 or C8.

Experimental analyses of the head–neck system are extremely common for whiplash injuries. These are constantly studied by the motor industry in order to improve safety standards. Simple mechanical 'spring' necks have been developed by manufacturers for crash studies [95]. The axis of rotation of the head depends on the direction of primary motion and the type of impact. Peak accelerations usually occur within the period of the actual impact or shortly after. Peak displacements typically occur between 100 and 300 milliseconds after impact [96].

Obtaining a detailed history and documenting the precise chain of events is essential. Include any pre-existing symptoms or injuries. Record the exact mechanism of injury, the immediate symptoms or signs and delayed symptoms or signs. The physical examination must include a description of any abnormal posture of the neck, degree of limitation of motion and in which direction, site of localized tenderness, degree of involuntary muscle spasm, any neurological findings and low back injuries. A key to estimating the extent of the injury is to estimate how far the patient can extend her neck. Ask the patient to put her head back, and then gently pull the head a little farther. If pains radiate down the arm, be more guarded in outlook and treatment. This type of pain is much more likely to be radicular and/or discogenic in origin. Also check for lower back injuries, with the usual method described in Chapter 11. Other factors to be evaluated are emotional shock, musculoligamentous strain, injury to the disc, fractures or dislocation of the spine, injury to the nerve roots and injury to the spinal cord. Severe injuries may require an X-ray of the cervical spine, especially to view the odontoid process, and possibly oblique views of each side, to study the intervertebral foramen. If necessary, magnetic resonance imaging (MRI) scans may be requested.

HEAD PAINS RELATED TO NECK DYSFUNCTION

As well as causing local pain in the neck, problems arising within the structures of the neck can be responsible for pains in the head. Head pains or 'head aches' arising from the neck can be extremely painful and debilitating. The neck contains many pain-sensitive tissues in a relatively small area. Pain may arise from any of the contained tissues caused by irritation, inflammation or even infection. The posterior longitudinal ligament is innervated by fibres of the recurrent meningeal nerve of Luschka. Pressure upon the ligament causes lower back pain as well as neck pain [97]. The nerve root within the spinal canal and in its course through the intervertebral foramen is also pain sensitive. The exact mechanism of pain production in nerve-root irritation still remains largely unknown. The three sites which have been indicated, however, are:

- The nerve fibres of the dural sheath of the nerve root.
- The sensory/dorsal root.
- The sensory fibres of the motor root.

Stretching the nerve and its dural sheath impairs the vascular circulation, therefore local ischaemia may cause pain. Pain can originate from muscle tissue in several ways:

- Ischaemia of muscle tissue.
- Accumulation of metabolic waste products.
- Forceful contraction as well as sustained contraction exerts a traction force at the myofascial junction to the periosteum. Irritation of the periosteum results in local pain and tenderness. In addition, the movement of passively stretching the muscle, or actively contracting the muscle bellies, results in pain, if the muscle is already sensitive because of a previous irritation. Small muscle fibre tears or tears of the fibrous element within the muscles can have the same effect [98].

THE UPPER CERVICAL COMPLEX

The upper two cervical functional units formed by the occiput and the atlas and the atlas and the axis are anatomically dissimilar to the functional units below.

The occipito-atlantal complex

This complex can be likened to a bubble of air in a spirit level – all intricate movements performed by the body are ultimately counter-balanced by the gliding occipital movements. There are two such joints which are symmetrically and mechanically linked. Their articular surfaces are the superior articular facets of the lateral masses of the atlas and the occipital condyles. Mechanical dysfunction at this level can be divided into two major groupings. For convenience they shall be referred to as primary and secondary problems:

- A primary lesion is one which is directly associated with a direct trauma or injury.
- Secondary lesions will follow a postural condition or follow functional abuse from occupational/habitual postures.

A lesion at this level can be defined as a dysfunction of the articular surface of the atlas in relation to the condyles of the occiput [99]. This working model was first proposed by C. H. Downing in 1923. Although his work was first published over 70 years ago, these simple working models are a useful way for the student to visualize some of the events which occur at the joint level.

Clinical evaluation of the upper cervical complex

The initial clinical task is to evaluate the subjective account of the patient. The chronological story will differentiate a primary from a secondary presentation.

Primary problems have an accentuated cervical lordosis. Secondary problems are related to straightening of the cervical spine. A precise delineation of the symptom pattern will localize the pain site. The first two cervical nerves (C1 and C2) are primarily sensory. After leaving the spinal canal, they travel for the most part through soft connective tissue, mostly muscle. The sensory distribution of these nerves is the posterior and lateral portion of the scalp (Figure 8.9).

Branches of C3 join the first two branches in forming the greater and lesser occipital nerves. The sensory pattern extends forward to the frontal supraorbital area, so that irritation of the nerves at the base of the skull can cause pain that may mimic 'sinus problems'. The nerves in this area are close to the vertebral artery just before entering the skull through the foramen magnum. These nerves are thus vulnerable to irritation and injury from the myofascial attachment of the neck muscles to the base of the skull, muscles which they traverse.

Suboccipital pain can arise from the periosteal site of the attachment of the suboccipital group of muscles. Traction exerted by these muscles can cause pain and tissue tenderness. Pain can originate in the joints of the neck with manifestation of joint pain from stretching of the capsular tissue. This is particularly seen when capsular tissue is thickened and contracted as a result of osteoarthritic changes.

Once a temporary hypothesis is formulated around the presenting history, the exact nature of the mechanical aetiology should then be established clinically. This is usually confirmed with the presence of a trauma or gradual build up of excessive mechanical use of the area. The symptoms are usually movement related.

A thorough examination is carried out to establish the relationship between the skull and the upper neck. Pay particular attention to the degree of sustained flexion/extension of the head. Next, look for any sustained rotation/lateral flexion of the head. The patient is asked to nod the head and to perform small turning movements. A record is made of any movement which increases the level of symptoms and of which movement is particularly difficult to perform.

The passive examination can be carried out with the patient both in the sitting position and supine. Initially the tone and tightness of the scalp is noted, particularly over the suboccipital area. Next palpate for any uneven suboccipital muscular tone. Does it feel tight or slack on one or both sides? Having gained a static impression of the contractile tissue tone, we need to familiarize ourselves with the passive, dynamic state of the area. This is achieved by applying a local palpatory pressure onto the skull, to project an overall movement in certain directions. The aim here is to test the known ranges of the joint movement, i.e. 10 degrees flexion and 35 degrees extension, as well as slight lateral shift. Both joints are tested in turn in order to determine the presence of joint dysfunction. This dysfunction is determined by noting an increase in tension due to irritation of the tissues.

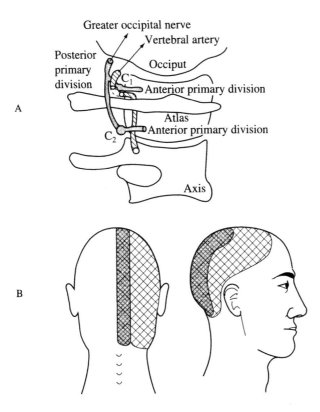

Figure 8.9 The upper cervical functional unit. A. The course of the C1 and C2 nerves as they merge into the occipital nerve; the relationship to the vertebral artery in the atlas–axis region is also shown. B. The shaded areas represent hypoaesthesia, hyperaesthesia or anaesthesia from pressure or irritation of these nerve roots.

Conceptual classification of 'occipito-atlantal lesions' (based on C. H. Downing)

1. *Flexion:* when the head is flexed resulting in a relatively posterior position of the occipital condyles on the superior facets of the atlas.
2. *Extension:* the reverse of the above.
3. *Lateral flexion:* the head will be tilted to one or other side with *no* anterior or posterior displacement.
4. *Pseudo-rotation:* when one occipital condyle rotates anteriorly and the other posteriorly.
5. *Impacted:* there is a closer than normal approximation of the articular surfaces.
6. *Unilateral displacement:* there is a unilateral anterior or posterior displacement with consequent fixation of the occipital condyles in relation to the superior facets of the atlas.

In *Principles and Practice of Osteopathy* [99], no less than 11 possible combinations were described by C. H. Downing. These illustrated the importance which was placed on positional factors at that time. Although this definitive classification is rarely used in modern practice, it offers a useful aid to a student of osteopathy to visualize the potential combination of mechanical dysfunctions.

Table 8.2, detailing Downing's possible classifications, is included more for historic interest than factual information.

Table 8.2 Conceptual classification of 'occipito-atlantal lesions' (according to C. H. Downing)

1. Unilateral anterior occiput on the left (torsion lesion)
2. Unilateral anterior occiput on the right (torsion lesion)
3. Bilateral anterior occiput (extension lesion)
4. Left lateral occiput (side-bending lesion to the right)
5. Right lateral occiput (side-bending lesion to the left)
6. Bilaterally posterior occiput (flexion lesion)
7. Unilateral anterior occiput on the left, posterior on the right (pseudo-rotation lesion)
8. Unilateral anterior occiput on the right, posterior on the left (pseudo-rotation lesion)
9. Impacted posterior occiput on the right/left (torsion lesion)
10. Unilateral posterior occiput on right (torsion lesion)
11. Unilaterally posterior occiput on left (torsion lesion)

On a practical note, the operator uses palpatory findings with reference to bony points on the cervical vertebral bodies. Having located the bony points, primarily the transverse processes of C1 and C2, mastoid processes, angle of the jaw and the spinous process of C2, any deviation from the anatomical normal position is noted.

Next, function is assessed. In other words, a directional force is applied to the cranium whilst a palpatory hand is retained on the suboccipital joint space.

In the non-fixation state, an approximate 10 degrees of flexion and 35 degrees of extension should be achieved by 'rolling' the cranium backward and forward in relation to the occiput.

A small range of side-shift should also be achieved using a sideward direction to the driving movement.

While flexing the osteoarthritic joint, a tensing of the soft tissues is initially felt. The movement gradually comes to a halt and the limiting force gradually builds up with a feeling of increasing resistance. This increase in resistance should seem equal on both joints. The same procedure is carried out for the other ranges.

From knowledge and understanding of normal movement a mental library should be compiled of any anomalous movements. Therefore, for example, lesion 6 above, according to Downing, a bilateral posterior occiput or flexion lesion, is evaluated as follows: static findings will include taut posterior soft tissues; the transverse processes of the atlas will be approximated to the mastoid processes posteriorly on both sides. Passive palpatory findings will show that any attempt to move the cranium further forward will be resisted; precise movement, however, applied in order to attempt any extension movement will be possible in some cases. On occasions, the fixing spasm of muscular protection is so strong that only a few degrees of extension can be achieved and not the total range of 35 degrees. In essence, the occiput will have travelled to its furthermost flexion position and on palpation only some of the extension range can be reproduced.

Such differentiation of specific movements requires careful and repeated practice. The movements are small and sometimes difficult to appreciate. A firm and confident palpating hand is required at all times to allow the patient to be as relaxed as possible, in order to reduce overlying muscular tone.

As with any physical assessment and diagnostic procedures, it is essential to remember that the presence of any or indeed all positive findings, which indicate a particular dysfunction, does not necessarily prove that the problem can be resolved by correcting the dysfunction alone. This is particularly important when dealing with head pains. Almost all of us have at some stage experienced head pains. We have self-diagnosed the problem by isolating a tender point at the base of our head. We must, however, always be aware that any underlying reason for head pain will be accompanied by muscular signs. Before commencing on a course of mechanical treatment, the absence of any other pathological state must be determined.

How can this be done satisfactorily? Often the patient feels far from well and is not keen to answer too many questions. A skilled practitioner allows the patient to be comfortable and performs one task at a time. Questions should be simple and follow a train of thought. For example, an elderly patient complaining of head pain, particularly over the temporal musculature, should be carefully screened for symptoms related to vision and any noted impairment, also for pains related to chewing particularly on the side of the facial/head pain. The questions should be directed at the present episode and restricted to conditions which could constitute a medical emergency. Cranial arteritis should be either eliminated or referred on immediately if suspected. The patient in this example is more likely to respond with certainty if asked direct and relevant questions. Vague or ambiguous questions, which don't 'ring any bells' with the patient are likely to lead to an uncertain diagnosis. What is more, a missed case of cranial arteritis will not only involve the risk of sudden blindness but will be severely aggravated by any physical pressure to the affected vessels. Unfortunately, most patients with arteritis also have a certain degree of cervical spondylosis which in turn can result in headaches. It is therefore vital to evaluate the entire condition and not stop at merely the tissues that are causing the symptoms.

OTHER CAUSES OF HEAD PAINS

Headache pain is a universal ailment of mankind and in any year will be experienced by 65–80% of the population. This pain represents the chief complaint of approximately 2% of the population seeking medical care. There are many causes of head pain, but relatively few ways in which it can be produced. The primary pain-sensitive structures within the skull are the cranial arteries. There is ample documentation to suggest that these vessels are the cause of most common, benign headaches. Among the other important pain-sensitive structures are the sensory nerves and the nerve roots. As briefly described above in this chapter, they are responsible for the various forms of neuritis, neuralgia and radiculitis. Pain in the head may be referred, either from structures within the head itself, primarily the eye, nasal sinuses, temporomandibular joint or teeth, or occasionally from one of the thoracic or even pelvic viscera [100].

Although ways of taking the history and examining the patient with neck pain and neck and head pains have already been looked at, particular attention must now be paid to patients presenting solely with the complaint of head pains.

Taking the history

The exact location of the pain must be established together with any related, associated symptoms. Often headaches present in a pattern of distribution, starting typically in one site then migrating along the same pathway every time. A full descriptive account of the type and character of pain must be thoroughly investigated, as many descriptive terms can be used to determine the origin of the symptoms. For example, a classic psychogenic headache is often described as 'like a wedge being driven into the skull'. This severe and definite picture is often accompanied by other symptoms of depression and distressed state of mind.

The general state of the patient may alert the practitioner to an underlying reason for her presenting head pain. For example, a diagnosed hypertensive may clinically present with headaches. In general, benign hypertension does not usually cause headaches, although a patient who knows that she has hypertension may complain of headache. Headache, however, is a striking feature of malignant hypertension. Such headaches are characteristically at their worst in the early hours of the morning. They are certainly vascular in origin, but their precise mode of production is unclear. The extra- as well as the intra-cranial vessels are involved, although whether the pain is due to contraction or dilatation of the vessels is uncertain.

Potential causes of head pain are given in Table 8.3; however, the table is not totally comprehensive and the reader is advised to consult specialized books for detailed explanations of the various problems.

Table 8.3 Potential causes of head pain

Space-occupying lesions
Meningeal irritation
Toxic headaches
Headaches in hypertension
Cranial arteritis
Neuritis and neuralgia
Referred pain
Cough headaches
Psychogenic headaches
Migraines
Migranous neuralgia

Psychogenic versus space-occupying lesions

Perhaps the most difficult patient to handle is the one with a long history of head pains, who has not been given an adequate explanation of what exactly is the problem. It is remarkable how many varieties of painful sensations in the head are the subject of complaint by patients who show no organic basis for them. However, to distinguish (and identify with confidence) between the two ends of the 'head pain' spectrum, i.e. the psychogenic headache and the space-occupying lesion, is perhaps the greatest challenge to the practitioner. Sometimes the psychogenic headache is fuelled by the anxiety of a potential space-occupying lesion. In rarer cases, this anxiety can be the sole cause of the headache.

Some psychogenic headaches can be attributed merely to increased tension of the scalp and neck muscles, which usually occurs as a sequel to the patient's tense state of mind. Each individual will have a personal, often elaborate, description of sensation which varies from a constant, nagging sense of pressure at the back of the head to a violent feeling of a 'drill being driven into the skull'. The severity of the clinical picture can make it difficult to locate the exact origin of the pain. This distinction can be particularly difficult in examples such as middle-aged to elderly women in whom a specific organic or mechanical dysfunction cannot be found. There is a disproportionate disparity between the symptom picture found, and the clinical, mechanical findings. The complaint can become a dominant feature of personality.

The symptoms of headache as a result of a space-occupying lesion have been established as arising from traction upon the intra-cranial blood vessels. The mode of onset of symptoms of a cerebral tumour is extremely variable, hence headaches alone are not of much localizing value, although, in the early stages, it has been long regarded as one of the classical triad of symptoms together with vomiting and papilloedema.

Migraine

There must be very few people who at some stage of their life have not suffered with, been diagnosed as having, or believe they have had a 'migraine attack'. The real victims of migraines will have no sympathy toward the occasional headache sufferer who recurrently has days off work because they wake up with a 'migraine', but feel much better by lunch time! It appears that at some time most of us experience a headache which shows some of the features of migraine.

Let us consider the cardinal features of a migraine. It is a paroxysmal headache which commonly, but not invariably, occurs unilaterally. It recurs at irregular intervals, and is often associated with visual disturbances and other disorders of cerebral function and vomiting. It has been commonly agreed that the headaches in migraine are due to stretching, by dilatation, of the branches of the external carotid artery and possibly to a lesser extent of the internal carotid artery. Constriction of one of the vessels supplying an area of the cerebral cortex seems to be the most likely explanation of the visual and other symptoms, such as numbness and tingling of the lips and tongue. Heredity seems to be the most important causal factor. Those who suffer from migraine often have a conscientious or obsessional personality [100].

In the predisposed individual an attack may be precipitated by emotional stress, by eating some particular food product, by alcohol or by menstruation. A childhood history of car-sickness and a family history of various allergies is not uncommon.

Migraines usually begin with or soon after puberty, much less frequently in middle age or later life. The main exception is an onset at or about the menopause.

The symptoms vary both in frequency and severity. A classic attack of migraine begins with a visual disturbance, which is usually localized to one side. This disturbance is usually described as misty or shimmering. There is often an accompanying spread of cutaneous symptoms, numbness and tingling, most frequently involving the lips, tongue and hand. Rarely there is a transitory loss of speech co-ordination and/or unilateral and transient paralysis. The headache usually begins as the visual symptoms are passing off, as boring pain in a localized area on one side, often the temple, and gradually spreads to the whole of the affected side. Gradually the headache acquires a more throbbing character, being intensified by stooping and all forms of exertion and by light. The superficial temporal artery on the affected side shows a vigorous pulsation.

In milder cases the headache passes away with sleep. In more severe cases it persists for days. Nausea is usually present during the stage of headache and vomiting may occur.

Avoidance management, based on experience of circumstances which precipitate attacks, seems to have the best results. Migraine does not shorten life, but in severe cases a state of chronic exhaustion may occur. Migraine usually ceases spontaneously in middle life.

A logical and progressive approach must be shown in trying to evaluate neck pain, with or without associated head pain, or upper limb pains or indeed head pains alone. Initially environmental influences on the person must be taken into consideration. Does the work generate the stress which leads to the headache? Or does the work environment cause the neck to be in a position of mechanical disadvantage, resulting in headache? This is seen as an initial differentiation of mechanical or organic versus psychogenic problems. How does the person feel when the pains are not present? This is also valuable information. A general state of exhaustion, with recurrent episodes of headaches, needs investigating to see if the headache is merely a by-product of the general state.

In summary, an intra-cranial cause, be it of a space-occupying nature, vascular disease or systemic disorder, must be identified and differentiated from an extra-cranial physical/skeletal or environmental and/or psychogenic cause. However, the intra-cranial may easily be masked by any overt physical signs such as degenerative changes in the neck or altered joint function. Psychological stress can easily be involved as a major player in the symptom picture.

Therefore, all the detectable components of the problem must be categorized clinically. This can be done by taking a thorough history, performing a detailed physical examination and maintaining an open-minded approach, being prepared to refer to other fields if some of the presenting components cannot be reasonably supported.

Case study 8.3 demonstrates how a multi-factoral problem can easily be categorized as a 'tension headache', until some profound signs and symptoms suddenly develop.

Case study 8.3

Martin, a 22-year-old final year university student, currently sitting his final exams, had every reason to believe that his headaches were purely 'tension' related. The accumulation of hours spent with his head buried in books invariably resulted in joint dysfunction of the neck resulting in a 'stiff neck'. During the history, however, it was established that he had noticed a deterioration of vision, with a mild, unilateral squint. These signs with this history, as well as the recent bouts of vomiting, were more indicative of an intra-cranial hypertensive state than the stresses and strains of university life!

9 The upper limbs

In order to achieve fine movements of the hand, the control of the whole upper limb must be accurately co-ordinated. We need only observe an artist in action to see the complex 'total' body co-ordination that is executed. A precise stroke of the brush can only occur when the whole body is poised; the arm is suspended in the air and the hand slowly applies the brush on the canvas. To complete this sequence accurately, the individual is dependent on an intact central as well as peripheral nervous system; fit musculature; pliable joints and a certain amount of acquired manual dexterity.

Seeing beyond the simplistic 'hand pain' or 'arm ache' will ensure that the practitioner does not overlook the less obvious causes of disorders of the upper limb. The muscle state of the palm of the hand can be a significant sign of some degenerative conditions of the central nervous system. A fine tremor of the arm can be a pointer to a metabolic imbalance; central nervous system disorder or a state of chronic alcohol abuse.

Commonly known disorders such as angina pectoris can be observed as pains in the arm. The first signs of disturbances in the gallbladder are sometimes pains at the tip of the right shoulder. These are some examples of referred pains experienced in the upper limb. Irritative lesions of the brachial plexus often extend from the base of the neck, over the top of the shoulder and thence into the arm.

Injuries to and disablement of the arm and hand have such great practical and economic consequences that prompt assessment must be made and appropriate treatment started as soon as possible.

ASSESSING THE UPPER LIMB

For ease of assessment, in this chapter the upper limb will be viewed as three separate sections:

1. The shoulder complex.
2. The upper arm and elbow.
3. The forearm, wrist and hand.

It must be remembered, however, that this is clinically artificial. Although the presence of a specific condition is sought, the following points must be kept in mind:

- The wider implications of the diagnosed conditions, in other words, the

levels of adaptation which the body has to undergo in order to continue
functioning – secondary somatic dysfunction.

- The direct effect the diagnosed condition has on the immediate,
surrounding structures – the local somatic dysfunction caused.

Examples are used to illustrate these two points:

The wider implications of the diagnosed conditions

A patient presenting with the signs, symptoms and clinical findings associated
with a 'frozen shoulder' will need to have their neck, elbow, wrist and hand
looked at very carefully, as the function of the arm will have been greatly sac-
rificed while suffering the condition. Also, the protection given to the affected
shoulder may alter the whole weight-bearing pattern. This alteration of
weight-bearing may result in patterns of adaptation which are alien to the
patient's posture and thus ultimately result in a dysfunction elsewhere in the
body, which may be remote from the painful arm. Therefore, a full postural
assessment is also called for even when the presenting problem may seem to
be clearly defined as a frozen shoulder.

Somatic dysfunction caused by a defined condition

Equally important to the osteopath is the aspect of local dysfunction. A patient
may present with a clearly defined case of osteoarthritis of the shoulder, as
shown on radiographs. However, the main point to address is why has the
patient become aware of the pains at this point in time. After all, osteoarthritis is not a sudden process. Therefore, one can argue that the 'condition' was
present long before the symptoms became apparent. One explanation is that it
is not the arthritis for which the patient is seeking treatment, but the inability
of the local tissues to cope with a new and unusual movement for them. An
example is given in Case study 9.1.

Case study 9.1

An elderly man decides to use his old 'push and pull' lawnmower, while his modern, light-weight lawnmower is
being serviced. The sudden strain on the muscles causes him severe 'pain in the shoulder'. On examination, he has
tenderness of all the muscles in the shoulder area and pain on resisted movements in all ranges. The passive examination did not cause any pain, other than discomfort at the end of range of movements. The overall range was less
than in his other shoulder and crepitation was present throughout the range; however, the movement was 'comfortable'.

This illustrates that the sudden demand on the shoulder muscles resulted in pain arising from those tissues, probably because of an inflammatory reaction in the muscles. Those same muscles were not causing the pain until
excess demand was placed on them. This extra demand was too much to cope with, given that they were already
under greater load because of the osteoarthritis in the joint.

Case study 9.1 is an example of somatic dysfunction. Injury to one or more
tissues around any part of the musculo-skeletal system will lead to similar response in the surrounding tissues. This is clearly seen in the arm condition
described above where hyperaesthesia was not only present around the rotator

cuff surrounding the gleno-humeral joint but also altered muscle tension was felt in the periscapular muscles and in the rotator cuff muscles.

Clinical assessment: observation and palpation

As in all thorough clinical examinations, the assessment is started with the first contact. Ordinary, daily movements can start to indicate the degree of hand control and co-ordination of the patient. Shaking hands can reveal accuracy of control, temperature discrepancy, excessive sweating and also coarseness of skin, which in turn can show the type and amount of workload on the hand. Indeed a simple handshake can afford insight into the patient's self-confidence.

The undressed arm is closely examined for any skin lesions. Many fungal infections or skin irritations are particularly prevalent in the axilla and elbow creases. Any overt areas of swelling or bruising are noted.

A systematic overview of the upper limb should start by looking at the tips of the fingers and then working upwards. Look and feel for any obvious superficial or deep anomalies of the soft tissues or the joint surfaces or contours of the long bones of the arm.

Having observed the limb statically, feel for the general flexibility of passive movements. Without becoming too involved in specific joint movement, a great deal can be learned from putting the various joints through their natural ranges. Gently but firmly gain an insight into the amount of joint 'tolerance' and compare with the other side. This is a useful exercise in trying to build up a general picture of joint flexibility, as well as a comparative study of the two limbs. Examination procedures in the early stages are best kept general and simple. A useful way to observe general active movements is to request a demonstration of daily actions, for example, combing the hair from the front of the head to the back, trying to fasten a zip at the back and reaching across the body to the back of the neck are all very good indicators of how the shoulder, elbow, wrist and hand act in co-ordination (Figure 9.1).

THE SHOULDER REGION

Mechanically, the shoulder movements are complex and intricate. The reason for this is that the region is made up of three components – the shoulder joint proper, known as the gleno-humeral joint, the acromio-clavicular joint and the sterno-clavicular joint. The gleno-humeral joint allows a free range of abduction, flexion and rotation, under the action and control of the scapulo-humeral muscles. The other two joints in combination allow 90 degrees of rotation of the scapula, upon the thorax, and a moderate range of antero-posterior (AP) gliding of the scapula under the action of the thoraco-scapular and cervico-scapular muscles. Disorders of the shoulder joint include most types of arthritis. Osteoarthritis, however, which is common in most other joints, is rare in the gleno-humeral joint. This joint is prone to conditions which seem to be particular to itself, notably to tears of the musculo-tendinous cuff, and the commonly termed 'frozen shoulder'. Pain in the shoulder is notoriously prone to misinterpretation, and special care must be taken to differentiate intrinsic pain arising in the shoulder from extrinsic pain arising from the cervical spine, the thorax or the abdomen.

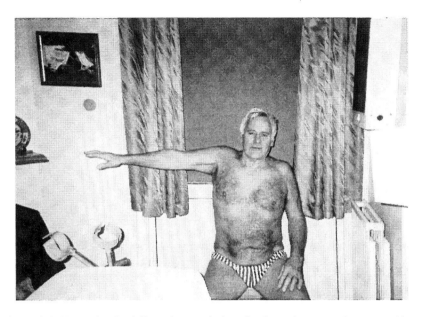

Figure 9.1 Example of a daily action carried out by the patient, seen here stretching out to reach out for his crutches. This highlights limitation of the gleno-humeral joint.

Taking the history

True shoulder pain is seldom localized to the shoulder itself. It is, therefore, essential to find out exactly the area and the associated distribution of pain. Typically, the pain radiates from a point near the tip of the acromion down the lateral side of the upper arm to about the level of the deltoid insertion. It occasionally extends below the elbow. Pain arising from the acromio-clavicular joint or sterno-clavicular joint is localized to the joint itself and does not radiate down the limb.

Referred pain in the shoulder from an irritative cause in the brachial plexus often extends from the base of the neck, over the top of the shoulder, and thence into the base of the arm. Unlike true shoulder pain, it frequently radiates below the elbow into the forearm or hand, and it may be accompanied by paraesthesiae or numbness. It must be remembered that pain may also be referred to the shoulder from a lesion in the thorax or upper abdomen.

The examination (Table 9.1)

The shoulder must be suitably exposed and it is advisable to stand behind the patient in order to observe the movements of the scapula.

Table 9.1 Routine examination in cases of a suspected disorder of the shoulder complex

---

Observation
    Surface markings
    Colour of skin
    Bony contour

Palpation
    Confirm bony contour
    Soft tissue contours
    Local tenderness

Movements (both passive and active ranges)
    Distinguish between gleno-humeral and scapular movement during:
        Abduction
        Flexion
        Extension
    ? Pain on movements
    ? Presence of muscular spasm
    ? Crepitation

Assessing the listed movements must be done in both the active and the passive ranges. When assessing the active ranges it is important to note the 'quality' of the movement, that is, whether it is smooth throughout the range or shows interruption in the flow. If the movement appears to be interrupted, the patient should be asked if it is the pain that is causing the loss of flow or simply that they feel a structural obstruction. In some cases intracapsular adhesions interrupt the free flow of the movement; chronic cases can be totally free of pain (Figure 9.2).

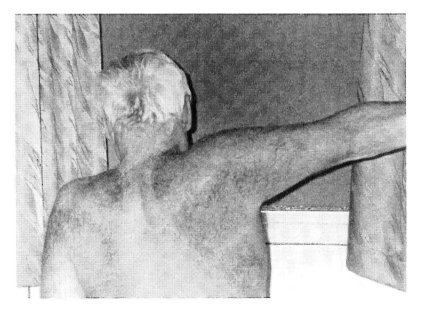

Figure 9.2 Characteristic raising of the shoulder seen in a case of a 'frozen' shoulder.

Muscular spasm is identified as an intense form of protection causing marked limitation of movement at least in one or more ranges of movement, depending on the tissues damaged.

Crepitation is a dry, crackling sound or sensation which is felt both by the patient, when moving the arm actively, and by the practitioner, when assessing the shoulder passively.

In addition, the upper thoracic spine as well as the cervical spine are examined for any local vertebral, somatic dysfunction.

Disorders of the shoulder joint (gleno-humeral)

The shoulder joint is prone to four main types of arthritic disorders, all of which are fairly uncommon.

Osteoarthritis of the shoulder

Unlike most other joints, the shoulder is very seldom affected by osteoarthritis. When it does occur, there is usually a clear predisposing factor such as a trauma or disease, avascular necrosis of the humeral head or simply old age. The rarity in presentation is probably due to freedom from all pressures of weight-bearing. When it does occur, there is an obvious hypertrophy of the joint margin, with osteophyte formation. Clinically, the presenting case is an elderly patient (younger patients are exceptional) with pain in the shoulder and down the upper arm. On examination the only obvious signs are localized soft swelling due to effusion of fluid into the joint and generalized muscle wasting around the joint. Movements are restricted.

Rheumatoid arthritis of the shoulder

Often both shoulders are affected by rheumatoid arthritis simultaneously with several other joints. The peripheral joints such as hands and wrists and feet are affected by rheumatoid arthritis more commonly than the shoulder joints. The main clinical features are local pain and swelling from synovial thickening.

Pyogenic arthritis of the shoulder

This condition is uncommon. It occurs most often in children, where the infection has spread to the shoulder from a focus of ostoemyelitis in the upper metaphysis of the humerus [101]. There is a rapid onset of pyrexia; the shoulder is typically swollen, restricted in movement and abnormally warm.

Tuberculous arthritis of the shoulder

Once again this is a relatively rare condition, which is less frequent than tuberculosis of the spine, hip and knee. The pathological features correspond to those of tuberculous arthritis of a major joint. Pain is usually the predominant symptom, and examination may reveal diffuse swelling with increased warmth, and marked reduction of gleno-humeral movement. An abscess may form.

Five mechanical conditions affecting the gleno-humeral joint

- 'Frozen shoulder' (adhesive capsulitis).
- Painful arc syndrome (supra-spinatus syndrome).
- Recurrent dislocation of the shoulder.
- Tenosynovitis of long tendon of biceps (biceps tendonitis).
- Tear of the tendinous cuff (supra-spinatus).

'Frozen shoulder'

Although this is a commonly seen disorder, it is ill understood and seen with a variety of clinical presentations. It is characterized by pain and uniform limitation of all movements. The cause is generally unknown and there is no evidence of infection. Injury is not always evident.

Although the exact pathological mechanism is not understood, there seems to be a general loss of resilience of the joint capsule. Clinically the patient complains of severe aching pain in the shoulder and upper arm, with a history of gradual or spontaneous onset. On examination the only finding is uniform reduction of movement in all ranges of shoulder movement. The scapular movement remains unimpaired. Other causes of painful limitation of gleno-humeral movement, particularly the various other types of arthritis, must be excluded with careful examination, and radiographic evidence if necessary. Along with the characteristic uniform limitation of all gleno-humeral movements, the condition does not have any evidence of inflammatory or destructive changes. There is a general tendency towards spontaneous recovery within 12–18 months. However, if movements are not encouraged actively and aided passively, there can be some permanent restriction of movement.

Painful arc syndrome (Figure 9.3)

When the supra-spinatus muscle is involved, it is also known as the 'supra-spinatus syndrome'. This is a clinical syndrome characterized by, as the common term suggests, pain in the shoulder and upper arm during the mid-range of gleno-humeral abduction, with freedom from pain at the extremes of the range. Pain is produced by the mechanical entrapment of a tender structure between the tuberosity of the humerus and the acromion process.

Even in the normal shoulder, the clearance between the upper end of the humerus and the acromion process is small in mid-abduction range. Therefore, if a tender structure present beneath the acromion becomes nipped causing inflammation, there will be consequent pain. In the neutral position and in full abduction the clearance is greater, and therefore the pain is less marked or even absent.

Five known causes of pain resulting in a painful arc syndrome

1. Injury of the *greater tuberosity* such as a bruise or undisplaced fracture.
2. Subacromial *bursitis*, where the bursal walls are inflamed and thickened from mechanical irritation.
3. Calcified *deposit in the supra-spinatus tendon* occurs when a chalky deposit forms within the tendon, and the lesion is surrounded by an inflammatory reaction.

4. Supra-spinatus *tendonitis* is believed to be a condition where an inflammatory reaction is triggered by the degeneration of the tendon fibres.
5. Minor *tears of the supra-spinatus tendon* commonly causes an inflammatory reaction with resultant local swelling. The power can be markedly lost with complete tear of the tendinous cuff.

Clinically, whatever the primary cause is, the presentation has the same general features. The arm can be assessed hanging freely, without pain in the patient, unless there is protective hypertonia due to increased neurological stimulation from a recent injury, for example such as a bruise of the greater tuberosity from a fall. During abduction the pain becomes painful at about 45 degrees and persists through the arc of movement up to 160 degrees. Gradually the pain disappears completely by full elevation. The descending movement will show the same pattern.

Differentiation of the five possible causes comes from a thorough history and can be confirmed with radiography. A sudden traumatic onset is more likely to cause injury to the greater tuberosity or a strain or tear of the supraspinatus tendon. Gradual unprovoked history is more likely to be a tendonitis, calcified deposit or subacromial bursitis. The onset of symptoms resulting from a calicifed deposit, however, can be very sudden and painful without trauma.

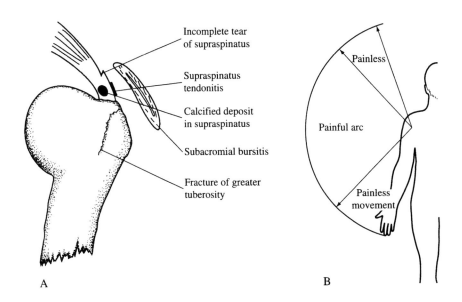

A. Incomplete tear of supraspinatus
Supraspinatus tendonitis
Calcified deposit in supraspinatus
Subacromial bursitis
Fracture of greater tuberosity

B. Painless
Painful arc
Painless movement

Figure 9.3 A. Five causes of painful arc syndrome. B. The different stages where pain is felt during abduction of the arm. Clinically, the middle arc of abduction is painful, the extremes are painless.

Recurrent dislocation of the shoulder

Some cases will present with an initial history of trauma to the shoulder, resulting in dislocation. Thereafter, recurrent cases of dislocation occur with little provocation. Classically this occurs during combined external rotation with abduction, for example, the simple action of putting on a shirt. On examination no apparent abnormality is shown. Patients with this typical presentation are advised to seek orthopaedic advice. Alternatively, extensive stabilizing exercises have been shown to be effective if carried out under good supervision over several months.

Tenosynovitis of the long head of the biceps

Known as biceps tendonitis, this is a common condition which results from overuse of the shoulder joint, frequently seen during 'Wimbledon week' when all spectators develop high aspirations! This condition is ascribed to frictional irritation of the tendon within its groove. Clinically, the complaint is of pain in the front of the shoulder, which becomes worse on active movement of the arm. There is often local tenderness in the course of the long tendon of the biceps. Resisted supination of the arm can sometimes aggravate the pain.

Tear of the tendinous cuff

The supra-spinatus can tear partially, as seen above, in the painful arc syndrome, or can sometimes tear completely. The clinical effects are different. The tendon can give way under a sudden strain which is usually caused by a fall or from saving the impact of a fall by grabbing with the hand. The resultant force will cause tearing, particularly of a degenerate tendon.

Clinically the presenting case is often a man of 60 years or above, with a traumatic history involving the arm. Although the passive range of movement is full, there is a painful inability to initiate any abduction. Younger subjects should be immediately referred for a repair operation. The older patient tends not to respond to operative repair due to the degenerate condition of the tendon. Spontaneous repair occurs gradually as the patient notices the disability less and less.

Case study 9.2

Ann is a 66-year-old retired machinist. Three years ago she slipped on the ice and dislocated her left shoulder joint at the gleno-humeral joint. This was successfully rectified at her local accident and emergency department on the same day. X-rays showed no other abnormality. Nine months later she heard a loud 'clank' when she was putting her coat on. Although it was painful, she was able to '… put it back …'. When she was seen, by the osteopath she complained of general aches in the left shoulder.

Although careful history taking and the physical examination can usually detect the specific conditions listed as seen in a case like Ann's (Case study 9.2), we are often confronted with a puzzle of multiple presentations.

In the example in Case study 9.2, all relevant clinical tests were carried out and none of the above categories of injury suited the case completely. The initial diagnosis of a dislocation was successfully treated. The clanking sound was probably the start of recurrent dislocation of the shoulder. As for the general aches in the left shoulder, it was concluded that she was suffering from chronic muscular fatigue in the shoulder. All ranges of movement were uncomfortable and a slight struggle ic achieve fully. All the symptoms came on after any prolonged unaccustomed activity using her arm.

On observation, the rounded contcur of the shoulder had been reduced and the tone of the muscles had a distinct lack of resistance to palpatory pressure. Ann's problem resolved after a course of stretching techniques to improve the partially adhesive capsular structures, and exercises to improve the muscular tone.

Combined presentations, with varying degrees of contributions from the syndromes, can confuse the clinical picture. It is advisable to try and identify the contributing components of the various syndromes, and then piece together the diagnostic puzzle.

Disorders of the sterno-clavicular and the acromio-clavicular joint

Localization of the pain and tenderness can usually differentiate and identify problems of these two joints. A common sequel to dislocation of either joint is subluxation, persistent or recurrent dislocation. Both joints are subject to arthritic conditions, with the acromio-clavicular being more prone to osteoarthritis than the gleno-humeral joint; this is rarely seen in the sterno-clavicular joint. Osteoarthritis of the acromio-clavicular joint is characterized by a localized pain over the joint, which can be felt as an irregular bony thickening of the joint margins, due to the osteophytes forming. There are none of the other cardinal signs of inflammatory processes. Active movements are characterized by pain arising locally toward the end of ranges of shoulder movements with an increasing severity. This is in sharp contrast to the picture seen in the painful arc.

The clinical picture of dislocation or subluxation is characterized by varying degrees of pain. There is a characteristically persistent upward displacement of the lateral end of the clavicle at the acromio-clavicular joint, while the sterno-clavicular joint is characterized by the medial end of the clavicle being displaced in a forward direction.

'Compression syndromes'

The next group of conditions is often described by patients as being a 'shoulder complaint'. In fact, they are a group of complaints whose causal origin is found to be compression of the neurovascular bundle in the region of the cervico-thoracic outlet. They can be classified as 'compression syndromes' [98]. These conditions include the scalenes anticus syndrome, claviculocostal syndrome, and the pectoralis minor syndrome.

Scalenes anticus syndrome

Case study 9.3

Evelyn is a 56-year-old secretary with a 5-year history of neck pain arising from a generalized condition of degeneration of the cervical spine. In the last 6 months she has developed a worrying set of symptoms, including constant neck pain, shoulder pain and difficulty in swallowing. She feels a tightness of the front of the neck as well as numbness and tingling of the arm, hand and fingers of the left hand. She has had extensive investigations from both a cardiologist and a gastroenterologist. They have both passed her fit in their respective fields.

Pain in the neck, shoulder and arm often has no local cause, but is referred from an extrinsic site. Such a possibility must always be considered in differential diagnosis. In a case such as Evelyn's (Case study 9.3), we must first of all consider the resultant effects of the degeneration in the neck. In this case the osteoarthritic changes have resulted in narrowing of the intervertebral foraminal space, thus causing pressure of the roots of the brachial plexus. This is found to be radiating the pain from the base of the neck, across the top of the shoulder, and down the front of the arm, extending into the forearm and fingers. The pain was descibed as a deep, dull, vague 'aching' in the arm and hand. All these symptoms appeared worse in the morning and woke her up. At first they calmed down, only to return after several hours of sitting and clerical activities. There were no objective changes found during the examination. A positive 'Adson test', however, was elicited for the anterior scalenes. This consists of turning the head to the side of the symptoms, *extending* the head, *abducting* the arm, taking a deep breath, and therefore obliterating the radial pulse in that arm, thereby reduplicating the symptoms complained of by Evelyn.

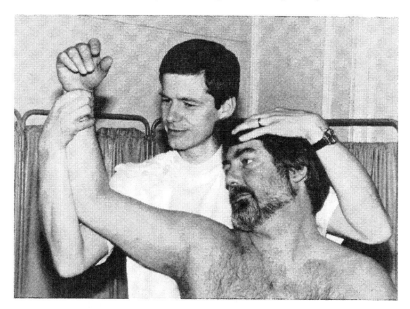

Figure 9.4 Adson test: consists of turning the head to the side of the symptoms, extending the head, abducting the arm and taking a deep breath. The test is positive for brachial artery compression if the radial pulse is obliterated.

It was concluded that the scalenes were responsible for the symptoms including the difficulty in swallowing. In the absence of a cervical rib it was thought that scalene spasm [102] was the most probable cause.

Claviculocostal syndrome

Case study 9.4

Josephine is a 62-year-old housewife, who has recently rediscovered her love of tennis. Up to the age of 30 she used to play to a competitive standard. Family commitments and a torn Achilles tendon forced her into early retirement. Two months ago she joined a local tennis club and has been gradually getting back into the game. Unable to miss the opportunity of joining in a league game, she played vigorously for three sets. That night she woke with severe paraesthesiae, numbness and pain in the right arm. The symptoms gradually eased during the day. On examination, unbeknown to her, her right hand and arm, despite being the dominant one, was objectively weaker in all testing of muscle power. The arm was slightly wasted and the hand seemed dryer and paler all round.

The history and combined vascular and neurological symptoms in Case study 9.4 indicated to the osteopath a compression of the neurovascular bundle. Analysis of the forehand action shows how the shoulder is speedily pulled back and downward. Reproducing this action by the patient resulted in obliterating the radial pulse. This was confirmed when the examiner pulled the shoulder back and down. He simultaneously noted the disappearance of the radial pulse and the return of the numbness and paraesthesiae. Palpation of the cervico-thoracic outlet showed an asymmetry in shape. X-rays confirmed this finding and showed that the clavicle was compressing the neurovascular bundle against the first rib. It was concluded that the change in posture with age and different activities had altered the space in the thoracic outlet. The recent strains from tennis resulted in a clinical presentation of claviculo-costal syndrome.

Case study 9.5

In contrast to the patient in Case study 9.4, Peter is a recently retired bank clerk, aged 58, who has never exercised before. In order to pacify his family he decided to 'get fit'. He joined a local gymnasium and was greatly impressed by the fitness of members of the club. His first aim was to build up his chest muscles. Ignoring all warnings of safety and instructions, he took it upon himself to lift free weights upwards and backwards until 'his arms dropped'. A strict regimen of daily repetition resulted in severe early morning pain in the hand and arms. The pain was accompanied with paraesthesiae and numbness of the hand. The osteopath reproduced the symptoms by pulling the hands and arms overhead, abducting them and pulling them slightly backward.

The pectoralis minor muscles originate from the third, fourth and fifth ribs in the anterior mid-costal area and insert into the coracoid process of the scapula. The pectoralis minor covers the brachial plexus and the axillary vein and artery as it descends over the rib cage. Vascular compression occurs from compression of the bundle between the muscle and the ribs (Case study 9.5).

Shoulder–hand syndrome

This is a painful shoulder with limited movement and symptoms of swelling, pain and stiffness, also sweating, with occasional colour changes. Initially the patient is aware of a 'burning' feeling of the hand. This is often accompanied by a moist hand which is also stiff and superficially sensitive. In the later stages the fingers diminish their range of movement, muscle atrophy then develops. Ultimately, the hand becomes pale and thin with marked muscular wasting. The joints become 'contracted' and osteoporosis is seen on X-ray. The causes of shoulder-hand syndrome may be myocardial, post-traumatic, post-herpetic, or secondary to cervical discogenic disease and periscapulitis.

Extrinsic disorders simulating disease of the shoulder

Disorders within the thorax

On some occasions, in a small proportion of cases, *angina pectoris* is felt predominantly in the shoulder region, usually the left and it is aggravated by exercise.

Basal pleurisy is sometimes a cause of shoulder pain [103]. This is explained by irritation of the phrenic nerve endings, with referred pain in the distribution of the cutaneous branches C4. The shoulder is clinically normal. Other features of the disease are usually sufficiently clear to indicate its true nature.

Disorders within the abdomen

The phrenic nerve endings under the diaphragm can be irritated from a diseased gallbladder. *Cholecystitis* can commonly cause referred pain to the right shoulder. The associated abdominal symptoms and signs, and the lack of clinical abnormality in the shoulder should prevent diagnostic errors. *Subphrenic abscess* is also an occasional cause of referred shoulder pain. Constitutional symptoms and pyrexia, with normal clinical findings in the shoulder, exonerate the shoulder from blame.

THE UPPER ARM AND ELBOW

The most common disorders of the upper arm and elbow are those of traumatic injury. These can be complex and often result in long-term disability, even after complete resolution of the initial injury. The humerus is subject to ordinary infections of the bone and occasionally to bone tumours, especially metastases. The elbow is liable to every type of arthritis, although none is particularly common. Together with the knee, the joint is affected by osteochondritis dessicans and loose body formation.

Taking a history

Ascertaining the exact site and distribution of the pain and its nature constitutes the main requirement of history taking. Pain arising locally in the humerus is easily confused with pain arising in the shoulder, which characteristically radiates to a point about halfway down the upper arm. Elbow pain is localized fairly precisely to the joint, although diffuse aching pain is often felt in the forearm. A history of previous injury, often in childhood, can be significant. Injuries in this region can often be seen to give clinical problems in later years.

Table 9.2 Routine examination of the elbow joint

Test the following:	
Humero-ulnar joint:	flexion and extension
Radio-ulnar joint:	supination and pronation
Power of the:	flexors, extensors, supinators, pronators
Stability of the:	lateral ligament, medial ligament
Ulnar nerve:	sensory function; motor function; sweating

The examination (Table 9.2)

Once we have satisfied ourselves, from a general survey of the body, that the local symptoms are not a manifestation of a widespread disease, we must begin an examination of the arms themselves. Both arms and shoulders must be exposed for comparison.

Close *inspection* of the joint alignment and bone contours must be carried out. Observe for any scarring, colour and texture of the skin, as well as soft tissue contours.

Follow this with a *palpatory* assessment of these points.

The *active* and *passive* movements are tested individually, taking special notice of any pain or crepitation.

The elbow movements can be separated into two distinct components. Flexion and extension movements are carried out by the hinge joint between the humerus above and the ulna and radius below. Rotation of the forearm is carried out at the pivot joint between the upper ends of the radius and ulna. It is important to ensure that the shoulder is kept totally still while examining rotation of the forearm and flexion-extension of the elbow.

The ulnar nerve

This is commonly known as 'the funny bone'. In fact, it is the vulnerable part of the ulnar nerve. It runs behind the elbow and testing its function should be part of the routine examination of the elbow. Test for any obvious changes seen in the sweating function of the nerve. This is done by comparing the texture of the skin on the palm of the hand, paying particular attention to the little finger and half of the ring finger. Any difference in the sweat distribution indicates ulnar nerve damage. The sensitivity of the hand must also be tested using pin-prick and cotton wool in the usual way.

So far the appearance of the upper arm, elbow and forearm has been examined. The function of the ulnar nerve has been assessed, and the elbow put through its movements and its muscular ability to perform the normal function tested.

Once this basic and simple scanning procedure is complete, the findings must be interpreted. The most important aspect of this procedure is comparing and contrasting the two arms. Allowing the elbow to move within its range, and then gently but firmly stretching the end of ranges, gives an indication as to what the limiting factors are to the joint movements. For example, an osteoarthritic elbow joint will show marked crepitations during examination of the flexion and extension range. Rotation is often full and unimpaired. The ranges of flexion will be limited, roughened, and gradually show an increasing resistance to full movement. The joint margins will show palpable thickening of the joint margins.

Friction neuritis of the ulnar nerve (Case study 9.6)

Case study 9.6

Reg has a 58-year-old body, regulated by a 25-year-old mind. His love for dangerous sport started in his youth and he suffered a supra-condylar fracture of his right humerus when he had a moto-cross accident at the age of 12. More recently he took up squash, playing 'vigorously' four times each week. He had been suffering with a self-diagnosed 'tennis elbow' for 6 weeks and was under the common illusion that it would 'work itself right', once his arm became used to the newly acquired squash racquet. His wife forced him to seek help when she noticed that he was becoming increasingly clumsy in performing fine finger movements such as drying wet glasses. At the same time he was puzzled as to why, despite his hand strengthening exercises, the palm of his hand was looking markedly wasted.

On examination, the carrying angle of the right elbow was increased. This was probably the result of the childhood injury. There was blunting and loss of sensibility along the ulnar border of the hand, as well as the little finger and medial half of the ring finger. There was obvious wasting of the small muscles of the hand innervated by the ulnar nerve. The skin in the ulnar territory was drier than on the other hand.

On further questioning, Reg volunteered that he had changed his job at work. He had been promoted to a much more desk-bound job from previously being a shop floor supervisor. This new position required him to spend many hours at a desk, leaning on his right elbow whilst problem solving on the phone. It was concluded that in fact it was not tennis elbow that Reg was suffering from, but a friction neuritis of the ulnar nerve. With the cause of the problem found, he was referred to the local orthopaedic consultant.

Tennis elbow and golfer's elbow

Despite the title it is not unusual to find tennis elbow occurring in the absence of sporting activity. It is believed to be caused by strain of the forearm extensor muscles at the point of their origin from the bone. This is a particularly painful condition, as the region of the attachments of the muscle fibres is plentifully supplied with nerve endings. Clinically, the pain is at the lateral aspect of the elbow, often radiating down the back of the forearm. The examination shows tenderness precisely localized to the front of the epicondyle of the humerus. Pain is aggravated by putting the extensor muscles on stretch, as clearly demonstrated by Peter in Case study 9.7 (Figure 9.5). It is also aggravated by active resisted wrist extension. Movements of the elbow are full. X-rays are normal.

Case study 9.7

In sharp contrast to Reg in Case study 9.6, Peter is a 30-year-old accounts manager who firmly believes that we are all born with a given number of heart beats, so why waste them by doing strenuous activity such as sport? He was horrified to find that his GP had referred him to an osteopath with suspected 'tennis elbow'. 'I wouldn't know the difference between a tennis racquet and a golf bat', he said in utter horror. Peter had developed a pain at the lateral aspect of the elbow, frequently radiating down the back of the left forearm. On examination there was localized tenderness to the front of the lateral epicondyle of the humerus. Pain was aggravated by putting the extensor muscles on stretch, as well as actively resisting extension.

On further questioning about his job, he mentioned that his firm is in the process of entering all of the old invoices onto a new computer program. This means that he spends many hours flicking through all of the old invoices by hand. He demonstrated this position, which showed how his wrist and fingers are held in full flexion whilst his hand is pronated.

Apart from the clinical findings mentioned, the rest of the examination was unremarkable. Even though Peter was successfully treated for his 'tennis elbow', he would not believe that he of all people was cursed by this 'sport-related' injury.

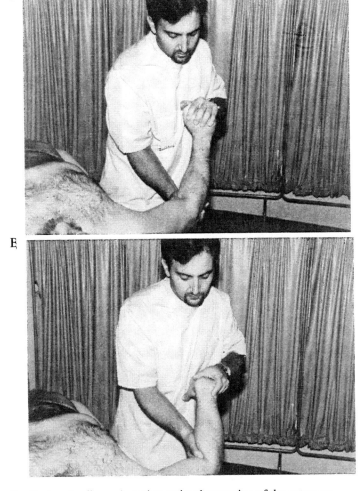

Figure 9.5 Testing for tennis elbow: A. active resisted extension of the extensor muscles; B. placing the extensor muscles in full stretch.

Golfer's elbow occurs due to strain of the forearm flexor muscles at the point of their origin from the bone. Clinically the pain is at the medial aspect of the elbow, radiating down the medial aspect of the forearm. It is aggravated by active resisted flexion of the wrist, as well as putting the flexor muscles on stretch.

Although these conditions have been viewed as local isolated problems, it must be remembered that they may be influenced by mechanical factors arising in other parts of the arm, or neck and upper back. It should also be noted that the sympathetic nerve supply to the arm derives from the upper four thoracic segments. Problems in this area of the spine or in other parts of the limb may therefore affect the recovery of the disturbance around the elbow.

THE WRIST AND HAND

Developing the natural progress of investigating the upper extremity, the points mentioned above must always be considered with respect to disorders of the neck causing hand pain, particularly with involvement of the brachial plexus.

The examination

Examination of the area includes close *inspection* of the colour and texture of the skin and soft tissue contours as well as looking out for any scars. *Palpation* of the hand is not complete until the skin temperature is noted. The bone contours are felt, the soft tissue contours are felt and any local tenderness is investigated. Movements of the wrist are conveniently divided into flexion and extension as well as adduction and abduction. These all occur at the radiocarpal joint, the inferior radio-ulnar joint allowing supination and pronation to occur. Placing the hands together in the praying position tests for extension range (Figure 9.6A). In contrast, flexion can be tested by touching the outer side of the two hands together whilst the wrist is fully flexed (Figure 9.6B).

A problem with these two ranges will suggest a dysfunction of the wrist. The inability of the patient, however, to carry out rotation at the wrist, will only localize it to a problem at the wrist or elbow.

Power testing

When testing the power, each muscle group must be tested individually. The thumb needs to be tested by actively using the abductors, the adductor, the extensors, the flexors and the opponens. In the fingers test the flexors, the interossei and the lumbricals. Testing the power of the grip is a useful way of assessing the combined action of the flexors and extensors of the wrist and the flexors of the fingers and thumb.

Nerve function testing

The nerve function of the median, ulnar and radial nerves is assessed by tests of the sensory function, motor function and sweating.

A

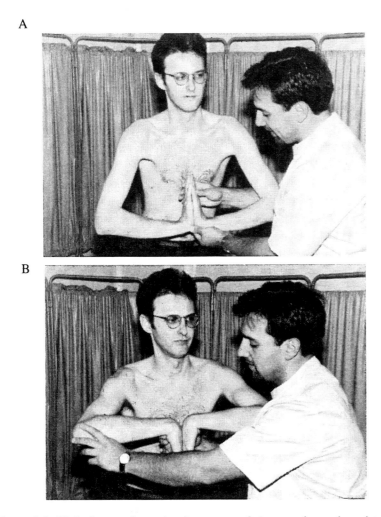

B

Figure 9.6 Clinical test to determine the amount of: A. extension at the wrist; B. flexion at the wrists.

Circulatory tests

Circulation is assessed by observing the general appearance of the fingers and hand, noting any colour differences and/or any changes in temperature of the hand. The arterial pulses are then palpated. It must be remembered that nerves require a blood supply to enable them to conduct impulses, and therefore any interruption of the blood supply will quickly diminish sensibility of the fingers.

Once the individual components are carefully assessed, that is, the individual movement of the wrist, fingers and thumb, these movements must be integrated to movements of the elbow and shoulder joint. First of all, with the patient sitting, carefully flex and pronate the wrist and follow this with flexion and pronation of the elbow. This combined movement will illustrate if there is partial contribution of problems from both the wrist and the elbow. Taking this a step further, elevation of the shoulder joint while carrying out the above combination, will illustrate why a patient may have pains when executing an overhead shot in tennis (Figure 9.7)!

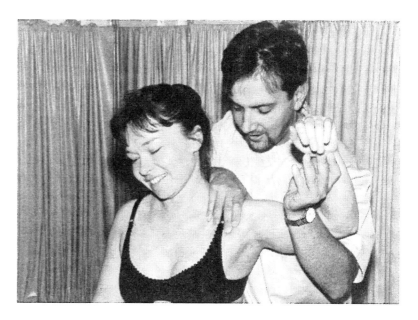

Figure 9.7 How the osteopath assesses the shoulder joint whilst carrying out a series of manoeuvres of the upper limb.

This highlights the possibility that it is a reduced internal rotation of the shoulder that is overloading the elbow and thus causing undue strain at the point of origin of the extensor muscles of the forearm; with the possible consequences of a tennis elbow developing.

The limply held wrists can be simultaneously oscillated in order to compare relative tension or laxity of the two upper extremities. This can be done by loosely holding the palm of the hand whilst the arm is dangling directly below the wrist. A slow and deliberate oscillation is generated by moving the palm back and forth. The oscillations must take into consideration generalized movements of all of the joint components of the arms. Lastly, in this general 'trend' of arm movements, it is important to apply a separating/tractioning force on the gleno-humeral joint (Figure 9.8). This can show up any adhesions at this level.

Disorders to consider in the wrist and hand

A systematic consideration of the possible causes of pains in the wrist and hand will highlight any local symptoms which may be only a manifestation of a more widespread disease. These will include not only those caused by the disorders of the neck or brachial plexus. A more general examination will show the classic signs and symptoms of acute or chronic infections. Any type of benign tumour may occur in the forearm bones. Osteochondroma is the most common. Clinically it is the long bones of children and adolescents that are mainly affected. Swelling, which is sometimes painful, is the main complaint. A common radiological appearance is a mushroom-like or cauliflower-like radiopaque mass [104]. The forearm bones are seldom affected by malignant bone tumours, whether primary or metastatic.

There are many disorders which can present clinically and are attributed to either articular or extra-articular disorders of the wrist and hand. However, in practice, there tends to be a 'handful' of commonly occurring ones. Generally the common *articular* problems are osteoarthritis and rheumatoid arthritis. *Extra-articular* disorders which are commonly seen include compression of the median nerve in the carpal tunnel and paratendonitis.

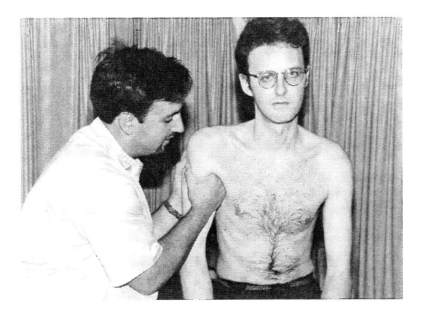

Figure 9.8 Localized separation of the humeral head from the glenoid cavity.

Tendonitis (Case study 9.8)

Case study 9.8

'Macker' is a part-time builder whose primary love in life is tug-of-war. 'I'm in love with "Tug", he proclaims, 'because once women have seen my hands they keep their distance!' On examining his hands, it all became very clear. The callosities on the palms were thick and infected from the combined activities of building and tugging. His main complaint was severe pain felt at the back of the wrist and lower forearm. The pain was aggravated by use of the hand. As well as the callosities, the examination showed localized swelling in the line of the affected tendons. The main ones were the extensors of the hand and wrist. A typical crepitation was felt over the tendons, when Macker flexed and extended his wrist.

Wrist degeneration

Case study 9.9

Hilda is a gentle 65-year-old, who has devoted her life to her cottage garden. Sadly, the severe winter frost one winter almost totally ended her gardening. She suffered a nasty fall and landed on her left forearm. Radiographic evidence confirmed a fracture of the lower end of the radius, with involvement of the articular surface and fracture of the scaphoid bone, complicated by avascular necrosis of the distal fragment. She was advised to rest the arm until the following summer. With great disappointment she presented at the end of the summer with a gradual return of pain and stiffness of the wrist. This followed some activity in the garden. The examination showed a normal presentation of the superficial tissues with normal skin texture and temperature. However, movements were markedly limited, and painful if gently forced at the extremes. New radiographs were advised, and they showed narrowing of the cartilage space and spurring of the bone at the joint margins. The scaphoid was seen to be un-united.

Cases like Hilda's in Case study 9.9 are commonly seen. In other cases, metacarpo-phalangeal and inter-phalangeal joints arthritis can occur in the elderly, even without trauma. Depending on the severity and spread of the wear and tear, the patient will experience pain and stiffness which is most marked at the end of ranges and particularly after activity and exposure to cold weather. These cases respond very well to osteopathic treatment which improves the overall function of the wrist despite the presence of degeneration.

Apart from cases of degeneration, the lunate bone in particular, as well as other carpal bones, can become displaced following trauma. The displaced bone can be seen with the wrist held in extreme flexion or extension; usually a pit forms where the bone has become displaced. The history usually records a trauma, with the wrist held in extreme flexion or extreme extension. Manipulating the displaced bone, with the wrist held in traction with some degree of flexion or extension, can give immediate relief. A common presentation is a fall on the outstretched arm, with the wrist and hand extended. The forced extension displaces the lunate in the palmar direction. The examination shows swelling of the wrist and careful palpation reveals a central depression at the wrist where the lunate should be.

Treatment approach for a displaced lunate

The wrist is initially placed in an extended position. The osteopath then iso-
lates the lunate on the palmar side of the wrist and applies a firm 'fixing'
pressure by crossing his two thumbs over it.

Then, with a single action, the osteopath tractions the wrist and moves it
through the full range until full flexion is reached. At the extreme end of flexion, a short and sharp thrusting movement is applied to the lunate to relocate
it in its rightful place. The end position should be held for about 10 seconds
once the procedure is complete (Figure 9.9). An audible 'click' may be heard
when the lunate slots back in line with the rest of the carpal bones. The patient
will feel the immediate benefit of a successful relocation.

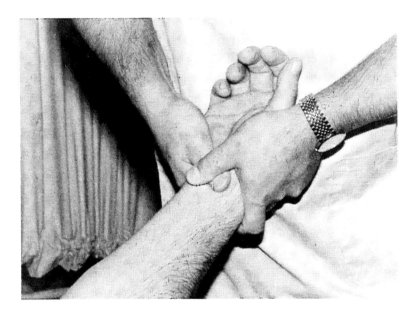

Figure 9.9 Relocation of the lunate.

10 The thorax and ventilation

And now I see with eye serene
The very pulse of the machine;
A being breathing thoughtful breath,
A traveller between life and death.

(Wordsworth, *She was a Phantom of Delight*)

Such expressions as 'He breathed his last' or 'He expired', have been used for centuries. This link between life, death and breathing has been the centre of many religions and philosophical beliefs. The book of Genesis declares:

And the Lord God formed man of the dust of the ground,
and breathed into his nostrils the breath of life
and the man became a living being.

Prana, the basic force of life, mediated by meditation, which is a process in which breathing plays a singularly vital role, is the centre of Eastern philosophical tradition.

Strangely, however, though breathing behaviour is central to physical and mental well-being, its clinical importance seems to have escaped the attention of many forms of clinical practice. It is hoped that with a more comprehensive approach to the mechanical functioning of the thorax and a deeper understanding and appreciation of the importance of breathing patterns, during the general assessment of the patient, the osteopath can improve the pattern of the patient's breathing and hence influence the physical, physiological and psycho-pathological processes.

The thoracic cage is the main vehicle which allows the vital interchange of gases. The principal function of the respiratory system is the ventilation of the body. A complex mechanism extracts oxygen from the atmospheric air in the lungs. This air is introduced to the lungs by creating a subatmospheric pressure when the thorax expands during inspiration. The oxygen is transported to the body tissues, and finally the excess carbon dioxide and water vapour is expelled out, back into the atmosphere.

Ventilation of the body is thus dependent also on the mouth, nose, trachea, bronchi, and bronchioles by which the air enters the lungs. Although these structures are merely the conductors of air in and out of the lungs, any dysfunction at this level can begin to alter the processing of air.

Case study 10.1

Paul has been suffering from constant vague facial pain, mild but irritating. He is 36 years old and works hard as a cartographer for the Ministry of Defence. The problem started about 2 years ago. Although this was initially intermittent, it has become more prolonged in the last 6 months. Over this period he has also noted a general deterioration in his well-being. His ability to concentrate has diminished, he is much more tired and he has developed generalized paraesthesiae in his limbs. He visited a neurologist who found no serious illness. A consultant general physician diagnosed ME. Paul was not totally convinced by this diagnosis and decided to have his facial pain investigated. He was convinced that it was soon after visiting his dentist that the problem became worse. The dentist assessed Paul's teeth again and noted that his occlusion had reduced over the last 6 months. The dentist then suggested consulting an osteopath.

The history reported here is remarkably like one would associate with a generalized lack of oxygen supply to meet metabolic needs. The patient was tired after effort, lethargic, uninterested in social activities and generally miserable. During the history taking, Paul repeatedly stretched his thorax, yawned quietly and apparently almost needed to think about his breathing. Curiously he spoke almost without moving his lips and his nostrils flared regularly as if to take in air. When asked about his peculiar way of breathing, while talking, he admitted that this was a newly adopted way of taking in sufficient air to cope. This also resulted in his nostrils being very dry and a slight whistle could be heard during quiet breathing. 'Nobody will take me seriously', he remarked, with desperation mixed with excitement that a practitioner had actually noticed it without prompting.

The examination showed severe restriction of jaw joint movement, particularly on the left side. His thorax was flexed and all the anterior neck muscles showed signs of excess workload and fatigue. Despite the absence of any respiratory disease, he had all the signs of a dysfunctioning ventilatory system. On the basis of these findings Paul was treated successfully with a regimen to improve his respiratory mechanics, starting at the point of entry, his ability to open his jaws fully. His long term management incorporated a regimen of breathing retraining, with exercises to help him use the diaphragm correctly. Physically the treatment was directed at releasing the excessive tone of the anterior neck muscles, particularly the scalenes. His pectoral muscles were stretched to allow better rib movement. His lower ribs and inter-costal muscles were worked on to improve the mechanics of the lower part of the thoracic cage.

VENTILATION – THE PROCESS OF EXCHANGE OF AIR BETWEEN THE LUNGS AND THE AMBIENT AIR

Breathing is a complex interaction of involuntary and voluntary physiological processes resulting in the ventilation of the lungs. Breathing brings oxygen to the body and removes excess carbon dioxide. Another major role of breathing is the maintenance of the acid–base balance, on which all metabolic processes depend. The principal role of the respiratory system is the ventilation of the body. The body has various sites of organization by which the air enters and exits the lungs. Initially air enters the mouth and nose, then, via the trachea and bronchi, it enters the bronchioles and alveoli, where gas exchange takes place.

Breathing by contracting the inter-costal muscles

Under normal and healthy circumstances the inter-costal muscles, when contracted, lift the rib cage upward and outward. The rise in the rib cage and the outward movement of the lower segment of the thorax create space in the thoracic cavity. This space causes negative pressure to occur, which is equalized by the air coming into the lungs and inflating them. This is the inspiration phase of breathing. In the expiration phase, the inter-costal muscles relax because of the release of air from the lungs and the rib cage falls back to its original state. Some schools of thought maintain that this phase is purely passive, others feel that there is some assistance from inter-costal contraction. Hughes [105] showed that abdominal (diaphragmatic) breathing is physiologically superior to breathing by the use of inter-costal muscles. He concluded that, in the absence of abdominal breathing, some segments of the lower lobes of the lungs may remain relatively unaffected by the process of chest breathing alone.

Breathing by contracting the diaphragm

The diaphragm is a dome-shaped muscle. It separates the thorax, containing the heart and the lungs, from the abdominal/visceral region of the body. When the diaphragm is relaxed, it is vaulted upward into the space filled by the lungs in the expiration phase of the breathing cycle. When the diaphragm is contracted, in the inspiration phase, the upward arching is reduced. This reduction creates a negative pressure that causes the lungs to expand. It has also been shown that this negative pressure aids venous return of the blood to the heart, thus reducing the amount of work required of the heart in blood circulation [106]. When the diaphragm contracts, the abdominal region below is pushed downward and outward, exerting pressure on the rectus abdominis muscle.

That is why, during abdominal breathing, the abdomen moves outward. The diaphragm relaxes in the expiration phase of breathing, and the rectus abdominis returns to its original configuration.

EXAMINATION OF THE VENTILATORY SYSTEM

To ensure that the whole system is assessed properly, the patient must be closely observed during the history taking, whilst unaware of such scrutiny, as well as formally during the examination.

There are two broad aims:

1. Ensure that the patient's metabolic needs are being met by the respiratory system. Listen and look for signs of unexplained fatigue, heaviness of the chest or generalized mild aches in the musculo-skeletal system, general restlessness and inability to retain concentration, when this has not been a problem in the past. Although all these symptoms are highly subjective and non-specific, they can be significantly indicative of a lack of proper or adequate ventilation. These symptoms should alert the practitioner that all may not be well in the system.
2. Assess all the components of the system, starting with the nose and mouth and proceeding systematically downwards.

Once again, begin observing during history taking:

- Is the patient able to tell her story with clear and uninterrupted speech? Or is her manner vague? Does she break off to breathe deeply or sigh? Is she showing obvious signs of confusion and uncertainty?
- Does the breathing seem natural and rhythmical or erratic and forced?

- Observe the way the neck is held. Is the patient comfortable or does she strain the front of the neck by protruding the jaw forwards, thus appearing to lift the upper part of the chest with the neck muscles?

These simple and yet obvious signs can sometimes initiate the suspicion that the respiratory system is struggling. They may occur in the presence or absence of a respiratory disease. If the patient has already been diagnosed as having a history of, say, asthma for example, then these signs are seen within the context of the known disorder. Other disorders such as chronic bronchitis or allergic reactions can have a similar system. In cases where the patient is not aware of any underlying condition, then the history must proceed accordingly. The symptoms which point specifically to the respiratory system as the seat of respiratory disease are a cough (with or without expectoration), breathlessness and, more rarely, pain. Occasionally the patient may report such objective features as cyanosis and clubbing of the fingers, but more often these are observed by the examiner. These symptoms are not always of respiratory origin, and the possibility of cardio-vascular, nervous and haemic causes must not be overlooked [107]. The reader is advised to consult Chamberlain's *Symptoms and Signs in Clinical Medicine* [107] for a comprehensive overview of the respiratory system.

The biomechanical examination of the thorax is carried out with the patient suitably undressed to observe the subtle movements of the rib cage. This should be done in a warm room and initially with the patient sitting. Begin by standing in front of the patient. It is important to maintain constant communication. It is, however, useful to talk 'at' the patient rather than trying to carry out a conversation. The purpose of this is to calm and to reassure them that this is a passive part of the examination. You are only observing, so it is better that they relax and try not to talk, as this interrupts the breathing rate.

- Look at the method used to breathe. Does the patient breathe through the mouth, nose or both? Is the rhythm regular or erratic? Do the nostrils flare out markedly? Does there seem to be nasal congestion? These are possible indicators that there is nasal or sinus obstruction to the normal breathing passage.
- Next observe the anterior cervical muscles. In quiet respiration there should be no effort in the movement. Signs of thoracic dysfunction are excessive contraction of the anterior neck muscles, particularly during inspiration. This indicates that extra effort is needed to lift the rib cage.

The problem can be a visceral respiratory disease or a mechanical one. The latter can range from an acute episode of spinal or thoracic cage pain, where the patient struggles to brace herself from moving excessively, thus aggravating the pain, to a chronic condition which has markedly reduced the overall movement of the thorax. A good example is seen in a case where a childhood organic scoliosis, which is particularly marked in the upper thoracic cage, has substantially reduced the thoracic expansion capacity. In such instances the patient is seen to 'lift' the cage using the anterior cervical muscles.

The observation procedure continues by scanning the front of the body, observing the distribution of thoracic to abdominal movement. At the same time the general morphology of the patient is taken into consideration. The size of the breast in women can dictate the mode of breathing. Large breasts, particularly in women of small stature, will result in an exaggerated thoracic kyphosis and often show a fast and shallow breathing pattern (Case study 10.2).

Case study 10.2

Tracy is a 32-year-old mother of two young children. After the birth of her 5-year-old daughter, Tracy's breasts remained large. This was attributed to her having fertilization treatment to assist with her pregnancy. When her daughter was about 18 months old, Tracy noted pains and numbness in both of her arms. The physical examination showed that she was unduly stretching the neurovascular bundle hence showing the clinical picture associated with these findings. The postural changes which accompanied the pregnancy and excessive enlargement in her breasts were considered to be the main contributory factors to the symptoms. Another set of symptoms, however, started at the same time as the arm-related ones. These were generally non-specific, and varied according to the amount of activity. They consisted of tiredness, loss of concentration, pitch changes in her voice, generalized pins and needles in her body and dizzy spells. At first she assumed that it was 'natural tiredness and disturbed nights'. A careful examination of her breathing pattern showed erratic changes in patterns, varying from shallow fast breaths to deep ones, with long pauses in between them. 'Breathing can be a real effort sometimes!', she exclaimed. Unable to make any real impact on her arm symptoms with treatment and exercises, Tracy was referred to a consultant neurologist. He, in turn, agreed that the only long-term solution was for her to have a surgical breast reduction procedure. She was delighted at the suggestion. Soon after the successful procedure her breathing pattern was drastically altered. Her thoracic spine was more erect, her thoracic expansion was greater and her breathing pattern was stabilized. She was made aware of her breathing variation and advised on some exercises to keep up a good pattern. Within 2 weeks of the exercise regimen and physical treatment to restore thoracic function, all of her symptoms disappeared. She felt 'full of life and fun'.

Continuing with the assessment of the front of the body, the respiratory movements should be constantly observed. The patient is asked to take a deep breath to reveal whether the proper method is used. That is, during inspiration, the abdomen should be allowed to expand outward, swiftly followed by flaring out of the lower ribs to increase the antero-lateral part of the lower thorax. This stage should be followed by expansion of the upper ribs in an upward and forward direction, thus expanding the antero-posterior (AP) part of the cage.

Palpatory analysis

Having observed the various but continuous stages of movements, the palpatory stage begins (Figure 10.1). Standing behind the seated patient, place the flat, examining palms on the lower ribs. The hands should be placed so that the sides as well as part of the front of the abdomen can be felt at the same time. First feel during quiet respiration. Then ask the patient to take a deep breath and maintain a constant and firm pressure. This method is repeated while moving the palpating hands upwards along the sides of the chest. When the top is reached, the examining fingertips should be placed up in the axilla to feel for upper rib motion. The front of the upper ribs can be felt by placing the flat hands over the upper ribs.

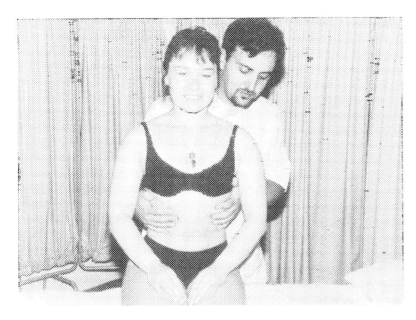

Figure 10.1 Examination of the thorax in the sitting position. Note how the osteopath compares the two sides of the lower thoracic cage by palpating the rib movements.

It is important to decide at the onset what the hands are feeling and to keep both hands at the same palpating level at all times. That is to say, choose either the surface of the ribs as a point of contact or choose the inter-costal space. It is important to maintain continuity. The former will indicate the amount of travel that the ribs under assessment will allow. The latter will indicate the amount of separation between the ribs, thus indicating the amount of 'give' that these muscles will allow. This distinction is particularly important when trying to isolate the presence or absence of movement of the individual ribs. This will be further explained later in the chapter.

Having assessed the thorax as a whole, palpate the clavicle and the muscles of the front of the neck. The information gained should be related to the findings of the observation procedure. Note particularly any altered muscle states (see Chapter 6). These should give clues as to whether the muscles have undergone changes due to the chronicity of the situation.

Having carefully gained an idea of the overall shape and flexibility of the thoracic cage, the next step is to re-evaluate the range and quality of movement which occurs at the individual levels. That is to say, individual ribs, which may be under suspicion from the history, are judged on their individual performance in terms of movement. Muscle groups involved in the mechanism of breathing can also be easily assessed.

The starting point is the established knowledge of functional anatomy. During normal quiet breathing the external inter-costal muscles actively contract; the ribs and sternum move upwards and outwards; the width of the chest increases from side to side and from front to back. The diaphragm contracts and descends. The depth of the chest increases. This in turn increases the capacity of the thorax. During the quiet expiration stage the external intercostal muscles relax; the ribs and sternum move downwards and inwards and thus the width of the chest diminishes.

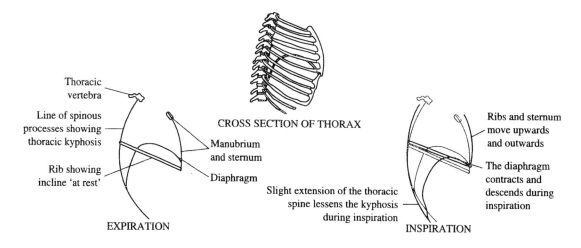

CROSS SECTION OF THORAX

Thoracic vertebra

Line of spinous processes showing thoracic kyphosis

Rib showing incline 'at rest'

Manubrium and sternum

Diaphragm

Slight extension of the thoracic spine lessens the kyphosis during inspiration

EXPIRATION

Ribs and sternum move upwards and outwards

The diaphragm contracts and descends during inspiration

INSPIRATION

Muscular contraction is responsible for the changes in the capacity of the thorax—the changes in the lung volume with intake or expulsion of air follows passively

EXPIRATION
External intercostal muscles relax
Ribs and sternum move downwards and inwards
Width of chest diminishes
Diaphragm relaxes and ascends
Depth of chest diminishes
Capacity of thorax is decreased
↓
Pressure between pleural surfaces
is increased (from –6mmHg to –2mmHg)*
Less pull is exerted on lung tissue
↓
Elastic tissue of lungs recoils
↓
Air pressure within alveoli is now
greater than atmospheric pressure
↓
Air is forced out of alveoli to the atmosphere

NORMAL QUIET INSPIRATION
External intercostal muscles actively contract
Ribs and sternum move upwards and outwards
Width of chest increases from side to side and
from front to back
Diaphragm contracts and descends
Depth of chest increases
Capacity of thorax is increased
↓
Pressure between pleural surfaces is reduced
(from –2mmHg to –6mmHg)*
Elastic tissue of lungs is stretched
↓
Lungs expand to fill thoracic cavity
↓
Air pressure within alveoli is now
less than atmospheric pressure
↓
Air is drawn into the alveoli from atmosphere

IN FORCED BREATHING
Neck muscles contract and aid by lifting first rib upwards
Sternum moves further upwards and forwards
Abdominal muscles contract to pull diaphragm
Muscles of nostrils and around glottis may contract
to aid entrance of air to lungs
Internal intercostals may contract

Figure 10.2 Mechanism of breathing – the different stages of chest movements during: (1) expiration; (2) inspiration. *Refer to McNaught and Callender [108].

The diaphragm relaxes and ascends with an associated lessening of the thoracic capacity. In forced breathing the muscles of the nostrils and round glottis may contract to aid entrance of air to the lungs. The extensors of the vertebral column also aid inspiration by helping to 'straighten out' the kyphosis. The anterior neck muscles contract, moving the first rib upwards and the sternum upwards and forwards. The external inter-costals may contract during forced expiration, moving the ribs downwards more actively; the abdominal muscles contract, which actively aids the ascent of the diaphragm (Figure 10.2).

The key areas to assess during rib movement are at the two extremities as well as the intervening portion – the posterior or vertebral, the anterior or sternal and the body or shaft. The vertebral extremity can be palpated deep beneath the paravertebral muscles. This part is called the head of the rib. A carefully positioned applicator which also keeps contact with the neck of the rib will register a pivoting movement of the head, with an associated upward movement of the neck of the rib during inspiration and a downward movement during expiration. This is the movement of the head of the rib in relation to the posterior part of the related transverse process. The shaft can be felt to be moving upward and forwards in the upper ribs (ribs 1–7), and sideways and outwards in the lower ribs. These conform to the characteristic 'pump-handle' movements of the upper ribs and 'bucket-handle' movements of the lower ribs. At the anterior or sternal end, the attachment can be felt as a slightly raised and flexible joint line. The movement here is directly linked to the sternal movement upwards and downwards accordingly.

Next, the palpating applicator is moved along to the shaft of the rib. This is thin and flat and presents two surfaces, an internal and an external and two borders, a superior and an inferior. A little in front of the tuberosity, on the external surface, there is a prominent oblique line which gives attachment to a tendon of the ilio-costalis muscles. This is called the angle of the rib. From this point the rib is bent in two directions, so that its shaft as a whole is curved and slightly twisted upon its own axis. The internal surface is concave and smooth. The interval between this ridge and the inferior border has a groove for the inter-costal vessels and nerve. The superior border is thick and rounded for the attachments of the external and internal inter-costal muscles.

Evaluation should take place at each of the above stages. The practitioner should be familiar with the more peculiar ribs: the first, second, tenth, eleventh and twelfth. The first is short and broad. Its upper surface is marked by two parallel grooves, separated by a tubercle for the scalenus anterior muscle. In the posterior groove runs the subclavian artery and in the anterior the subclavian vein. The second resembles the first in that it is flattened and not twisted. The tenth has only one facet for articulation with the tenth thoracic vertebra. The eleventh has a slight angle, but no tubercle. The twelfth has no angle, tubercle or neck.

COSTO-VERTEBRAL JOINT DYSFUNCTION – 'RIB' DYSFUNCTION

For many years osteopaths have been assessing clinical conditions which are related to abnormal rib functions according to their 'fixed' position within the respiratory movements. That is to say, if a rib is found on examination to be held in forced or exaggerated inspiration it has been termed an inspiration lesion. Alternatively, if a rib is found to be immobilized in the expiration position, it is known as an expiration lesion. Early literature by Downing does not clearly define the term 'lesion' in this context. He does, however, describe at length the various axes of rotation which are related to the particular ribs in question [99].

Acute fixation of rib joints occurs commonly, most frequently in the upper half of the thoracic region, and shows all the usual characteristics of synovial joint locking [109], that is to say, the features seen in cases of synovial joint dysfunctions.

Once the clinical analysis as set out above has been followed, particular attention should be paid to the way that any suspect rib is positioned. Because of their functional anatomy, some of the ribs possess intrinsic characteristics, specifically the first, eleventh and twelfth.

First rib

If held in inspiration, this would depend upon the muscles attaching it to the cervical spine to be maintained in a state of contraction. Although theoretically possible, it would be difficult for the muscles to lift the whole weight of the thorax which is suspended beneath it. If the first rib is held in inspiration, characteristically, the rib is elevated anteriorly with a downward backward rotation posteriorly on the transverse process of the first thoracic vertebra. An expirational lesion is more commonly found, where the rib is found to be depressed anteriorly with an associated upward movement posteriorly on the first thoracic transverse process. This is encountered following traumas such as those seen on the rugby field or following a long-term depressed posture or after prolonged periods of sitting at a computer terminal.

On observation, the upper trapezius fibres are in some spasm, and palpation reveals increased tenderness of the muscle mass. Cervical rotation towards the painful side is restricted, and lateral flexion to the opposite side feels tethered. Extension hurts the painful side and movement of the shoulder on that side may be moderately painful at extreme ends of range. There are no neurological signs.

The eleventh and twelfth ribs

These are known as floating ribs. They have no anterior attachments. As a result of this free-floating state they can be found to be held in a multitude of positions. There is no set pattern observed clinically and all that can be said about them is that their ultimate position of fixation depends upon the force applied by the muscles which attach upon them. They may be elevated or depressed, in or out, or rotated upon their long axis.

The second to tenth ribs

These are usually held in a position dictated by their articulating spinal facet attachments. As a rule of thumb, the upper ribs (first to sixth) are characterized by an inspirational, pump-handle lesion or expirational, pump-handle lesion. In the inspirational lesion, the rib in question is elevated and slightly immobilized in this position. The neck of the rib is found to be held downward and backward. The expirational lesion in the same ribs occurs by means of reverse rotation, causing the rib to be depressed anteriorly, with an upward, backward rotation of its neck on its long axis.

A combined pump- and bucket-handle lesion may occur in any rib from second to sixth inclusive. Movement takes place on both the pump- and bucket-handle axes, causing a combined lesion with diagnostic features of the above two.

The lower ribs, seventh to tenth inclusive, can present as an inspirational bucket-handle lesion, or an expirational bucket-handle lesion. In an inspirational lesion the rib bulges laterally, the outer surface moves outward and upward, the lower border is everted and the upper border is inverted. There is separation from the adjacent rib below and approximation to the rib immediately above. The gross malposition of the rib can be better ascertained during exaggerated inspiration. The reverse clinical findings will be noted in an expirational bucket-handle lesion.

Although considerable detail has been given concerning the ultimate position of fixation in which specific ribs are found, it must be emphasized that the overall findings from the rib cage as a whole are equally important. The concertina arrangement of the thoracic cage is responsible for the drawing in and expelling out of air. The component parts, therefore, the ribs, are expected to conform to the general movement of the cage. Malposition, however, with or without fixation at any point of its range, can cause considerable local pain and discomfort to the patient. In addition, specific rib problems found particularly on the left side of the chest, can cause immense anxiety-related problems, as they can easily be mistaken for cardiac pains.

TWO CONDITIONS ASSOCIATED WITH 'THORACIC DYSFUNCTION'

Hyperventilation

Breathing is a complex interaction of physiological processes which are both voluntary and involuntary. The end result is the ventilation of the lungs approximately every 5 seconds in normal, healthy adults. The purpose of this ventilation is to bring oxygen to the body tissues and remove excess carbon dioxide. Simultaneously it contributes to the maintenance of the acid–base balance of the blood, on which all metabolic processes depend. Some people show an increase in the rate of breathing which is excessive to their metabolic need. When this increased ventilation results in a change in the level of carbon dioxide in the blood, the person is said to hyperventilate. This state may be accompanied by physical and/or mental symptoms due to changes in the oxygen transport system and changes in circulation to the brain, as well as neural and cardio-vascular adjustments to the low carbon dioxide.

The initial diagnosis of hyperventilation is by symptomatology. A fair impression can be gained during history taking. The typical thoracic breathing pattern is observed and often conversations are abruptly and irregularly interrupted by sighs and gasps for breath. With a little practice anyone can learn to recognize the signs. Lum [110] listed the signs in Table 10.1 as symptoms of hyperventilation.

Table 10.1 Symptomatology of hyperventilation (according to Lum)

Breathing is predominantly thoracic
Little use is made of the diaphragm
Breathing is punctuated by frequent sighs
Sighing has a peculiar 'effortless' quality, with a marked 'forward and upward' movement of the upper sternum but little lateral expansion
Normal breathers can imitate the breathing chest movements used by hyperventilators only with difficulty

Table 10.2 Signs and symptoms associated with the hyperventilation syndrome and psycho-pathology (compiled by Huey and Sechrest [111] at the Centre for Research on the Utilisation of Scientific Knowledge, Institute of Social Research of Michigan)

Light-headedness, giddiness, dizziness, faintness
Fainting, syncope
Headache
Blurred vision
Tremors, twitching
Numbness, tingling, prickling
Chest pain, pressure
Nausea
Vomiting
Abdominal pain
Gas and abdominal extension
Lump in the throat
Dry mouth
Dyspnoea, difficulty breathing
Weakness, exhaustion, fatigue
Apprehension, nervousness

Huey and Sechrest [111] compiled the list in Table 10.2 from reports in the clinical literature. Although the list in Table 10.2 is incomplete, it is a useful guide for practitioners to use in the recognition of the hyperventilating patient. In practice it is unlikely that the patient will present with these symptoms alone. Many of the above, however, will be seen as part of the general clinical picture. The presenting problem may be an accentuated form of any of the above, with particular emphasis on a musculo-skeletal symptom.

Jacqueline's case, in Case study 10.3, is a fairly typical presentation of a hyperventilation/panic attack. Although her arm symptoms were the main reason which prompted her to seek advice, it soon became apparent that they were not caused by the obvious neuro-muscular causes. The history and anxious behaviour shown at the consultation indicated an improper breathing pattern. A prolonged regimen of breathing retraining, running concurrently with continued counselling sessions, should in time restore her confidence and reduce her arm symptoms.

Although this case was fairly self-evident, many patients present with symptoms which are partly caused by altered breathing patterns. Breathing can represent a small element of the overall picture, or, as shown by Jacqueline, it can be the predominant feature.

Case study 10.3

Jacqueline is a 50-year-old housewife who has been confined to her home because of a deep-seated 'fear of dying'. After many years of counselling and solid family support she manages to go out for 2 or 3 hours a day, as long as she is accompanied by a friend or member of the family. She presented with a heavy feeling in both arms, with associated prickling of her hands. A full clinical assessment did not show any signs which would indicate a musculo-skeletal cause for her complaint. She had been tested at the general hospital for both cardiac and neurological problems. Nothing abnormal was found. During the history and clinical assessment she became more and more agitated and restless. Her breathing became more thoracic and rapid. Close observation of her facial expressions showed a slight transient tremor of the eyelids and facial musculature. These tremors were gradually replaced by muscular rigidity of her face and gradually her hands were affected. As time passed she noted that her arms were becoming heavy and prickly. Her symptoms were becoming more and more evident as she went deeper and deeper into a state of hyperventilation. At this point she was reassured that the symptoms were a result of her high anxiety state and altered breathing rate. She was slowly talked through methods of slowing down her breathing. Then she was instructed to breath slowly into her cupped hands, to breathe back in some of her expired carbon dioxide. Within a few minutes her symptoms disappeared.

Thorough physical assessment, careful listening and close observation, during the history-taking as well as the examination itself, will, with practice, lead to successful differentiation of the component parts of the overall presentation.

Asthma

Bronchial asthma usually starts in childhood, but may not appear until middle age, when it is known as 'late-onset asthma'. Characteristically it is associated with attacks of wheezing and breathlessness, due to narrowing of the bronchi by spasm or mucous secretions. These attacks are brought on by a variety of factors, including allergy to certain inhaled pollens, respiratory infections, emotional upsets or physical exercise. Physical examination reveals laboured breathing associated with prolonged expiratory wheeze, activity of the accessory muscles of respiration and a 'pigeon chest' from overinflation of the lung, due to trapping air during expiration.

The key features dealt with by the osteopath are the changes seen in the muscles associated with breathing, primarily the accessory muscles, the scalenes and the sternocleido-mastoid. These are in a prolonged state of increased tone and hence are treated to relieve the tone. Hypertonia will also be noted in the diaphragm and the internal inter-costal muscles; the internal inter-costal muscles will be shortened and fibrotic due to reduced forced expiration.

Functionally, the ribs will be held horizontally and the thoracic spine rigid and extended, with an associated increase in the cervical lordosis.

Each individual sufferer will present with a unique pattern of physical findings. The age, condition and 'give' of the tissues will determine the techniques used to improve the function of the breathing pattern.

THE THORACIC SPINE

The thoracic spine is the least mobile part of the spinal column. The attachment of the rib cage, together with the thinner discs, combine to reduce its movement considerably.

Few people have a normal thoracic spine [19]; the presence of a reduced range of movement, owing to the rib attachments, localized tenderness and spreading pain on careful palpation is clinically demonstrable in most patients. The combination of spondylotic change and secondary arthrotic change, with costo-vertebral joint dysfunction, particularly in the middle thoracic segments, is probably the clinical state usually responsible for chest wall symptoms commonly simulating serious disease of thoracic viscera [15].

Arthrosis

In the thoracic spine, in common with all other synovial joints, there is a palpable stiffness and reduced range of movement. There will also be palpable joint irritability. (This will be felt as a localized reaction on palpatory pressure applied to the joint.) In the absence of visceral disease, including cardiac ischaemia or pulmonary involvement, pain in the thoracic spine can be confirmed by X-rays as being arthrosis. The signs observed will be visible chondro-osteophytosis forming at the facet margins which tends to reduce the transverse foraminal dimensions. However, there does not appear to be much evidence of nerve root interference on the scale observed in the cervical and lumbar regions.

The rib joints often also show a localized painful loss of movement. These become particularly irritated in even mild degrees of pre-existing spinal scoliosis, particularly when they are aggravated by cramped working postures or by carrying heavy objects. The oedema of the inter-spinous ligaments which is caused by these irritations can cause referred pain along the line of the rib or through the chest [112].

Spondylosis

This usually occurs at the middle and lower levels. Marked clinical features associated with acute disc prolapses are infrequent in the thoracic spine. Epstein [109] gives the incidence as 2–3 per 1000 cases, seen surgically, equally frequent in men and women. Stoddard [19], however, reported that post-mortem studies of the thoracic spine show that disc pathology is common in the thoracic spine, leading to spondylotic degenerative change. These changes are less overt and clinically noticeable in the early stages and therefore less recognized.

In terms of radiographic appearance, the thinning of the discs and associated bulging tends to produce bony outgrowths in the anterior lateral aspects of the vertebral bodies.

Vertebral osteochondrosis (idiopathic kyphosis, Scheurmann's disease)

Refer to Chapter 7 on spinal curves.

Miscellaneous complaints of the thorax

Cervical rib

This is a congenital overdevelopment, which can be bony or fibrous, of the costal process of the seventh cervical vertebra. It often exists without causing any symptoms. When it does present clinically, it is usually as a result of compression of the subclavian artery and the lowest trunk of the brachial plexus. When symptoms occur, they usually begin during early adult life. They may be neurological, vascular, or both. Sensory symptoms as a neurological presentation are pain and paraesthesiae in the forearm and hand, particularly on the medial (ulnar) side, often relieved by changing the position of the arm. Motor symptoms include increasing weakness of the hand, with difficulty in carrying out finger movements. The physical examination shows an area of sensory impairment which does not correspond in distribution to any of the peripheral nerves, but may be related to the lowest trunk of the brachial plexus. In chronic severe cases, there may be wasting of the thenar muscles or of the inter-osseous muscles. The vascular manifestations are absence or merely weakness of the radial pulse. The presence of a cervical rib can be confirmed by radiographs.

Unexplained pains of the ribs and sternum

Occasions may arise when pains occur in the ribs or sternum in the absence of any obvious injury or direct trauma. An alert practitioner must always remember that the sternum and ribs contain abundant red marrow, which is favourable to the development of blood-borne metastatic tumours. Any mysterious pains in these structures must therefore be referred for histological examination of the bone marrow.

In contrast, obvious blows to the rib cage may result in fractures. These must once again be spotted and passed on for radiographic investigation.

Acute and chronic costochondrosis (Tietze's disease)

This condition may simulate disease of the thoracic viscera or mimic the anterior referred pain from vertebral joint problems seen above. It is clinically recognized by the localized and acutely painful swellings of two or more costal cartilages on one side. These represent a traumatic or low-grade inflammatory response at these joints. It is important to recognize these conditions and explain their innocence to the patient, who is often fearful and anxious about them.

The thorax and abdominal regions are fascinating areas which can easily be overlooked when assessing the overall physical state of the patient. The supporting mechanism of the spine is intrinsically dependent on a strong anterior abdominal wall. This provides support for the trunk as well as containing the abdominal viscera. It is important to examine and advise appropriately on the function as well as importance of good abdominal tone. The examination should look out for localized bulges within the abdominal wall, indicating a weakness or a hernia within the abdomen or lower down in the inguinal area. These pockets of interrupted muscle tone must be monitored and referred on if appropriate. Lack of abdominal tone is often associated with poor ventilatory mechanics. As we have seen, this can often result in a poor sense of general well-being as well as disturbing symptoms associated with severe, moderate or even mild cases of hyperventilation. Often the patient needs only to be advised and alerted that a better state of general health is within reach. A tailor-made programme of stretching-toning, followed by stamina building exercises as well as some breathing retraining movements can make a considerable impact. These suggestions apply to each and every patient who consults the osteopath, irrespective of the nature of the complaint. A general state of good health must be promoted at every opportunity.

Lumbar region 11

The lumbar spine is the most commonly affected area of the spine, as it is vulnerable to physical strain, particularly the lower two segments. The spinal column has to combine two distinct roles; it provides weight-bearing and support to the trunk, but also allows mobility in a number of ranges.

The mechanical stress imposed on the lumbar spine can be resolved into three components: vertical compression, postero-anterior shearing and torque in the three planes of movement, i.e. rotation, side-bending and flexion-extension.

Compression is absorbed mainly by the anterior column of vertebrae and inter-vertebral discs. When standing vertically, however, the lower two vertebrae are tilted slightly forward. This causes a shearing force, which is resisted in part by the facet joints [33]. Because of this, up to 16% of the vertical compression may be carried by the facet joints in the standing position [113] and this will be increased greatly in a forward bent position, causing considerable strain on the posterior arch. If the spine is in a relatively flexed position while weight-bearing, then the compression force is taken entirely by the disc.

Shearing force is also restrained by the inter-vertebral discs, ligaments and muscles of the lumbar spine, particularly the deep lumbar multifidus muscles. This is evident in people with spondylolisthesis, where there is a defect in the pars interarticulares, and therefore the facet joints cannot restrain the shearing force. Although some with this condition do suffer symptoms, there are many who have very little, if any, problems. The shear strain is absorbed successfully by other structures.

Torque strain is also absorbed by the discs, facet joints, ligaments and muscles. In the lumbar spine the plane of the facet joints markedly limits the rotation available to approximately 1 degree in either direction at each level and this movement occurs mainly by lateral shearing of the disc. This prevents excessive rotation, which could cause severe strain on the disc structure. It has been observed that when facet planes are anomalous in the lower lumbar spine, degenerative changes are more common on X-ray [114].

Because of the relatively high strain imposed on this area, the lower lumbar spine is the most prone to degenerative change. As has been noted previously, however, there is no direct correlation between degenerative changes and clinical symptoms. There are many people with marked degeneration but no symptoms, and vice versa.

If there is restriction of movement at one or more levels of the lumbar spine, in theory there is likely to be more strain imposed on adjacent segments. So, for example, if there is osteochondritis in the upper lumbar or thoraco-lumbar area, then this will stress the lower segments more. Likewise if there is previous injury to the upper lumbar area, with residual joint restriction, then this may predispose adjacent segments to further strain.

The passive structures of the lumbar spine are essential to the maintenance of stability, but it is the muscles that are vital to postural balance and to dynamic control of movement. These muscles include posteriorly the deep and superficial erector spinae including multifidus, interspinalis, transverso-spinalis, longissimus and ilio-costalis. Laterally there are the quadratus lumborum, anteriorly the psoas and abdominal muscles. A major function of the transversus abdominus muscle is to tense the thoraco-lumbar fascia, which acts to support the posterior muscles [115] (Figure 11.1).

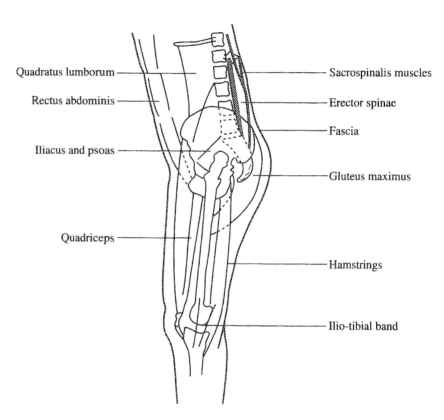

Figure 11.1 Lumbar spine structures.

MECHANICAL FACTORS THAT MAY PREDISPOSE TO LOW BACK STRAIN

Tissue damage occurs when the imposed physical strain is greater than the capacity of the weakest part of the structure to resist that strain. Symptoms therefore occur at the weakest part. The imposed strain may be a single large force or cumulative repetitive loading. When a load is applied to a mechanical system, it is absorbed by the whole system. If one part becomes more rigid, the strain may be transferred elsewhere. Thus mechanical strain may be increased on the lumbar spine by altered functions in other parts of the body. These may cause static strain when the body maintains a particular posture or dynamic strain when the body is performing particular movements.

Static strain

Lumbar spine function is closely related to pelvic and lower extremity function. In a lateral plane, if there is asymmetry of the legs for any reason, then a tilt of the sacral base plane occurs. This imposes asymmetrical stress on the lumbar spine and may lead to spinal curvature throughout the spine (see Chapters 3 and 7). This may predispose the lumbar spine to strain. There is considerable controversy regarding the significance of leg-length difference. It is more likely to be of significance if the back pain sufferer's symptoms are worse when standing than at other times, since this would indicate that the problem is aggravated by this posture. Altering the leg length with a heel or foot pad may be helpful in these circumstances. The leg-length difference may be due to an anatomically shorter bone (femur or tibia), because of asymmetrical inversion/eversion of the feet, or because of varus or valgus of one knee. There may also be asymmetry of the bones of the pelvic bowl.

There is a natural lordosis in the lumbar spine resulting from the forward tilt of the sacral base. The lordotic curve may be altered by the balance of muscle tension of the hip muscles, including the ilio-psoas, quadratus femoris, tensor fascia lata, hamstrings and glutei. Shortening of the posterior muscles may lead to relative extension of the hip, a more horizontal plane of the sacral angle and a flattening of the lumbar lordosis, whereas shortening of the anterior muscles results in hip flexion, anterior tilting of the pelvis, and an increased lumbar lordosis. As mentioned in Chapter 3, the degree of lumbar lordosis and other postural factors may be affected by the patient's psychological state as well as the state of their muscle balance.

Anterior hip joint contracture due to injury or degeneration can also limit or even prevent hip extension and therefore increase lumbar lordosis. An increased lumbar lordosis has been shown to increase the incidence of low back pain [15]. Limited knee extension from habitual poor posture or from degeneration may lead to associated hip flexion, with similar effects.

Lumbar spine posture and function may be affected by abnormalities in the middle and upper spine. Because of the restriction of movement in an organic scoliosis it may cause both static and dynamic strain on the lumbar spine. Postural low back pain is commonly reported in people with this condition. Osteochondrosis in the thoracic spine will cause an increased thoracic kyphosis, with a compensatory increased lumbar lordosis (Figure 11.2). If, however, the upper lumbar area is affected by osteochondrosis, this results in flattening of the lordosis leading to relative posterior tilt of the pelvis, so long as the muscle balance of the hip muscles and the hip joints will allow this. Otherwise there is an accentuation of the lordosis in only the lower two or three lumbar segments, causing a hyperextension strain. These conditions cause both static and dynamic strain, since not only do they affect the posture but also they cause marked restriction of movement of the area concerned.

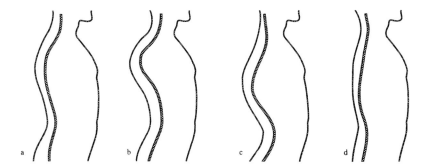

Figure 11.2 Effects of osteochondrosis on the shape of the antero-posterior spinal curve. A. Normal curve showing the typical thoracic kyphosis and lumbar lordosis. B. Upper thoracic osteochondrosis: this has caused a marked thoracic kyphosis but has minimal effect on the lumbar lordosis. C. Mid-thoracic osteochondrosis: the lumbar spine adapts for the increased kyphosis with an increased lordosis. D. Thoraco-lumbar osteochondrosis: the relative flexing of the area causing a reversal of the natural lordosis leading to a slightly flexed area in this region; the lumbar spine therefore seems flat.

Dynamic strain

Any cause of reduced mobility may increase the vulnerability of the body to mechanical strain. A number of causes were discussed in Chapter 6 (see Table 6.3).

Shortened hamstrings will reduce flexion of the hips, thus potentially increasing the strain on the spine (see Figure 6.7). Reduced extension of the hip joint, because of muscle shortening (psoas, quadratus femoris, tensor fascia lata), ligament contracture or joint degeneration, will cause shortening of the stride length. The lumbar spine may compensate for this by extending more when walking.

Dynamic function of the thorax may be reduced by respiratory conditions. For example, asthma may lead to hyper-inflation. Muscle contracture associated with this may cause restriction of the thoracic spine, with potential strain on the lumbar spine.

Even shoulder restriction may cause altered strain on the lumbar spine when attempting to reach up, especially in full shoulder flexion which causes the lumbar spine to extend.

Effect of local or distant dysfunction

In addition to the mechanical effect of restricted joint function resulting from dysfunction, it is conceivable that the altered reflex behaviour in a disturbed segment may have secondary effects on other distant segments via neurological connections within the spinal cord. Thus, in theory, an area of persistent somatic dysfunction in the thoracic area may interfere with the normal reflex behaviour of other areas of somatic dysfunction, for example in the lumbar spine. Therefore the co-ordination of the lumbar joint may be altered such that it becomes less efficient in its movement pattern. It is possible that this altered co-ordination may play a part in why somatic dysfunction develops in a segment suddenly, without any significant trauma.

SOURCES OF PAIN

Low back pain can be caused by damage or irritation of virtually all tissues in the low back region including the inter-vertebral discs, facet joints, ligaments, sacro-iliac joints, lumbar nerve roots, the dura and bone [11]. Pain results from stimulation of nociceptors in these tissues by chemical or mechanical factors commonly mediated by inflammation. It may also be caused by irritation of many of the viscera, particularly those attached to the posterior wall of the abdomen. These include kidneys, gastro-intestinal tract, gynaecological organs, prostate, pancreas and abdominal aorta.

Clinically it is important to differentiate between local spinal causes and those that refer to the lumbar spine (i.e. abdominal causes, etc.) (Figure 11.3). Although osteopathic treatment may be helpful for some functional disorders of abdominal viscera, if serious disease of a viscera is suspected then referral for medical evaluation is generally appropriate. Referral is also advised if serious pathology of spinal structures is suspected. If nerve root irritation or compression is present, then this has implications for treatment techniques: for example, forceful high-velocity thrust or articulatory techniques might aggravate the symptoms. If there are signs of serious neurological deficit, for example cauda equina syndrome or serious loss of muscle power, then early referral is vital. Otherwise treatment must be cautious to minimize the possibility of increasing the neurological damage.

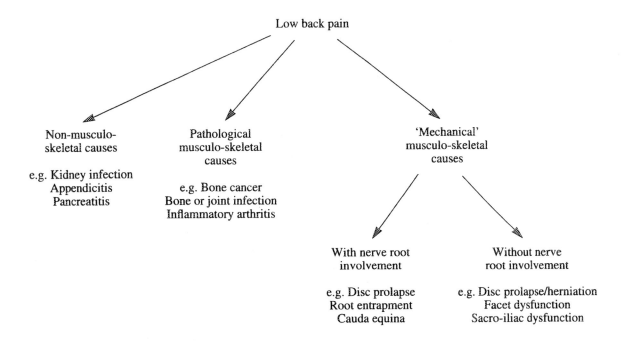

Figure 11.3 Differential diagnosis of low back pain.

HISTORY

The patient's history is often the most helpful tool in differential diagnosis. A mechanical problem is more likely if the symptoms of low back pain, with or without referred symptoms, are related to posture or spinal movement. Most mechanical low back pain is relieved by lying down, either supine or side-lying, though sometimes one or more recumbent positions may not bring relief, especially when there is marked inflammation. It is commonly aggravated either by standing or sitting; alternatively, the patient may be comfortable in one position, but pain is provoked by movement. When, however, the problem has become chronic, the pain may be less clearly related to position. Acute pain may be exacerbated by sudden spinal movement or attempting to bend too far (e.g. putting socks on in the morning), but careful movement is possible and walking may actually relieve it. Some non-musculo-skeletal structures, however, may be affected by movement, for instance gynaecological pain may be affected by walking. Generally speaking, however, the pattern of presentation of pain from internal organs is characteristically different, as will be described later in this chapter.

It is important to question the patient for symptoms from any of the internal systems that may refer to the lumbar spine, particularly where symptoms develop insidiously or are not related to specific activity at the onset. Past history may also be important. It is less likely that a serious, benign mechanical problem will develop in a patient over 50, in the absence of a history of low back pain, and there is therefore a higher likelihood of such symptoms being referred from the abdomen or having a pathological cause in the spine itself.

When considering spinal mechanical problems, it is important to explore with the patient the physical stresses imposed on their spine by their occupation and lifestyle, since these may be vital factors in the cause or aggravation of their symptoms. Excessive strenuous bending and lifting by a manual worker may predispose to back pain. Conversely, an office worker who is desk-bound most of the time may have a less fit spine and be vulnerable to strain when tackling physical tasks such as gardening or do-it-yourself.

As was discussed in Chapter 2, previous dysfunction may cause persistent restriction and abnormal reflex behaviour. Previous symptoms in a distant part of the body may indicate a predisposition to spinal injury and dysfunction. It is, therefore, important to probe carefully into other past musculo-skeletal symptoms, both below and above the presenting area. These may give a preliminary guide to where detailed examination will be appropriate.

The history may be helpful in differentiating the regional cause of symptoms. For instance, both the lumbar spine and the hip may cause pain in the buttock and thigh, either posterior or anterior. The low back region tends to be aggravated by sitting, whereas the hip tends to be more painful when standing and walking. Leg pain that is aggravated by walking or by twisting on the leg is much more likely to be from the hip.

REGIONAL AND LOCAL EXAMINATION

The broad examination of a patient was discussed in Chapter 6 in terms of general health, posture and active movements. The principles of examination of the patient in the passive state were also described. Here we shall consider the passive examination of the low back region and its anatomically related internal organs.

With the patient supine

If there is any pain or neurological symptoms in the lower limbs, neurological examination including muscle power, sensation, and reflexes should be carried out as described in Chapter 6. Straight-leg raising and femoral nerve stretch tests should be included.

The abdomen may be palpated for any tenderness or the presence of any masses. If specific organ infection or irritation is suspected, for instance in the case of the gallbladder or kidney, palpation of these organs may reproduce the presenting symptoms. It is quite common to find slightly tender areas in the bowel also and the presence of faeces within the bowel must be borne in mind, since these may be mistaken for tumours. Details of specific organ examination should be sought from specialized texts [69].

The psoas muscles may be palpated in the lower abdomen as they emerge from the pelvis into the front of the thigh. Abdominal muscle strength may be tested by asking the patient to sit up from the supine position with knees bent, without using the arms. This should not be attempted if the patient is in acute pain, particularly if there is the possibility of an unstable disc injury. The function of the diaphragm may be assessed by observing the breathing pattern at rest and by asking the patient to breath more deeply. The diaphragm tone may be palpated indirectly for tightness by gently palpating the upper abdomen bilaterally below the rib cage and, with the abdominal muscles relaxed, probing up and under the costal margin, sensing the resistance.

Because of the close relationship between the function of the lumbar and pelvic area, the pelvic joints should be examined. The detailed examination is described in Chapter 12.

With the patient prone

The muscle tone of the posterior muscles may be palpated including the erector spinae, quadratus lumborum and glutei (see Chapter 6). It is important to discover how reactive muscles are to palpation and also whether they are shortened. Very reactive muscle suggests a protective response, often with an underlying local joint disturbance. Shortened muscle results from more prolonged dysfunction and may require a different treatment approach to a recent acute injury.

Hip extension may be tested by lifting the thigh from the plinth. This tests both the flexibility of the hip joint and also the psoas muscle. Psoas is frequently shortened in the presence of a disc injury [116]. The tightness of rectus femoris may also be tested by extending the hip in this way, with the knee flexed at 90 degrees. This will also stretch the femoral nerve.

Springing

General and segmental joint movement may be assessed by gently 'springing' on the patient's spine (Figure 6.10). The practitioner places the heel of his hand on the spinous processes and gently leans on the spine and palpates the resistance to this pressure. If the heel of the hand is placed over a series of segments, with the fingers pointing away from the spine, then an impression of the general flexibility may be gained, whereas if the heel of the hand is placed with the fingers pointing along the spine, then a more localized force is applied and individual segments may be assessed.

Alternatively a springing force may be applied, using two hands. With the practitioner standing to one side of the table the thenar eminence of one hand is applied to the tranverse process of a vertebra on the opposite of the patient's spine, while the hypothenar eminence of the other hand is applied to the other transverse process of the same vertebra. A force may be applied vertically down towards the table and the resistance to pressure assessed. This tends to be a less uncomfortable technique since the spinous processes may often be particularly tender.

Specific aims of segmental palpation were discussed in Chapter 6. Any excessive muscle reaction to gentle springing may indicate underlying bone or disc pathology or damage. If, from the history, there is suspicion of fracture, then examining the patient in the prone position is likely to be very difficult and should be avoided. Reproduction of pain by localized springing is helpful in identifying the probable segment containing the source of pain. Hypomobility and hypermobility may be apparent. Any restriction of movement may be chronic or acute. Acute restriction, due to pain of one of the tissues within the segment, will cause a rapid rise in resistance under light pressure, whereas chronic restriction may be painless and will come to a more sudden endpoint without an increase in muscle tone.

Springing mainly tests spinal extension, though, by altering the direction of force, side-bending or rotation may be examined. Specific ranges of movement are, however, more easily palpated in the side-lying position.

With the patient side-lying

This is often the most comfortable position for an acute patient both to move into and to lie in. The spinal muscles may be palpated in this position and, by modifying the relative flexion and extension of the upper and lower parts of the lumbar spine, the tension of the superficial and deep muscles may be palpated. For instance, with the whole lumbar spine in partial flexion, the superficial muscles which traverse a number of segments will be stretched and feel tighter. To palpate the deeper muscles, the upper lumbar spine may be positioned in a neutral or even extended position, thus relaxing the superficial muscles.

Small movements of the lower lumbar spine may be performed by moving the legs in a rhythmic flexion-extension range (see Figure 4.3). The actual range of movement may be palpated by feeling the movement of the spinous processes as they move apart in flexion and approximate in extension. Also the adjacent muscles may be palpated as the spine is moved. The reactivity again can be palpated; if there is dysfunction for any reason, the muscles tend to tense actively during the movement and the increase in tone is palpable.

In the side-lying position, side-bending of the lumbar spine may be assessed. The patient is placed close enough to the edge of the table so that the knees and lower legs are not supported by the table. The hips are flexed so that the lumbar spine is in a neutral position. The practitioner then uses one hand to raise and lower the legs to create a side-bending movement in the lumbar spine, while the other hand palpates the movement in the lumbar spine.

From the general and local examination the body's mechanical function may be assessed. This will reflect both the current state of the musculo-skeletal system and how it has responded to the disturbance in the body. It may also reveal other areas of the musculo-skeletal system which have predisposed to the presenting problem. This will give important clues about appropriate osteo-pathic or other treatment to enable the patient to overcome the disturbance or injury. The examination will also provide information about the nature of the underlying tissue disturbance. This will be explored further in this chapter.

NON-MUSCULO-SKELETAL CAUSES

As was pointed out in Chapters 1 and 2, low back pain may be caused by many visceral structures when there is dysfunction or disease; conversely pain may be referred from the musculo-skeletal system to the related visceral region.

In addition, visceral dysfunction may cause abnormal reflex behaviour within a segment, leading to secondary segmental or even extra-segmental musculo-skeletal dysfunction, which will cause palpable movement restriction and changes in the texture of tissues in the related spinal joint.

Case study 11.1

A 53-year-old man had an inflamed gallbladder, which caused pain referred to the postero-lateral thoracic wall. The pain was aggravated after meals, especially if there was a high fat content. It was not related to spinal move-ment and was reproduced by gentle palpation of the upper right quadrant of the abdomen. On examination of the spine, however, there was restriction of movement in the mid-thoracic joints, where there was tenderness local-ized to two segments on the right.

It is likely that the somatic dysfunction observed in Case study 11.1 was a reflex response to the gallbladder dysfunction. In the past many osteopaths and others have considered the question of which came first, the somatic or the visceral dysfunction. At present there is not conclusive evidence to answer this question. It is not intended to infer that somatic dysfunction by itself will cause visceral disease, but it may be one of a number of causal fac-tors (see Chapter 2).

Clinically the significance is that there may be somatic dysfunction, particularly in the thoracic and lumbar spine, which is caused by visceral disturbance. This may cause some confusion in differential diagnosis. On the other hand there are many osteopaths whose experience suggests that treating the somatic manifestations of benign functional disorders, such as irritable bowel syndrome and gallbladder irritation, sometimes helps to relieve the visceral pain and dysfunction. It must however be emphasized that on many occasions the visceral symptoms are not relieved. Clearly more research is required in this area. Some diagnostic points are considered below. For more details see Borenstein and Wiesel [117].

Genito-urinary

Pain from the kidney is commonly experienced at the costo-vertebral angle, just lateral to paraspinal muscles at T12–L1, radiating around the flank towards the umbilicus. It is usually dull and constant. Pain is most common when the capsule is stretched rapidly, for example in the case of an acute infection, haemorrhage or of acute kidney obstruction from a stone. Where there is only gradual distension of the capsule, for example with a tumour or partial obstruction, frequently pain is not experienced. Pain is rarely aggravated by movement or relieved by rest.

With an acute infection there is usually severe constant aching pain over one or both costo-vertebral angles and this may radiate to the flank and lower abdomen, even to the iliac fossa. The patient may also report either present or recent bladder symptoms of infection including dysuria and frequency. There may be generalized symptoms and signs of infection including pyrexia. If a kidney stone is causing obstruction the pain is more often colicky rather than constant and frequently severe.

Acute prostate inflammation may cause pain in the low back, as well as the perineum and external genitalia, but there will always be associated symptoms of frequency, urgency, dysuria and nocturia. Prostate cancer, when localized to the prostate gland, does not generally cause referred low back pain. Low back pain may, however, result from a metastasis in a vertebra resulting from the primary prostate cancer.

Back pain secondary to a gynaecological disorder is almost invariably associated with symptoms and signs of the pelvic organs. Usually the low back pain experienced is a vague aching, which is not greatly affected by activity or rest. Visceral pain from these organs is experienced in the related segments T11–12 and S2–4 and is deep and diffuse. Somatic nerves, however, supply supporting structures of the pelvis, including muscles, ligaments, and peritoneum. Irritation of these structures causes more localized sharp pain that is felt in the supra-pubic area or sacrum. Period-related pain is associated with menstruation and not affected by posture or activity.

Uterine prolapse, fibroids and retroverted uterus may all cause low back pain, which may be aggravated by standing and walking and relieved by rest [118]. Back pain may occur with benign tumours, uterine malposition, endometriosis and pelvic inflammatory disease. It is rarely experienced with ovarian tumours.

Gastro-intestinal

The organs of the gastro-intestinal tract associated with back pain are those in direct contact with the retroperitoneum or those that refer pain to the back. These include the gallbladder, pancreas, duodenum and colon. Characteristically there is associated anterior pain and usually other symptoms of visceral dysfunction. Aggravating and relieving factors are usually distinctly different from musculo-skeletal causes, generally being unrelated to posture or movement and unrelieved by rest.

Pain from an ulcer in the upper gastro-intestinal tract may refer to the back at about the level of L1/2, though it may occasionally be higher. Referred back pain is rare without epigastric pain. It tends to come on 1–3 hours after a meal and may even awaken the patient from sleep. Pain can be referred from the colon to the back, for instance, in diverticulitis, which results from inflammation of pouches in the bowel wall which have become infected. The pain starts in the abdomen and radiates to the back; it rarely occurs with low back pain only. The pain is severe and griping. Pain may be relieved by bowel movement and increased by eating.

Vascular

A gradual enlargement of the aorta may occur through weakening of the vessel wall, leading to an aneurysm. This is usually asymptomatic until there is direct pressure on the vertebral bodies and surrounding structures, as a result of the increasing size of the artery. The patient complains of abdominal pain that is dull, steady, and unrelated to activity and eating. If back pain occurs it is usually associated with epigastric discomfort and may radiate to the buttocks and thighs. If an aneurysm is suspected, medical referral is essential. The development of abdominal and lumbar spine symptoms associated with an aneurysm is commonly a sign of an extension and worsening of the vascular wall weakness.

The blood flow to the legs may gradually become seriously impaired. The patient may therefore first complain of leg pain on walking, especially uphill; the pain is quickly relieved by stopping. This is due to ischaemia of the muscles supplied by the artery.

MUSCULO-SKELETAL CAUSES

Pathological

Neoplastic

The vertebral bodies are a common site of metastases from primaries in the breast, thyroid, lung, kidney, prostate, cervix and colon. Typically, local pain over a bone develops gradually over a period of a few months with a progressive and unremitting course. It is painful enough at night to disturb sleep and is unaffected by changing position or by treatment. There are, however, a significant number of patients with apparent mechanical back pain that responded to manual treatment, who have later relapsed and been found to have a metastasis after all. It is conceivable that in the early stages there was either a concurrent mechanical problem or in some way the metastasis presented in a similar way to a benign mechanical problem. Even if all patients were X-rayed or scanned (which is economically unrealistic as well as potentially harmful to many patients from exposure to radiation), it is still likely that some cases would be missed at an early stage. It is, therefore, imperative to use the minimum force necessary to achieve the required treatment.

Multiple myeloma is the most common spinal primary malignancy. Suspicion should be aroused if there is unremitting pain, especially in an elderly person with no previous history of back pain. Other primary bone tumours are rare in the spine, although sarcoma, chordoma, osteoid osteoma and Paget's disease occur occasionally.

Infective

Osteomyelitis is a relatively rare cause of low back pain. A history of recent infection (urinary tract, recto-sigmoid disease, soft tissue or post-dental extraction infection) or an invasive procedure is common. Although low back pain is typically persistent, continuing even at night, it may be intermittent. It may be present at rest and be exacerbated by motion. Acute systemic symptoms are usual. On examination there is decreased movement, muscle spasm and percussion tenderness over the vertebra.

Inflammatory

There are a number of sero-negative arthropathies that may affect the spine, the commonest being ankylosing spondylitis. Others include enteropathic arthropathy (associated with Crohn's disease and ulcerative colitis), Reiter's syndrome and psoriatic arthritis (usually developing only after the skin lesions). The last two more frequently affect peripheral joints rather than the spine.

The patient commonly complains of low back or unilateral sacro-iliac pain. This tends to be worse in the morning and there is marked morning stiffness, which may take an hour or two to subside. The onset is usually insidious, with no associated trauma. The patient may report previous episodes of backache over a period of years, which have tended to come and go, with or without treatment. The pain tends to increase when they are at rest and eases once they have become active. After inactivity they are again very stiff. There may be pain at night, the patient waking in the early hours, which is eased by getting up and moving about. The patient may also have one or more swollen and painful peripheral joints, for example hip, knee or shoulder.

Ankylosing spondylitis is a form of inflammatory arthritis which affects the pelvic joints and spine. It tends to develop in the second to fourth decade, particularly in men (males : females, 9 : 1). There is some inherited tissue sensitivity. Inflammation affects the facet joints and the spinal ligaments, often starting in the sacro-iliac or thoraco-lumbar areas. Initially stiffness results from local inflammation, but this may proceed to ankylosis, with irreversible fusion of spinal segments. X-rays show a characteristic appearance of a 'bamboo spine'.

On examination there is marked stiffening of the affected region and not just one or two spinal joints. Even at an early stage, when X-ray changes are not evident, widespread stiffness may be palpable. Furthermore, the development of ankylosis may be relatively asymptomatic; the patient may assume the stiffness is part of normal ageing and ignore it. They may eventually present because the neck has started to stiffen and this affects their ability to see over their shoulder. Examples are given in Case studies 11.2–11.4.

Case study 11.2

A 54-year-old man complained primarily of persistent neck stiffness and also some aching. On examination he had virtually no lumbar or thoracic spinal movement and he had only 40 degrees of cervical rotation and 20 degrees of side-bending. X-rays showed ankylosis from the lower lumbar to the lower cervical region. He reported also that he had suffered a serious episode of low back pain 10 years earlier, which, he recalled, had puzzled his orthopaedic surgeon and had eventually been diagnosed as a disc injury. Probably this episode had been related to the ankylosing spondylitis, but had not shown any X-ray changes at that time.

Case study 11.3

Frequently the erythrocyte sedimentation rate (ESR) is raised by inflammatory arthritis. A 42-year-old lady, however, presented with a typical history and demonstrated characteristic signs of ankylosing spondylitis, yet had an ESR of less than 5 mm per hour.

Case study 11.4

A 36-year-old lady who did heavy manual work complained of a long history of low back pain over a number of years. She used to do a great deal of sport, including weight-training, but due to a change in working pattern became less active about 18 months before. The back pain had worsened at this stage. At the time of consultation she was awakening most nights at about four to five o'clock and was very stiff when getting up. This was worse if she stayed in bed longer on her day off. On examination there was still quite reasonable lumbar movement, which suggested that there was inflammation without widespread ankylosis.

Rheumatoid arthritis can also affect the spine, but it is usually at a late stage, after the peripheral joints have been involved for some period of time, and therefore should cause little difficulty in differential diagnosis.

Acute problems

Dysfunction

Probably the vast majority of patients with low back pain fall into this category. They have low back pain, with or without referred pain in the leg, which is affected by different postures and movement. This will be associated with an altered range of spinal movements and there is no neurological deficit. There are a number of possible sites of the cause of pain, including the inter-vertebral disc, the apophyseal joints, the spinal ligaments and muscles and the pelvic joints. There are few objective, research-based, clinical criteria for any of the syndromes that have been described to date. As has been mentioned in Chapter 2, one reason for this is that frequently there is not just one tissue that has been damaged and we are therefore usually viewing a 'mixed' syndrome. In addition, it is the effects of the damage to the body that are observed, which include the results of inflammation and muscle spasm. Because there can be no objective differentiation between the various causes, specific treatments cannot therefore be applied to a particular tissue diagnosis. In practice, how-ever, most osteopathic techniques alter the function of an area rather than just one tissue.

Although there are no objective criteria for differential diagnosis, experience reveals there are some differences between various types of prob-lems.

Facet joint inflammation/irritation

Injury to the apophyseal joint may occur while bending, particularly with twisting, which leads to mild to marked intra-capsular and peri-capsular inflammation, with associated somatic dysfunction. Referred pain from the facet joints has been shown to spread into the leg from the lower lumbar spine and the pain may reach below the knee (see Figure 5.2). Mooney suggested that the extent of referral away from the site of pain seems related to the inten-sity of pain, thus, as pain increases in the back, the pain spreads further down the leg [119]. Referred pain from apophyseal joints has sometimes been found to extend even to the foot. Although the referral patterns shown are from the apophyseal joints, pain may be referred from other lumbar spine structures also, including muscles, inter-vertebral discs and peri-capsular tissues.

Symptoms typically result from a particular movement involving bending, twisting and possibly lifting. It may even be a trivial movement which precip-itates pain, such as reaching to pick up a piece of paper. Sometimes the pain may be experienced first on rising from bed; in this case frequently the pre-cipitating trauma occurred the previous day, but because the joint was predis-posed, for some reason the trauma required to cause damage was trivial and no pain was experienced immediately. Inflammation builds up over a few hours, particularly when at rest, stiffness develops and muscle spasm is initi-ated when the joint is moved.

Pain may be persistent initially, but gradually subsides over a few days to weeks. Pain is aggravated by movement, especially when rising from sitting or lying, but is eased by cautious movement. Sudden or incautious movements may cause sharp pain. Pain is usually eased by lying down, though when there is acute inflammation, pain may still persist.

On examination a spinal list is sometimes seen in the early stages or occa-sionally there is a flexion deformity. This is more commonly observed with a disc injury and if the acute posture is maintained more than a week or two, the likelihood is that the problem principally involves the disc rather than the facet joint.

When there is acute joint inflammation, all active spinal movements may be painful. However when the inflammation is less intense, the ranges most affected tend to be side-bending and extension, though flexion is commonly limited also. Combined ipsilateral side-bending with extension is particularly painful.

On examination of passive movement, there is usually relatively localized restriction of one segment, indicating the level of dysfunction. Commonly, passive movement is not painful, though there may be palpable increase of tone around the disturbed joint compared with surrounding segments during the movement. Associated with the movement restriction there is usually localized muscle tightness at rest that is frequently greater on one side than the other. Tenderness may be found over the joint, either over the spinous process, supra-spinous ligament or over the transverse process. Isolated tenderness, however, without other signs of segmental disturbance, is of little significance. If there is no palpable segmental restriction, then joint manipulation is not appropriate.

On the other hand, the presence of signs of somatic dysfunction does not inevitably mean that the cause is within the musculo-skeletal system. Visceral disturbance may cause signs of somatic dysfunction also, including tenderness, altered muscle tone and tissue texture and restriction of movement. Differential diagnosis will be facilitated by the presence of symptoms of visceral dysfunction, such as abdominal pain, diarrhoea or constipation from bowel dysfunction or dysuria from disturbance of the urinary system. Although signs of somatic dysfunction may be present, merely manipulating the disturbed joints does not necessarily resolve the visceral condition. Osteopathic treatment may be of benefit sometimes, using a wide range of techniques, for functional visceral conditions. It is of course essential to exclude, as far as is possible, the presence of a serious pathology before performing any treatment.

Apparent facet joint 'locking'

This may simply be a variant of the previous problem. It usually presents as acute or subacute low back pain (though similar problems occur throughout the spine, especially in the neck). It is commonly initiated by a trivial movement, often in the mid-range of movement, though quite frequently associated with some rotation or side-bending, and pain is felt immediately. Movement is suddenly restricted; for instance, if it occurs in slight flexion, then it may be difficult to straighten up fully again. Pain is mainly caused by attempts to move, while the patient is able to get relatively comfortable by remaining still.

There is usually no gross protective posture or widespread spasm. Active movements are limited, but not equally in all directions. When laid down, the muscles are able to relax, though often soft tissue massage is needed to assist this. Any attempt, however, to move the spinal joint involved meets immediate resistance. The joint feels very restricted but there is some 'give' if it is moved with care.

Theories of joint locking were discussed in Chapter 2. It is likely that various different mechanisms are involved in different people. The characteristic feature of a 'facet lock' is that it responds rapidly to manipulation, producing immediate improvement in the range of movement and relief from pain. Thrust techniques are often effective, but sometimes muscle energy or even functional technique can release the joint restriction.

Disc herniation

The inter-vertebral disc has received considerable scrutiny over the years since Barr first identified it as a cause of pain in the low back [120], and at some stages of history it was apparently considered by some as the only cause of low back pain. Many other structures, however, have now been demonstrated as causes also. Disc degeneration has been discussed in Chapter 2. Types of disc pathology have been described in a variety of terms. For purposes of clarity the following definitions will be used:

- There may be cracks within the annulus, which allow nuclear material to break through the inner annulus. If these cracks enlarge, so that the annulus bulges externally, this is described as an 'herniation'.
- The outer annulus may be breached allowing the nuclear material to form a 'protusion' or 'prolapse'.
- If the nuclear material remains attached to the remaining central nuclear material then this is known as an 'extrusion'.
- If the nuclear material becomes separated from the remaining central nuclear material, it is a 'sequestration' (Figure 11.4).

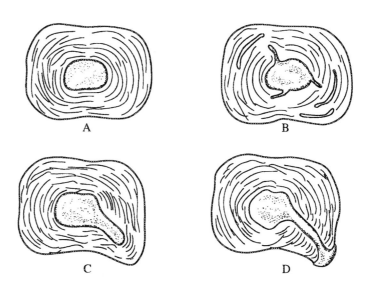

Figure 11.4 Disc injuries – structural changes. A. Normal. Intact nucleus (central), intact annulus. B. Circumferential and radial cracks and tears. C. Herniation: nuclear material has been forced into a weakened radial tear in the annulus, causing a postero-lateral bulge; the outer border of the annulus is still intact. D. Disc prolapse: nuclear material has breached the outer annulus and protrudes; this significantly reduces the size of the adjacent root foramen.

Disc pathology has been demonstrated in asymptomatic subjects, using imaging techniques such as myelography [121], discography [122], CT scanning [123] and magnetic resonance imaging [124]. Equally, disc pathology has been identified as the cause of pain in patients. This of course leads to confusion in diagnosis. There is still no definitive clinical test which can be used in isolation to identify the cause of low back pain. Modern X-ray and scanning techniques can be helpful in verifying the presence of a disc prolapse, but the significance of this must be related to the clinical symptoms and signs.

Even in normal inter-vertebral discs, the superficial part of the annulus is innervated by free nerve ending, and in abnormal discs up to one-half of the depth of the annulus has been shown to have a nerve supply [68]. Thus, when the annulus of a disc is cracked or torn, this may cause pain. If the disc bulges, this may cause irritation of adjacent structures, which include the posterior spinal ligaments and the spinal nerve root. Disc prolapse with nerve root irritation is discussed below. In the absence of nerve root pain it is very difficult to differentiate between various forms of disc injury.

Pain from disc injury may be local to the spine or referred to the buttock, thigh and, less commonly, below the knee. It is usually central, but may spread to one or both sides. Nerve root irritation will only occur if the disc bulge actually encroaches on the nerve root. Nerve root irritation will be unilateral unless there is a massive prolapse, which will inevitably involve the cauda equina also (see below).

Disc injuries are most common between 30 and 50 years of age [125], but may occur as early as the teenage years. Disc herniation and prolapse probably occur less with increasing age, but disc degeneration may predispose to strain of other tissues, particularly the facet joints.

The onset of symptoms from a disc injury is variable. Pain may develop suddenly and very acutely on bending, especially if lifting and twisting. This is when the disc is biomechanically most vulnerable. Some patients may merely experience a sensation that something has happened, that 'they felt a click' or that 'something seemed to give' but pain built up only gradually over a few hours, especially after having been inactive for some time. On occasion it may even be the next morning that they find that their back has seized up, when they try to get out of bed.

With a disc injury in a relatively young person (up to 40 years) pain is characteristically worse in the morning when rising from the bed and may only gradually ease with movement over a period of 1–3 hours. It may well increase again towards the end of the day. Pain is typically aggravated by sitting, increasing as time passes. With more intense pain, sitting may be unbearable for any length of time. Bending also is severely limited and dressing may be extremely difficult.

On examination there is sometimes a spinal list (see Figure 7.1) or less commonly a flexion deformity. A persistent deformity over a few weeks is more indicative of a disc injury. The mechanism underlying the deformity is unclear, but it is presumably the body's attempt to minimize the total nociceptive activity in the damaged area. Listing may occur with or without nerve root irritation.

With an acute disc injury, flexion is virtually always markedly limited, sometimes even to only a few degrees. In the extreme, even simply flexing the neck is painful. There may or may not be pain on extension. If there is a spinal list, then side-bending towards the concavity of the lateral curvature is usually limited, while side-bending to the convexity is painless. For instance, if the patient stands listing to the right they are usually able to side-bend further to the right, but side-bending to the left is very limited and accompanied by pain. If, however, there is no spinal list, then there may be full and painless side-bending.

Passive examination usually reveals localized or even multi-segmental restriction. Sometimes a group of segments feels almost rigid and any attempt to stretch the area too far causes pain and may also cause a reaction after treatment. This is best avoided. Gentle manual traction, however, applied to the pelvis may give pain relief. This is helpful both diagnostically and as a form of treatment.

Sacro-iliac joint

Although pelvic joint problems are discussed in Chapter 12, it is appropriate to mention the important differential diagnostic points here for comparison with the various lumbar spine problems. Sacro-iliac pain induced by injection by Fortin was characteristically located over the pelvic joint and lateral to it [67]. In asymptomatic subjects the pain radiated to the buttock and to the lateral thigh but not to the midline. Other authors have reported pain spreading to the posterior thigh and even into the calf. In practice it is wise to assume that low back pain which spreads from the sacro-iliac area to the midline comes from a spinal structure rather than a pelvic joint, unless clearly demonstrated otherwise.

An acutely painful sacro-iliac joint causes a nagging ache, aggravated particularly by changing position, and walking, particularly the commencement of walking.

Nerve root irritation

For osteopaths it is particularly important to recognize when nerve root irritation is present because of the potential to make matters worse with injudicious manipulation. Neural tissue, once inflamed, is very vulnerable to physical trauma. Manual treatment may still be beneficial, but more strenuous techniques are best avoided initially, particularly by inexperienced practitioners. High-velocity thrust techniques, therefore, which are potentially traumatic, and others that tend to narrow the intervertebral foramina on the affected side of the spine should be avoided.

Nerve root inflammation most commonly results from mechanical irritation by surrounding structures in the intervertebral foramen. In younger people the most likely cause of the irritation is disc prolapse and in older people it is encroachment into the nerve root foramen, resulting from degeneration of the disc and facet joint. The clinical presentation tends to be different and will be discussed separately. Other mechanical causes include spondylolisthesis and nerve root adhesion (following persistent nerve root inflammation).

The actual dimensions of the nerve root foramen vary significantly between people. The development of symptoms secondary to a disc prolapse depends therefore on the relative size of the disc prolapse to the foramen. Porter demonstrated that a large prolapse with a large foramen may not cause nerve root irritation, whereas even a small prolapse into a small foramen can cause problems [126]. Clinically it is important to identify the degree of nerve root irritation rather than establish the size of the prolapse, since this will dictate the clinical management.

Pain is initiated by inflammation of the nerve root. It has been demonstrated that simple compression of the nerve root causes only mild tingling or numbness, but does not cause pain [127]. If however the nerve is traumatized, then inflammation and swelling develop and ischaemia may complicate the tissue damage. The nerve root becomes sensitive to both pressure and to stretch [128]. Treatment is therefore directed to reducing the inflammation and ischaemia rather than moving the disc bulge. With severe foraminal trespass, surgery may be necessary but the majority of disc injuries will settle with conservative treatment.

As described in Chapter 5, typical nerve root pain is usually unpleasant or even sharp in character, in a relatively narrow linear band in the distribution of a dermatome, and worse distally, greater in the limb than in the spine. Nerve root irritation is more likely than somatic referred pain if it spreads below the knee [129]. Pain is often accompanied by dysaesthesia (numbness or tingling) and less commonly by muscle weakness.

Apart from disc prolapse and degenerative trespass of the root foramen, nerve root pain may be caused by other tissue pathology, including a tumour such as a neurofibroma, or infection such as a dural abscess, herpes zoster or vertebral body infection with bone destruction. A neurofibroma may simulate the presence of a disc prolapse because it is unlikely to cause systemic symptoms. It has sometimes even been found unexpectedly during an operation.

Disc prolapse

As mentioned above, disc prolapse may present with or without nerve root irritation. If nerve root irritation results from a disc injury, then there is usually a prolapse rather than a herniation present; in the absence of nerve root irritation it is clinically very difficult to distinguish between a prolapse and a herniation.

The behaviour of the back pain caused by disc prolapse is similar to that described above for disc herniation. As with the back pain, leg symptoms from nerve root irritation are also frequently aggravated by sitting and driving. It is also significant that in the younger age group (where the nerve root irritation is predominantly caused by disc prolapse) *leg* pain is particularly aggravated by coughing, sneezing and straining on the lavatory. Low back pain aggravated by coughing and sneezing is a non-specific symptom and not necessarily characteristic of disc injury. With severe nerve root pain standing and walking may also markedly aggravate the symptoms.

Many sufferers with disc prolapse and nerve pain stand with a spinal list, which straightens when the patient lies down. Porter reports that up to a third of all patients with this problem have such a list. He also reports no correlation between the position of the disc bulge found at operation and the direction of the list. The presence of a list appears to be no indication as to which level is affected.

As with disc herniation, flexion and extension are likely to cause pain, both in the back and the leg. Side-bending may be painful in one direction if there is a spinal list, otherwise it is often pain free.

Neurological examination may give evidence of deficit of nerve function (Table 11.1) if there is actual nerve damage. Straight-leg raising is usually markedly reduced, frequently to 30 degrees or less on the affected side. Positive crossed straight-leg raising is a particularly significant sign, since its presence correlates with a poor response to conservative treatment (see Chapter 6). The symptoms and signs listed for root lesions should be used only as a guide to the probable level, since there are many reasons for variations.

Table 11.1 Possible symptoms and signs of specific root lesions

	L4	*L5*	*S1*
Location of pain	Anterior thigh and leg to medial ankle	Lateral thigh and leg to lateral ankle	Posterior thigh and calf to heel
Nerve stretch test	Positive femoral nerve test	Straight-leg raising may be affected	Straight-leg raising often affected
Muscle weakness	Quadriceps, hip flexors	Ankle and toe extensors especially of hallux	Glutei especially maximus, triceps surae, toe flexors
Reflex affected	Patellar reflex	None	Ankle
Sensory loss	Anterior thigh	Lateral thigh and leg to lateral ankle	Posterior thigh and calf, lateral foot to fourth and fifth toes

Even with the patient in a comfortable lying position there may be marked spasm and there is relatively little if any passive movement (especially in flexion) of a number of lumbar joints, not just the immediately affected segment. Tenderness is a non-specific sign with regard to the level of disc injury.

Although disc prolapse is commonest in the fourth decade, Grieve points out that it is not rare even among teenagers. In younger people the signs are frequently more marked compared with the symptoms, with marked limitation of straight-leg raising and neurological deficit [15].

Conservative treatment over a period of 2–4 weeks is often worthwhile in an attempt to reduce muscle spasm and reduce foraminal congestion, thus allowing symptoms to ease. Other areas that are commonly affected by or contribute to the development of disc injury are tightness of the psoas muscles and alteration of the pelvic or thoraco-lumbar mechanical function. These should be carefully assessed and treated if necessary. If, however, there is no progress or there is neurological deficit, a surgical opinion may be appropriate. Surgery has been shown to be effective for disc herniation [130].

Sphincter disturbance

If a large central disc prolapse protudes into a relatively small spinal canal the bulge may compress the cauda equina. Typically this will lead to loss of bladder and bowel function, and saddle anaesthesia, known as cauda equina syndrome. Usually bladder retention and bowel incontinence occur. This may or may not be accompanied by root pain in one or both legs, since this will depend on the location and size of the prolapse in relation to the spinal canal. When disc injury is suspected, it is vital to ask about these symptoms, since some patients will not think to mention them or be embarrassed to discuss them.

In all cases of sphincter disturbance and saddle anaesthesia surgical opinion should be sought immediately, since delay may lead to poor recovery of visceral function. Even with an operation there may not be full recovery.

Foraminal encroachment

Narrowing of the root canal occurs by osteophytosis from the vertebral body and the facet joint, by thickening of the joint capsule, ligamentum flavum or posterior longitudinal ligament (see Figure 2.7). Delauche-Cavallier followed the progress of the size of disc bulges by studying their CT scans [131]. She observed that the disc bulge did not necessarily reduce in size over a significant period. It is probable that fibrosis of a disc sequestrum may further narrow the antero-posterior diameter, while disc thinning may reduce the vertical diameter. Loss of space in the root canal does not inevitably lead to symptoms. Indeed, significant distortion of the root has been seen without any evidence of nerve root irritation [132]. Encroachment, however, may clearly predispose the nerve root to damage and inflammation, with consequent symptoms.

Root entrapment becomes more common in middle and later life with the highest incidence in the sixth decade. A history of low back or leg pain is by no means invariable. Compared with root pain caused by disc prolapse, pain from root entrapment tends to be unremitting and more severe. Lying down brings little relief and sleep may be very difficult in the acute phase. While sitting is painful, standing is also painful, particularly aggravating the leg pain. Coughing and sneezing has very little effect. Contrast this with the intensified pain from coughing and sneezing from a disc prolapse.

A spinal list is rare with root entrapment. Spinal extension is the movement most affected by pain and is usually limited. Flexion however is frequently very good, causing little pain if any. Ipsilateral side-bending may be painful, particularly if combined with spinal extension. Neurological signs are usually absent; reflexes and muscle power are only rarely affected. Straight-leg raising also is commonly unaffected in the majority of sufferers [133].

Symptoms can be very persistent over many weeks or months even with treatment but in most cases they do settle, demonstrating that it is the inflammation of the nerve that triggers the pain, rather than the presence of structural changes encroaching on the foramen.

Spondylolisthesis

Olisthesis refers to the forward slippage of one vertebra in relation to the next. Though it is usually the upper vertebra that moves anteriorly, occasionally posterior slippage has been seen, especially when the defect is in the upper lumbar area. The commonest cause for spondylolisthesis is a defect of the isthmus between the articular processes of a vertebra. This may result from a fatigue fracture of the pars interarticulares, elongation of the pars without bone defect or acute fracture of the pars. Slippage is also seen as a result of degeneration which has led to segmental instability, also without pars defect. Disc degeneration allows greater shearing movement of the segment and the increased mechanical strain leads to gross alteration of the facet joints, which then fail to restrain the anterior shear force.

Isthmic spondylolysis and spondylolisthesis are both quite common findings on X-ray, but they are frequently incidental findings, unrelated to the reason for the X-ray. Thus the presence of a spondylolisthesis should not be assumed to be the cause of symptoms, especially in a patient over 40 years, who presents initially with back or leg pain.

It has been demonstrated that there are free nerve endings in the pars defect itself and therefore that it is potentially pain sensitive [134]. A pars defect, however, is a common structural abnormality that is *occasionally* associated with low back pain [135]. Although the pars is potentially a source of pain, other tissues may be affected by forward slippage, including the disc, which often suffers accelerated degeneration, the facet joints and their capsules, and spinal ligaments and muscles, which are required to restrain more shear force than in a normal spine. In addition nerve root and cauda equina irritation and compression may occur. Symptoms may result from each of these sources, leading to a variety of clinical presentations.

Low backache, sometimes accompanied by referred pain in one or both legs, is the usual symptom pattern in the younger age group. The pain may be quite acute but is often less intense but persistent or recurrent. A history of trauma involving extension may be recalled. Pain is characteristically aggravated by standing and relieved by sitting and walking.

Active extension is the most uncomfortable movement while flexion is usually full and painless. The lumbar erector spinae appear to stand out more, with a deep furrow between. A bony shelf may be visible in the lower lumbar spine and is usually palpable on standing and when lying down. If significant AP shearing is possible, then the shelf may be less apparent when examined in a side-lying position. The level of the shelf associated with a pars defect will be at the segmental level above the defective vertebra; i.e. with an L5 pars defect, the shelf will be at the L4/5 segment (Figure 11.5). This is because, while the L5 vertebral body slips forward, the L5 neural arch is restrained by the superior articular facets of the sacrum, while the L4 neural arch is drawn forward with the L4 and L5 vertebrae.

Symptoms may result from root involvement particularly with a patient with a recurrent or chronic history. With progressing defect or degeneration, root trespass becomes more likely. If nerve root symptoms develop (and they may not) they will occur in the third decade or later.

Finally, with severe trespass, cauda equina symptoms may result causing bladder dysfunction and sensory loss in the buttocks, posterior thighs and calves.

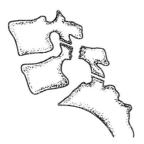

Figure 11.5 Spondylolisthesis: although anterior slippage of the body of L5 occurs, movement of the posterior arch of L5 is resisted by the facet surfaces of S1. The resulting shelf is palpated at the L4/5 level.

Fracture

Vertebral body fracture may occur as the result of significant trauma, particularly with vertical compression (e.g. a fall from some height on to the feet) or forced flexion or extension (e.g. rugby or riding injury or head-on collision in a car). Normal bone can absorb considerable force without damage. Bone may be weakened, however, by a number of conditions, making fracture more likely. For instance, osteoporosis is not uncommon in women, even in the sixth decade, and increases with age, particularly after an early menopause (i.e. before 40), though this is less likely if the patient has received hormone replacement therapy. Long term steroid use also causes osteoporosis. The presence of spinal metastases also weakens bone and may only become apparent when fracture occurs. For this reason the possibility of spinal fracture must be borne in mind when examining older patients.

The onset of pain is usually sudden and related to some trauma, though with a pathological fracture this may be relatively trivial, for instance as a result of bending down, without lifting anything. Pain is usually severe and disabling, making any spinal movement painful. It may be localized to the damaged area, but if bone damage leads to compression of an adjacent nerve, then root pain in the limb may result. Pain is worse when weight-bearing, but initially even lying down does not bring relief, because muscle spasm persists to protect the unstable area. On examination, spinal deformity with an angular kyphosis may be seen and there will usually be marked spasm and considerable restriction of movement in *all* planes. The limitation in all planes is a key feature indicating the likelihood of fracture.

Following fracture, pain gradually normally subsides over a period of 6–8 weeks. Even with a pathological fracture bone repair occurs, but is usually seen on X-ray to be abnormal in its structure.

Chronic problems

It must always be borne in mind when a patient presents with chronic low back pain (longer than 3 months' duration) that it may not be caused by a mechanical disturbance and a high level of suspicion of a non-musculo-skeletal cause is usually wise (Table 11.2).

Table 11.2 Common mechanical causes of chronic low back pain

Unresolved facet (capsular) or disc injury
Unresolved sacro-iliac strain
Postural myofascial strain
Facet arthrosis
Spondylolisthesis
Nerve root irritation secondary to disc injury or foraminal encroachment
Neurogenic claudication

Chronic mechanical pain often begins with an acute episode that does not resolve adequately. The emphasis in management of acute low back pain should therefore be on full rehabilitation and restoration of function rather than merely pain relief – the two are not synonymous. Chronic pain, however, does not always result from inadequate recovery from an acute injury. For instance, soft tissue fatigue secondary to poor posture or excessive postural strain imposed by occupation may begin as an intermittent ache, which becomes more persistent over a period of time, if the underlying ergonomic design of the workplace is not addressed. It is almost inevitable that there will be a number of factors contributing to chronic pain. There will be internal tissue changes (chronically inflamed tissues, residual damage, altered mechanical function of various tissues, including shortened muscles and ligaments), and altered or avoided movement patterns (bending, lifting, walking). There may often be external factors which prevent resolution by maintaining stress on the damaged or disturbed area (poor physical working conditions, soft bed, pressure of work). A sufferer's psychological state also may be affected by and contribute to her response to chronic pain (see also Chapter 1). Here we will now discuss some of the more common causes of chronic pain.

Dysfunction

All acute dysfunction may become chronic. Most research into the facet syndrome (one cause of somatic dysfunction) has been performed on chronic patients, since sufferers do not tend to be referred to specialist clinics in the early stages of a problem. Even when the symptoms have persisted for some months, it is still difficult to differentiate clinically between pain from a facet joint and from a disc. It has been argued that damage in one tissue may lead to disturbance in the other, because of the close mechanical relationship. This may well be the case, but it does not necessarily mean that the secondary tissue disturbance becomes symptomatic. Indeed Schwarzer explored the relative contribution of disc and facet in chronic low back pain by pain provocation tests, and he concluded that it was relatively rare to find both to be a pain source [136].

From an osteopathic viewpoint it may not be important to differentiate between the precise location of the source of pain, since the aim of treatment is not necessarily to initiate repair of the damaged tissue itself, but to restore normal function locally and in other parts of the neuro-musculo-skeletal system by manual intervention and by other physical measures, i.e. exercises. The potential success of management therefore depends on how amenable the tissue disturbance is to change.

Postural fatigue

This occurs when one or more tissues become sensitive, such that sustained postures cause aching to develop. The symptom pattern discussed in Chapter 3 includes:

- Aching or even pain that is aggravated by sustaining one or a range of postures, e.g. standing, sitting or even lying down.
- The ache gradually builds up while the posture is maintained.
- The ache is relieved by moving about or changing position.
- Prolonged postural ache is often associated with stiffness when the person moves after a period of inactivity.

Tissue sensitivity may often be caused by the presence of joint dysfunction rather than simply muscular fatigue due to poor fitness or poor postural positioning of the body. It will generally help to improve the sitting or standing posture that aggravated the symptoms by retraining, but treatment of specific dysfunction can frequently bring rapid relief.

Chronic pain secondary to degenerative changes

Lateral foraminal encroachment

There may be structural changes which are irreversible, due to previous trauma or degeneration; these were discussed in Chapter 2. Their most significant effects are on the spinal foraminae, including the central and lateral canals. As has already been discussed, narrowing of the lateral canals (the nerve root foramen) may predispose to nerve root irritation and compression, which can be acute (see above), and may then progress to a chronic state of inflammation. Signs of nerve root irritation may well be present, in addition to persistent leg pain in a dermatomal distribution. Low back pain may be absent.

Alternatively the nerve may be compressed gradually. In this case pain does not necessarily occur, but may lead to mild neurological deficit with parasthesiae, numbness and even muscle weakness. In these cases the symptoms are intermittent and not too troublesome for the patient. There is usually a history of previous episodes of pain and dysfunction in the related spinal area, with signs of degeneration on examination. It is most commonly found in the lower cervical region, causing tingling and numbness in the hands, although, if the lumbar spine is affected, similar symptoms may be experienced in the toes.

Central spinal stenosis – neurogenic claudication

Narrowing of the central spinal canal may occur as a result of encroachment anteriorly by osteophytosis from the vertebral body, bulging of the disc or posterior longitudinal ligament thickening, laterally by osteophytosis of the facet joint and capsular thickening, and posteriorly by thickening and folding of the ligamentum flavum. Further narrowing may occur if there is displacement of a vertebra with an intact neural arch. Distortion and displacement may result from vertebral collapse.

The presence of a narrow spinal canal does not necessarily cause symptoms, since the size of cauda equina also varies. It is the relative size of the nervous tissue to the space available that is critical. It has also been observed that the symptoms of neurogenic claudication rarely occur unless there is multisegmental involvement. Neurogenic claudication results from nerve ischaemia, induced by compression of roots of the cauda equina. Unlike the symptom pattern from a large central disc prolapse, the bladder and bowel functions are not affected since the nerve ischaemia is intermittent rather than persistent.

Symptoms are usually felt in the legs, though there is usually a long history of low back pain, which has since become chronic. The patient complains of marked discomfort in the legs when walking, usually in the thighs, calves and feet. It is not well localized nor in a dermatomal distribution. The patient does not experience severe pain, but usually describes the sensation as a heavy feeling or tiredness of the legs. Walking is commonly restricted to a distance of 500 metres, after which they have to stop and rest. Towards the end of the walk they will tend to stoop; this presumably opens the spinal canal slightly and maximizes the blood flow. Resting with the lumbar spine in a flexed position usually affords more relief; sitting on a wall, for instance, may bring more rapid relief. Often they find it easier to walk uphill rather than down because this flexes the spine rather than extends it. Similarly they may be able to cut the grass for half an hour with a lawn mower, since this requires a slightly flexed position, whereas they are normally unable to walk for more than a few minutes.

On examination there is usually a characteristic posture. The spine is either flat or even flexed, due to marked degenerative changes. To compensate for this the hips and knees are flexed. Spinal flexion may still be quite reasonable, but other movements are limited, indeed extension is absent. There are usually no neurological signs and straight-leg raising is normal.

Vascular claudication also causes leg pain on walking. Characteristically spinal flexion when walking does not help the leg pain. There will also be signs of inadequate blood supply to the limb including reduced or absent pulses and trophic changes in the feet. Neurogenic claudication is highly unlikely in a patient with a lumbar spine which will extend and is reasonably flexible. Difficulty in diagnosis sometimes occurs when there is both spinal degeneration and vascular deterioration.

Arthrosis

Apophyseal joints may be affected by osteoarthritis. The spine may be affected as a result of specific mechanical strain or as part of a generalized condition affecting a number of joints (i.e. primary osteoarthritis). It may occur secondarily to or in the absence of disc degeneration and may even be the late stage of chronic apophyseal joint dysfunction.

As with other osteoarthritic joints, symptoms may be intermittent over a period of years while there is still cartilage present on the joint surfaces and the symptoms result from soft tissue irritation. However the joint cartilage deterioration may progress until there is virtually complete loss of cartilage and eburnation of the bone underlying the joint. If this occurs, symptoms then tend to become more persistent, with night pain in the early hours and stiffness on rising from bed. Movement tends to relieve the pain, though long periods of standing or walking aggravate it, presumably because this causes compression of the joint surfaces. As with osteoarthrosis in other joints, osteopathic treatment is less effective in this late stage of the condition, though some relief may be afforded.

On examination there is generally loss of lumbar lordosis and limitation of all movements (especially extension) due to joint deterioration rather than by pain.

TREATMENT CONSIDERATIONS

The emphasis in the latter half of this chapter has been on differentiating between particular patterns of presentation of lumbar pain. This is essential to understanding the underlying tissue breakdown. The aim in treatment and management, however, as discussed in Chapters 2 and 4, is to restore normal function where possible and to relieve pain. A diagnosis of a specific tissue damage does not lead to a particular technique or techniques. For instance there is not a set treatment procedure for a disc injury. With a disc problem which has developed recently, the tissue response may be predominantly localized to the lower lumbar area and therefore treatment may be directed only to this area. If the problem has been present for some weeks, then there may well already be secondary somatic dysfunction occurring elsewhere, for instance in the pelvis or further up the spine, and therefore it may be important to deal with this also.

It is essential that the examination at the outset is as thorough as it can be to establish where any abnormal function may be found and to assess what may be causing it. There are occasions when a full examination is not possible, for example when the patient is in acute pain. It is not enough to discover areas of somatic dysfunction and treat them without consideration of the cause of the symptoms, since there may be a problem that requires other more specific treatment, particularly if there is serious pathological tissue breakdown in either viscera or the musculo-skeletal system.

As well as possible reflex interaction with other parts of the body, there may also be mechanical effects on the symptom area as discussed in Chapter 3. It is important to consider all the mechanical influences which may contribute to the problem. Thus, although pain may be caused by damage of a lumbar disc there may be dysfunction in upper lumbar, pelvic or hip areas. There may also be myofascial shortening which is contributing to abnormal function of the area. Treatment of these and other areas may allow more rapid recovery and restoration of normal function of the whole region, rather than merely the disturbed joint.

12 The pelvic ring

The pelvic ring is a key anatomical structure, which is not only responsible for supporting the spinal column, but also houses important organs. The descriptive use of the term 'ring' provides a useful model when studying this complex anatomical basin. It is made up of three component parts: the two large structures which join together anteriorly at the pubic symphysis, the iliac bones, and, posteriorly, the double wedged shaped sacrum. The sacrum is shaped so as to present the characteristics of a double keystone, which is both wider in front than behind and above than below. The obliquity of the joint surfaces means that the articulating parts of the ring are not suitable for weight-bearing. The integrity of the ring is dependent on the strong posterior sacro-iliac ligaments. These act in such a manner as to hold the sacrum between the iliac bones in suspension. In turn the stability of the sacro-iliac joints varies according to the contours of their joint surfaces; the smoother the joint surface, the more unstable the joint. Conversely, the rougher the joint surface, the more stable the joint. This variable also influences the mobility of the joint; the smoother-surfaced joints are the more mobile. The position and make-up of the ring mean that it is in constant mechanical equilibrium, whether it is under load from above or when the subject is recumbent and the soft tissues of the abdomen and thigh dictate the exact 'resting' position of the component parts of the ring. The powerful abdominal muscles attach onto the superior margins of the ring, and the anterior and posterior thigh muscles anchor onto the inferior surfaces. Other influential muscles which play a part in both stability and mobility include the psoas and the lumbar erector spinae. We can begin to see how important both position and soft tissue tone are to the mechanical well-being of the ring (Figure 12.1).

In assessing the causes of pain arising from the pelvis, it is convenient to consider *three* main possible causes:

- Visceral.
- Inflammatory (of the joints).
- Mechanical.

The main emphasis here will be placed on the mechanical causes of pelvic pain, or pain arising from the pelvis leading to remote symptoms.

In the early part of the century an appreciable percentage of low back pain problems were attributed to sacro-iliac disorders or disease. Fusion of the sacro-iliac joint as a form of specific treatment was popularized by Smith-Peterson [81]. Identification of sacro-iliac disease was dependent on the patient's subjective identification of a pain pattern in the posterior thigh, leg and groin, and early writers believed that the most important single diagnostic finding was the localization of tenderness around the inferior sacro-iliac ligaments and the sacro-sciatic notch, together with intra-rectal tenderness at the front of the sacro-iliac joint [137]. More recently, Coventry has reported instances of sacro-iliac laxity and pain, together with symphyseal symptoms which followed the removal of bone grafts from the posterior iliac crest [138]. Historically, dating back to Downing in 1923, osteopaths viewed biomechanical problems of the pelvis as specific lesions. These lesions were initially named on their anatomical findings and purely on a structural basis. Nowadays, however, osteopathic assessment is based on positional, functional and soft tissue findings.

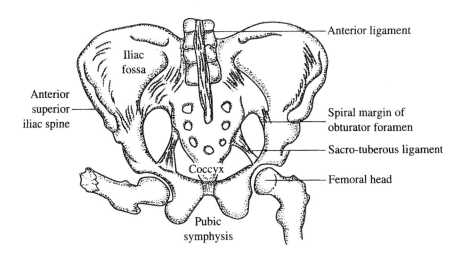

Figure 12.1 Anterior view of the pelvic ring.

The current concepts of dysfunction are clinically used when assessing the pelvic ring. The main identifying features of joint dysfunction are seen below:

- Changes in tissue texture of muscle/connective tissue.
- Altered muscular activity (contraction in the related muscles).
- Altered joint mobility (i.e. abnormal function).
- Altered position.

CLINICAL PRESENTATION

The history

As with any clinical assessment, begin with the patient's description of their problem. The exact location of the site and character of the symptoms are particularly important, as pains of mechanical pelvic origin tend to be precise and very localized.

Once the exact location of the 'primary' focal point of pain is localized, the other sites of discomfort or awareness of symptoms should be explored. Commonly a mild discomfort is felt in the other pelvic joints. For example, a primary injury of the left sacro-iliac joint will be associated with a mild ache of the right sacro-iliac joint, the L5/S1 joint and the pubic-symphysis joint. Patients have been successfully screened for sacro-iliac joint dysfunction based on comparison with a pain referral map generated from sacro-iliac joint injections causing pain in the above areas [67]. Common areas of referral include the postero-lateral aspect of the thigh and posterior knee, the groin region and, in men, the testicles. A slight feeling of 'swelling' is sometimes experienced by patients over the exact site of pain. This observation has been seen as a puffy focal point over the joints when examining the ring.

History of direct trauma is not always present. When present, it is usually linked with a fall directly onto the ring, post-partum injury, or is of a rotatory nature whilst pivoting on the other, weight-bearing limb. For example, the footballer may, with a long and powerful kick, strain one or other of the sacro-iliac joints.

The other major category of causative events is the repetitive minor trauma history. Often the patient recalls a recent period of time where their action was repetitive, biased to one side and mostly with one leg stretched out ahead. Raking garden leaves is a seasonal favourite to aggravate the pelvic ring. This may occur in conjunction with, or as a separate injury to the hip joints, also damage to the lumbar discs, ligaments or muscles.

The history may lead to the following hypotheses

⊗ A localized, primary injury of one of the joints of the pelvic ring with secondary associated mechanical disruptions of the other joints. The patient may or may not present with associated muscular protective posture.

⊗ A primary injury of the related muscle groups which originate from or insert onto the ring, which has ultimately resulted in the disruption of the normal physiology of pelvic ring mechanics.

⊗ Referred pain to the posterior part of the pelvic ring from dysfunction of the lumbar spine or referred pains along the posterior portion of the second and third lumbar dermatome.

⊗ Visceral referred pain. Visceral dysfunction causes pain experienced in related areas of the musculo-skeletal system. One example is seen in endometriosis. This is a disease which occurs when the endometrium that normally lines the uterus lies outside the uterus and causes pelvic pain in 42% of sufferers. The reason for the pelvic pain is attributed to the deposit of endometrial tissue onto the utero-sacral/round ligament. This in turn causes abnormal fixation of the uterus in the retroverted position.

Visceral dysfunction leading to disease of any of the following organs may give rise to referred pain experienced in the pelvic ring:
bladder
kidney, urethra
uterus, ovaries and tubes

lower bowel, rectum, anus.

⊗ Inflammatory condition of the joints such as ankylosing spondilitis, pyogenic arthritis and rheumatoid arthritis.

[handwritten: arthritides!]

The examination

The acute patient

As with any acute condition, the emphasis is placed on taking a thorough history and then allowing the patient to assume a comfortable recumbent position. Details of the recumbent examination will be given later in this chapter. The standing examination is omitted in these cases.

The non-acute patient

Standing

Once the patient is allowed to assume a comfortable standing position, the examiner should observe carefully the weight-bearing posture. In many cases, an apparent 'spiral' standing position is assumed; this posture combines anterior or posterior weight-bearing with left or right weight-bearing. These combined positions seem to offer the least pain, when standing, in cases of pelvic ring dysfunction. For example, if the pain is localized to the left side, the standing posture of choice may be right weight-bearing with an anterior tendency. These presentations are likely, but not invariable. It is, however, important to acknowledge their occurrence in order to assess fully the other musculo-skeletal structures associated with this adaptation.

[handwritten: Standing obs]

[handwritten: weight-bearing - antalgic?]

The static tone of the large muscle groups related to the pelvis is noted and compared for any changes in muscle states. Note any compensatory scoliosis (see Chapter 7). Focusing more locally, observe for visible signs of swelling or redness over parts that have been isolated as painful areas by the patient.

[handwritten: tone]
[handwritten: swelling]
[handwritten: pelvic levels]

The prime important point to establish is the level of the pelvis. This will be the first indicator of the underlying reason for any potential disruption of the ring. The patient should be barefoot when examined, with both legs close together and extended at the knees. The examiner places the fingertips of his hands on the pelvic brims on each side. By assessing the horizontal levels of his fingertips, the examiner can establish the level of the iliac crests. The following procedure is used to assess the posterior superior iliac spines (PSIS). The 'dimples' noted in most people in the region of the sacro-iliac joints can be lined up by the eye and provide a fairly accurate estimate of the pelvic level. Anteriorly, the levels of the anterior superior iliac spine (ASIS) must be noted (Figure 12.2).

*[handwritten: levels - crests
PSIS
ASIS]*

Once a difference is noted, the amount can be estimated by adding cards of known thickness under the apparently shorter of the two limbs. Using the landmarks as before (the levels of the iliac crests, the PSIS and the ASIS), cards are added under the shorter of the lower limbs until the levels become equal (Figure 12.3).

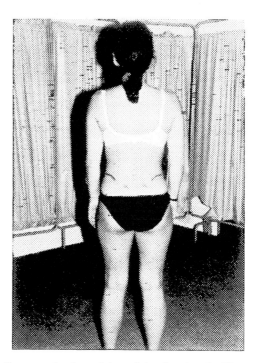

Figure 12.2 Standing examination of the pelvis, showing the iliac crests, the posterior superior iliac spines and the spinous processes.

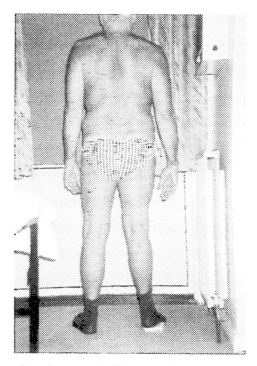

Figure 12.3 Illustration of how cards of known height can be inserted under the heel to equalize the level of the pelvis in cases where there is a discrepancy.

The articulations that must be considered in all pelvic examinations include the hip joints, the sacro-iliac joints, the pubic symphysis joint and the lumbo-sacral joint (Figure 12.4A).

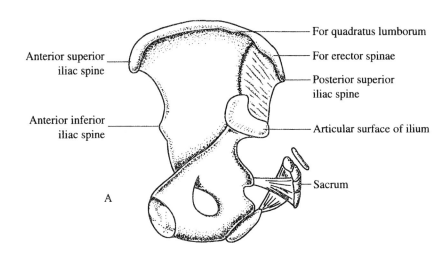

Anterior superior iliac spine

Anterior inferior iliac spine

A

For quadratus lumborum

For erector spinae

Posterior superior iliac spine

Articular surface of ilium

Sacrum

Interosseous sacro-iliac ligaments

Sulcus

Posterior superior iliac spine

Sacrum

B

Figure 12.4 A. Inner surface of ilium, showing the landmarks used in assessing the pelvic ring. B. Transverse section of the sacro-iliac joints.

The tone of the muscular attachments both from above and below must be carefully noted and compared. The relative position of the PSIS with reference to the posterior surface of the sacrum is established. The depression created by their relative position forms a 'sulcus' (Figure 12.4B).

The two sides are compared and any obvious difference should be analysed. As a rule of thumb, a deep sulcus is one indicator that the iliac on that side has rotated backwards. Vice versa, a shallow sulcus points to an anterior rotation of the iliac bone. The distance between the PSIS and the sacral spinous processes is also noted. Approximation of the PSIS to the midline on the posterior surface of the sacrum, which is made up of the fused spinous processes, is yet another indicator of a posterior rotation of the iliac bone on that side. The significance of these points of reference can be appreciated more when we

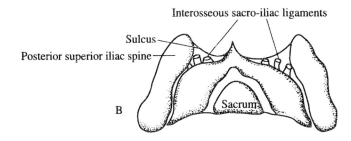

assess

- deep SI sulcus suggests posteriorised ilium
- shallow SI sulcus suggests anteriorised ilium

look at the classification of pelvic ring dysfunction according to Downing, later in this chapter.

The patient is then seen under uneven load. This can be easily done by asking her to stand with one foot forward and then transferring her body weight from one leg to the other. This diagonal transference introduces a torsional twist to the pelvic ring, which then highlights any lack of or excessive movement in any of the components of the pelvis.

Having established the influence of gravity on the pelvis, now assess what happens in the recumbent posture.

Recumbent

Initially the patient is asked to assume the supine position. Here the lower abdomen can be viewed and palpated. Next focus on the femoral triangle. Any localized swellings can be palpated and assessed. Commonly inguinal hernias are noticed. It must, however, be remembered that small ones may disappear when supine. Swollen lymph nodes can also be found.

The hips can be examined by rolling them, that is, gently rotating them internally and externally. The pubic symphysis can be palpated for any differences in levels and for any excessive movement. The anterior sacro-iliac ligaments are tested by fixing the inner surfaces of the ASIS and gently pushing them outwards (Figure 12.5). Any excessive movement on one or other side will indicate ligamentous laxity and damage.

The reverse compressive action of the iliac bones tests the posterior sacro-iliac ligaments (Figure 12.6). This test is also diagnostically positive when pain is reproduced locally to the ligaments.

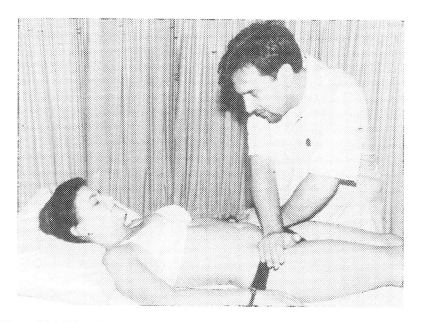

Figure 12.5 Clinical testing of the anterior sacro-iliac ligaments can be achieved by gently pushing apart the inner surface of the anterior superior iliac spines.

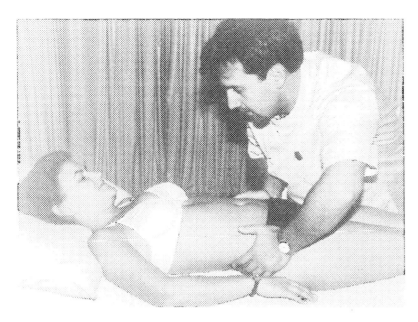

Figure 12.6 Clinical testing of the posterior sacro-iliac ligaments can be achieved by gently approximating the anterior superior iliac spines.

To test the individual movement of the sacro-iliac joints, the patient should be positioned side-lying and asked to grasp gently the flexed hip of the side they are lying on. This flexes the lumbar spine and minimizes the spinal movement. A rotatory movement should be applied by the practitioner, while gently grasping the iliac crest of the uppermost side. This is done by extending the uppermost hip, using the thigh as a lever. The palpating finger should gauge the amount and quality of movement of the joint. The travel at this joint is very small. Careful palpation, however, will reveal some 'give' in the joint. An additional finite movement can be felt by moving the sacrum relative to the ilium. Again the fingertips will act as both the generators of movement and as the monitors of the actual range. A freely moving joint should allow a definite springing sensation of the sacro-iliac ligaments. The movement will be that of the sacrum moving in relation to the ilium and vice versa. Once both sides are assessed and compared, the patient is then asked to assume the prone position if able to do so. A light palpating hand presses down on the apex of the sacrum. This has a resultant flexing action on the base of the sacrum. The relative movement of the L5 on the sacrum is then felt.

Amongst the soft tissues to be examined are the quadratus lumborum, the ilio-psoas, the gluteals and the thigh musculature.

MECHANICAL DYSFUNCTION OF THE PELVIC RING

Having looked at ways of assessing the moving parts of the ring, it can be seen that there are many potential sites of mechanical dysfunction. The sacro-iliac joints are among the most common sites of problems within the ring. Being a highly ligamentous mechanism and naturally playing a key part in childbirth, the sacro-iliac joints are particularly vulnerable during pregnancy. Problems can occur, however, at any other time, especially when a pivoting action is carried out whilst weight-bearing on one leg only.

Downing [99] described a wide variety of sacro-iliac 'lesions'. It is not clear whether these were meant to be absolute or merely an abstract interpretation of functional anatomy. The term 'lesions' was then used generally to describe a fixation of the joint and more modern schools of thought place a wider, balanced view on both joint dysfunction as well as soft tissue involvement. Downing's classification is, however, a very useful way of creating a mental image of how clinically a pelvic ring may be functionally disrupted.

The various types of pelvic dysfunctions classified below may present clinically with very similar sympton patterns. We aim to differentiate the dysfunctions as follows: Using Downing's classification, we work on the basis that sacro-iliac joints should allow a limited amount of movement. When a normally moving joint is found to be fixed at its extreme end of movement, the fixation is classified according to the position of the end point of the ilium in relation to the sacrum.

So, when one of the iliac bones has travelled in a forward direction and becomes fixed at its anterior-most end of range, it is called a unilateral anterior innominate. This same condition has also been termed a unilateral sacral counter-nutation.

Working with the concept of the 'pelvic ring', how the related bony structures are influenced with each permutation can easily be deduced. An anterior innominate, therefore, will have a shallower sulcus between the posterior surface of the sacrum and the posterior superior iliac spine (PSIS). The PSIS will be further from the midline/sacral spines. The contour of the buttock will appear larger on the same side. The pubic symphysis will be stepped, being lower on the side of fixation. In practice some of the conditions below are found more commonly than others, but it is important to be aware of all of them.

Classification of pelvic ring dysfunction (according to Downing, 1923 [99])

- Unilateral anterior innominate (unilateral sacral counter-nutation).
- Unilateral posterior innominate (unilateral sacral nutation).
- Bilateral posterior innominates (bilateral sacral nutation).
- Bilateral anterior innominates (bilateral sacral counter-nutation).
- True twisted pelvis: combined unilateral posterior/unilateral anterior innominate on the opposite side.
- Pseudo twisted pelvis: apparent asymmetry of the pelvis due to imbalanced lumbar muscle tension and L5 rotation. There will be a resultant compensatory functional scoliosis (see 'Spinal curves in practice' in Chapter 7). This is probably due to the tension pull of the ilio-lumbar ligament and the contracted state of the surrounding musculature.

The main significance in identifying these positional lesions is that in some osteopathic techniques, different lesions are corrected in specific ways (see Chapter 4).

The isolated hypermobile joints are probably the most difficult cases of sacro-iliac joint dysfunction to manage clinically. These are identified by their excessive travel, even with gentle and light palpatory pressure. The clinical picture can vary greatly in the same patient, with the end point of the joint movement changing from anterior innominate to posterior innominate, with a mere change in weight-bearing. These extreme changes in end point are often accompanied by repeated episodes of inflammatory changes within the joints. They are experienced as episodes of severe pain and tenderness localized to the joint, with occasional referred pain into the thigh.

Practical application

Once the pelvis is assessed within the criteria listed above, manipulative corrective techniques can be applied to correct and restore the imbalance back to the 'normal' position. This 'correction' will take into consideration the state of the associated soft tissues as well as the joint disfunction. On a broader scale, the postural adaptation may also be worked on and any lower limb length difference may have to be made up using inserts in the shoe or building up the sole of the shoe.

Other causes of sacro-iliac pain

Ankylosing spondylitis

Although it may affect a larger part of the spine, this condition usually begins in the sacro-iliac joints and the patient may present initially with sacro-iliac pain. In a related condition, sacro-ileitis, the radiological changes resemble those of ankylosing spondylitis, but the remainder of the spine is unaffected.

Tuberculosis of a sacro-iliac joint

The patient is a child or a young adult. The condition is usually confined to one side, but it may be bilateral. As in tuberculous disease of other joints, there is destruction of articular cartilage and thickening of the synovial membrane, often with erosion of bone and abscess formation. Clinically, the main feature is pain in the affected joint and in the iliac fossa and groin. A diffuse, ill-localized pain may be referred down the lower limb. Examination shows restriction of lower spinal movements, and side to side compression of the pelvis aggravates the pain. An abscess is often palpable posteriorly or in the iliac fossa. Radiographs show local rarefaction, with loss of definition or 'fuzziness' of the joint outline.

Other forms of sacro-iliac arthritis [85]

Pyogenic arthritis

This is relatively uncommon. Its general features conform with those of pyogenic arthritis elsewhere. The joint becomes infected by bacteria of one of the pyogenic groups. Typically there is acute joint infection of rapid development, but the infection may be subacute or even chronic.

Rheumatoid arthritis

The sacro-iliac joints may be affected in common with the other joints of the spine, usually in the later stages of the condition.

Osteoarthritis

This is uncommon and seldom, if ever, the cause of serious disability.

The coccyx

There are many variations found in the structure of this bone. Although they are not of great practical significance, anomalies in the region may tend to confuse palpation findings. This is particularly so when coccydynia is of recent traumatic origin, but the coccyx had been deviated from birth. Referred pain and referred diffuse tenderness frequently occur in the coccygeal region from joint problems at the lumbosacral segment and in ankylosing spondylitis. A traumatic periostitis can occur after a force is applied to the bone tip. Similar traumas can be responsible for strain of the soft tissues; these strains are also seen in childbirth.

The pubic symphysis

The two pubic bones are united anteriorly by the strong arcuate ligament at the pubic symphysis joint. As with all synovial joints, it undergoes small changes at the surface and joint margins. These changes can be responsible for dull, deep aching symptoms and present with marked tenderness on palpation. Dysfunctions of the pelvic ring can be reflected at this joint by palpating an uneven level anteriorly at the joint margin. Although changes at the joint itself do not present any great clinical significance, the adjacent parts of the joint are important anchoring points for large adducting muscles of the thigh. Traumatic periostitis can occur in forced movements of the lower limb, as seen in football or dancing injuries. In dancers this is a common site of pain, characterized by sudden or maybe gradual onset of discomfort in the fleshy part of the inside of the leg below the crotch. Possible causes include a change of technique, for example from ballet to modern dance. When this is a traumatic injury it may be caused by violent acceleration or deceleration, with no previous stretching or inadequate warm-up.

The lower limbs 13

The lower limbs are primarily seen as the providers of locomotion, but another major role is their supportive role in spinal mechanics. That is to say, the lower limbs are responsible for the way in which the spine settles on top of the pelvis, in both the static and the dynamic state. Proprioceptive messages conveyed from the lower limbs are responsible for the postural adaptation of the spinal musculature and spinal curves to maintain the body balanced in the upright position. It is therefore extremely important to examine the effect of the local area of dysfunction on the whole lower extremity; the postural adaptation to the local dysfunction as well as the actual site giving rise to pain within the lower extremity.

In terms of clinical presentation, the symptoms in the lower limbs can be divided into two major groups: the 'primary' or 'local' problems of the limbs themselves, and the 'secondary' or 'referred' problems, which are felt in the limbs, even though their site of origin is distant.

LOCAL PROBLEMS

A standard diagnostic thought process can be applied to this group. Initially problems which arise as a result of local pathologies of the bones themselves must be considered. The group will include bone disorders, for example osteosarcoma. This is the most common of the primary bone tumours. Joint problems, which vary according to their altered physiological state, will be considered individually later in the chapter. The soft tissue injuries will also be considered individually, followed by the congenital defects of the limbs themselves. Finally, vascular problems, which include local varicosities, ulcerations or obstructions, will be considered.

Neurological problems of primary origin are seen when nerve trunks are compressed and damaged; for example, a peroneal nerve damaged in a horse riding accident. This will show the classic signs of nerve damage to all structures, supplied by the nerve, beyond the site of injury.

REFERRED PROBLEMS

These can be defined as any problem which has its aetiology or source of origin at a site distant from the limbs themselves. A general metabolic problem, for example gout, may prompt a patient to present to an osteopath with a painful and swollen joint in the foot. A generalized ischaemic vascular disease may present clinically as pain in the calves.

Nerve root pain, somatic referred pain or visceral referred pain from a distant site can present with solely lower limb pains. In a case of pain in the thigh, the examination will often have to include a study of the spine, abdomen, pelvis and genito-urinary system, as well as local examination of the hip and thigh.

REASONS FOR EXAMINING THE LOWER LIMBS

The lower limbs should be examined for *two* reasons. The first is to gain a general impression of the limbs in respect of the rest of the body. This may reveal evidence of any general medical problems, trophic changes of the skin, vascular problems and so on. Measurement of the limb length is often necessary, where the discrepancy between the two sides is important. Measurement of the circumference of a limb segment on the two sides provides an index of muscle wasting, soft tissue swelling or bony thickening.

The second reason is to identify a primary problem of the limb itself.

'A general impression'

It is essential that the part to be examined should be adequately exposed. A systematic inspection should include the following points: the bones should be observed for general alignment and position, to detect any deformity and shortening or unusual posture when in the standing position. The soft tissue contours should be compared on the two sides; noting any evidence of general or local swelling, or of muscle wasting. A close examination of the pelvic levels should be carried out to detect the influence of the lower limbs on the pelvis and spine. The reader is advised to read Chapters 12 ('Pelvic ring') and 7 ('Spinal curves') to achieve an integrated and coherent understanding of these areas.

'Identification of the primary problem'

There are four main points to consider:

1. *Skin temperature.* By careful comparison of the two sides judge whether there is an area of increased warmth or of unusual coldness. An increase of local temperature denotes increased vascularity. The usual cause is an inflammatory reaction, but it should be remembered that a rapidly growing tumour may also bring about marked local hyperaemia.
2. *The bones.* The general shape and outline of the bones should be investigated. Feel in particular for thickening, abnormal prominence, or disturbed relationship of the normal landmarks.

3. *The soft tissues.* Direct particular attention to the muscles (are they in spasm, or wasted?), to the joint tissues (is the synovial membrane thickened, or the joint distended with fluid?) and to the detection of local swelling (cyst?; tumour?) or general swelling of the part.
4. *Local tenderness.* The exact site of any local tenderness should be determined and an attempt made to relate it to a particular structure.

CLINICAL ASSESSMENT

Determining the cause of a diffuse joint swelling

Palpation of the joint is probably the most accurate way of determining the cause of joint swelling.

For practical purposes, a diffuse joint can have only *three* causes:

1. Thickening of the bone end: this is detected by deep palpation through the soft tissues, the two sides then being compared.
2. Fluid within the joint: this gives the feeling of fluctuation of fluid between the two hands.
3. Thickening of the synovial membrane: this gives a characteristic boggy sensation, which can be described as a layer of rubber between the skin and the bone.

Sometimes two or all three causes may be combined.

Movements

In the examination of joint movements certain information must be established:

- What is the range of active movement?
- Is passive movement greater than active?
- Is movement painful?
- Is the movement accompanied by crepitation?

In measuring the range of movement it is important to know what is the normal. With some joints the normal varies considerably from patient to patient, so it is always wise to use the unaffected limb for comparison. Limitation of movement in all directions suggests some form of arthritis, whereas selective limitation of movement in some directions, with free movement in others, is more suggestive of a mechanical derangement. Except in two sets of circumstances, passive movement will usually be found to be equal to the active. The passive range will exceed the active only in the following conditions:

- When the muscles responsible for the movements are paralysed.
- When the muscles or the tendons are torn, severed or unduly slack.

Stability

The stability of a joint depends partly upon the integrity of its articulating surfaces and partly upon intact ligaments. When a joint is unstable there is abnormal mobility; for instance, lateral mobility in a knee joint. It is important, when testing for abnormal mobility, to ensure that the muscles controlling the joint are relaxed. A muscle which is in strong contraction can often conceal ligamentous instability.

Peripheral circulation

Symptoms in a limb may be associated with impairment of the arterial circulation. Time should be spent in assessing the state of the circulation by examination of the colour and temperature of the skin, the texture of the skin and nails, and the arterial pulses. This examination is particularly important in the case of the lower limbs.

THE HIP

The hip region presents probably the most fascinating problems in the lower limb. It is the most difficult joint to examine accurately in the lower limb. This is because of the large and strong muscular tissues which act upon it. Problems within the hip can lead to complications in gait and spinal mechanics.

Points to note in evaluating hip pain

The characteristics of hip pain

- Pain in the region of the hip is notoriously misleading as it is often referred from the spine or pelvis and has no connection with the hip joint itself. Therefore, one must always be cautious in attributing such pain to a hip lesion without first investigating the possibility of a distant cause.
- Pain arising in the hip is felt most commonly in the groin and in the front or inner side of the thigh. Pain is often referred also to the knee, and frequently this is the predominant feature. In contrast, the 'hip' pain that is felt mainly in the gluteal region and radiates down the back of the thigh is referred from the spine.
- Pain arising from the joint itself is made worse by walking, whereas buttock pain referred from the spine is aggravated by activities such as stooping and lifting, and it is often eased by walking.

Many of the important hip disorders occur in childhood, and often at a particular period of childhood.

Clinical examination of the hip

Gait

Observe the patient walk and stand still. A patient using a walking stick will always use it on the opposite side of the painful hip. Look out for any altered weight-bearing or preference to walk more on one or other leg.

Recumbent examination

As a preliminary step, it is important initially to *set the pelvis square* on the examination table. It is customary to use the anterior superior iliac spines as guides. If it is impossible to set the pelvis square, it means that there is an adduction or abduction deformity of one or other hip. This should be noted and taken into consideration in later stages of the examination.

Measuring the length of the limbs (Figure 13.1)

Accuracy in measurement of the lower limbs is in most cases of academic significance. Estimated differences, however, are important when compiling a total evaluative picture. Measure from the anterior superior iliac spine to the medial malleolus.

If discrepancy is found, determine the site of shortening:

- Above the trochanter; this indicates an intrinsic hip problem.
- Below the trochanter; one must determine which of the bones are causative.

Measure the lengths from the greater trochanter to the line of the knee joint for femoral length. Determine the length of the tibia by measuring from the line of the knee joint to the medial malleolus on each side. This may show a true shortening arising from a congenital defect of development or the result of a previous injury or trauma.

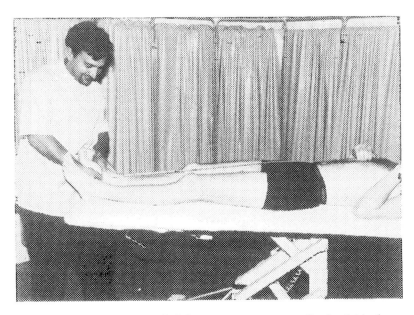

Figure 13.1 Measuring leg length. It is customary to use any fixed point in the midline, for example the xiphisternum to the medial malleolus.

'Apparent' or false discrepancy in limb length is due entirely to incorrectible sideways tilting of the pelvis. The usual cause is a fixed adduction deformity of the hip, giving an appearance of shortening of that side, or a fixed abduction deformity, giving an appearance of lengthening. Occasionally fixed pelvic obliquity is caused by severe lumbar scoliosis. To measure this discrepancy it is usual to use any fixed point in the midline of the trunk, for example, the xiphisternum to the medial malleolus.

Determining 'fixed' deformities

Contractures of the joint capsule or of muscles prevent the hip from being placed in a neutral position.

Normal movements

The normal movements of the hip joints must be assessed carefully and accurately, to ensure that the movement assessed is coming from the hip joint, and not from the pelvis and lower back. This can be achieved by placing one hand on the pelvis, to detect any movement there, whilst the other, guides and supports the limb (Figure 13.2).

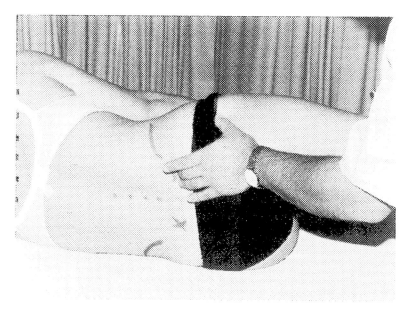

Figure 13.2 Clinical assessment of true hip joint mobility whilst ensuring that there is no lower back or pelvic movement.

Flexion

The normal amount of flexion is about 120 degrees. This is tested with the patient supine; one hand grips the ilium to detect incipient rotation of the pelvis, while the other hand flexes and supports the limb.

Abduction
The limb to be tested is supported by one hand, while the other forearm spans from one anterior superior spine to the other anterior superior spine; this resting forearm is used to stabilize the pelvis and keep it flat on the examining table. In this way true abduction at the hip can be determined. The normal range is between 30 and 40 degrees.

Abduction in flexion
This is often the first movement to suffer restriction in arthritis of the hip. The normal range is about 70 degrees.

Adduction
The limb to be examined is crossed over the other limb. The normal range of adduction is about 30 degrees.

Lateral and medial rotation
The distance travelled should be judged from an imaginary line taken axially from the patella and not from foot travel. This combined range is about 80 degrees.

Extension
Contrary to what has often been written, the range of extension at the hip joint is negligible. Apparent, backward movement of the thigh is almost entirely by rotation of the pelvis and extension of the spine, not by extension at the hip joint.

Examination for postural stability: the Trendelenburg test

The manoeuvre is a test for stability of the hip, and particularly of the hip abductors (gluteus medius and gluteus minimus), to stabilize the pelvis upon the femur. This works on the principle of the hip abductors' ability to lift the pelvis up when the leg on the same side is lifted off the ground. If the abductors are inefficient they are unable to sustain the pelvis against the body weight and it tilts downwards instead of rising on the side of the lifted leg.

There are three fundamental causes for a positive Trendelenburg test:

1. Paralysis of the abductor muscles.
2. Upward displacement of the trochanter – as seen in severe coxa vara. This results in marked approximation of the insertion of the muscles to their origin.
3. Absence of a stable fulcrum – as seen in an ununited fracture of the femoral neck.

Osteoarthritis of the hip and capsular strain

Osteoarthritis, as well as all its pre-clinical and associated sequences of events related to hip disease, is by far the most common of the hip conditions seen in osteopathic practice. Although it is often thought of as a disorder of the elderly, many younger patients present with symptoms associated with osteoarthritic changes.

Classification of disorders in the hip region (Table 13.1) [85]

Table 13.1 Articular disorders of the hip

Congenital deformities
Congenital dislocation of the hip
Arthritis
Transient synovitis in children
Pyogenic arthritis
Rheumatoid arthritis
Tuberculous arthritis
Osteoarthritis
Osteochondritis
Perthe's disease
Mechanical disorders
Slipped upper femoral epiphysis
Capsular overstrain

In younger patients, it is particularly seen in those who have suffered previous damage from injury or disease. It is generally caused by wear and tear. Any injury or disease that damages the joint surface accelerates wear and tear. However, commonly seen in practice are conditions which are very similar to classical osteoarthritis of the hip. The fundamental difference is that there is *no* radiographic evidence of changes of the architecture of the joint surface. Careful and specific examination of passive hip joint movements will reveal particular limitations. These problems can be attributed to injuries of the hip joint capsule. For diagnostic convenience, instances of capsular strain can be subdivided into those of sudden traumatic origin and those of repeated minor traumatic origin.

Sudden traumatic origin

In this type the patient will have suffered one specific trauma to the hip, as seen in a football injury. The pain can be localized to the buttock and groin area and can be very severe at first. This subsides with rest. After a week to 10 days, the patient becomes aware of a deep and nagging pain, which is aggravated with certain movements. The aggravating movements are particular to the part of the joint capsule which has been overstrained in the original injury. There may or may not be associated referred pain to the knee.

Repeated minor traumatic origin

This injury is the sequel to a repeated mechanical injury to the hip joint, particularly as a result of unaccustomed movements. The most striking example is seen in horse riders. Regular riding, particularly for the novice rider, may excessively strain one or both hip joint capsules. The pain is often felt deep inside the groin. It may also result in buttock pain. The degree of discomfort can be regulated by altering the joint position at rest.

Both of these groups will have associated changes to the related muscle groups.

Clinically, in osteoarthritis, the pain is in the groin and front of the thigh, often also in the knee and sometimes exclusively in the knee. The pain is made worse by walking and eased by rest. Later stiffness becomes the main complaint and eventually the patient develops a painful limp.

On examination, all hip movements are impaired. Limitation of abduction, adduction and rotation is marked, but a good range of flexion is preserved. Forced movements are all painful. A fixed deformity (flexion, adduction or lateral rotation, or a combination of these) is common.

Radiographic examinations will show the characteristic changes seen in osteoarthritis. There is diminution of cartilage space, with a tendency to sclerosis of the surface bone. Osteophyte formation is usually seen at the joint surface.

A developed sense of palpatory accuracy can allow the osteopath to make specific decisions as to which part or parts of the joint capsule are affected in the presenting complaint. The quality, range and end feel of joint movement can reveal the presence of even mild changes within the joint itself. The 'quality' can be defined as the resistance felt during the range of movement and 'end-feel of joint movement' is the mounting resistance felt towards the end of range, which then comes to a sudden and definite stop. Radiographic confirmation of joint surface damage will only contribute to the prognosis of the case.

The management will be directly related to:

- Type of onset.
- General physical state of the patient.
- Degree and nature of muscular adaptation to the condition which the hip, thigh and lower back muscles have undergone.
- Effect of daily habits and occupational demands on hip joint function.
- Patient contribution to rehabilitation programme.

Snapping hips

This is another common complaint, particularly among young and active people. Although it is a harmless condition, it can often lead to great anxiety. A distinct snap is heard and felt on certain movements of the joint. It does not denote any underlying injury or disease and it is of no practical significance. The snap is attributed to slipping of a tendinous thickening in the aponeurosis of the gluteus maximus over the bony prominence of the greater trochanter.

Extrinsic disorders giving rise to pain in the hip

For diagnostic ease, these can be divided into three main categories:

Disorders of the spine or sacro-iliac disease

The pain of a slight or moderate disc injury is commonly referred to the gluteal region or lateral aspect of the thigh. On examination there is usually evidence of a spinal disorder, whereas the hip itself will be clinically and radiographically normal.

The pain caused by arthritis of the sacro-iliac joint, whether it be tuberculous, pyogenic osteoarthritis or the early stages of ankylosing spondylitis, spreads diffusely over the gluteal area and may simulate an affection of the hip.

Disorders of the abdomen and pelvis

Inflammation involving the side wall of the abdomen may mimic a hip problem. The condition responsible is usually a deep peri-appendicular abscess. The hip symptoms arise partly from irritation of the obturator nerve, causing referred pain in the thigh, and partly irritative spasm of the hip muscles, namely the psoas, iliacus, pyriformis and obturator internus.

Differentiation from a hip lesion depends on a careful history and on examination which includes the pelvis and abdomen.

Occlusive vascular disease

Thrombosis of the lower aorta may cause ischaemic pain in the muscles of the buttock or thigh. This is from occlusion of the aorta or its main branches. Diagnosis should not be difficult. In occlusive vascular disease the pain is brought on immediately by activity and quickly relieved by rest. The femoral pulses will be weak or absent. The hip movement will be full and painless.

THE KNEE AND THIGH

The knee joint is a technically interesting area as it is a site where many of the principles of bone and joint disorders may be represented. The stability of the joint is highly dependent upon the quadriceps muscle as well as its four main ligaments. A rapid and striking wasting of the quadriceps can be observed in many presenting knee injuries. The efficiency of the quadriceps is particularly observed when the muscles can be seen to maintain stability of the knee, even in the presence of considerable ligamentous laxity. Apart from its vulnerability to traumatic injury, the knee is prone to almost every kind of arthritis.

Investigation of the knee and thigh

The precise history is of particular importance in assessing the disorders of the knee. In the event of a previous trauma, the exact sequence of events at the time of the injury as well as afterwards must be ascertained. There is a need to know the detail of the mechanism of the injury. What was the patient doing at the time and was it possible to carry on afterwards? If the patient suffered a football injury, was she able to finish the game? If not, was she carried off the field or was she able to walk?

Clarifying the terms used is also important. For example, 'locking' is often used to mean stiff and painful. True locking in a meniscus injury, means that the knee cannot be straightened fully, although it can usually be flexed relatively freely. Locking, however, which arises from a loose body within the joint, means that the joint cannot be flexed or extended.

Examination of the knee

A complete knee examination necessitates full exposure of both knees, with the patient lying recumbent.

Suggested clinical examination

The history will have suggested the presence of knee symptoms as a result of local injury or as one manifestation of a widespread disease.

Mechanical investigations of the hip and spine will have revealed any associated symptoms and dysfunction.

Inspection

Colour, texture and scars on the knee are surveyed.

The contours of the soft tissues, particularly of the quadriceps, are carefully assessed. The bone contours and alignment are also examined.

Palpation

Palpate for general temperature, skin and soft tissue contours as well as local areas of swelling. Measure equivalent places for soft tissue bulk comparison or for diffuse swelling within the knee. The knee can swell for three main reasons:

1. Thickening of bone caused mainly from osteophytes at the joint margin or perhaps from a bone infection or tumour.
2. Fluid within the joint. This develops slowly from 12 to 24 hours after an injury. The tension is never as great as with a haemarthrosis. This effusion of blood appears within an hour or two of injury. An effusion of pus is usually associated with general illness and pyrexia.
3. Thickening of the synovial membrane. A thickened synovial membrane is always a prominent feature of chronic inflammatory arthritis. A suprapatellar pouch develops, which characteristically feels boggy on palpation and has a warm area of overlying skin.

Movement

There must be accurate assessment of movement together with the amount of accompanying pain and crepitation. The normal range of flexion varies with the build of the patient. The range of the sound knee must be taken as the norm for that individual. Use the sound knee as the yardstick for extension, note that even a slight impairment will indicate a deformity.

Stability of the knee will depend on the integrity of the main ligaments. The ligaments should be tested in turn. Medial, lateral, anterior and posterior ligaments are usually tested when the patient is in the supine position.

The McMurray test is used in cases of suspected tears of the menisci. The manoeuvre will result in an audible loud click, which is heard and felt as the knee is straightened.

Intra-articular disorders of the knee

Because the knee is so exposed to injury, it is the most common joint to be subjected to pyogenic infections. Pyogenic arthritis is typically experienced as acute pain and swelling, with marked loss of function; there may or may not be a history of trauma and there may or may not be a visible site of infection. When both knee joints present with severe pain and stiffness, simultaneously with other joints, rheumatoid arthritis must be suspected and further tests performed.

Osteoarthritis

Probably the most common form of arthritis to be presented in practice is osteoarthritis. The knee is affected more often than any other joint. Overweight is the most common factor for the wear and tear, but previous trauma, or fractures causing irregularity of the joint surfaces and malalignment of the femur on the tibia, can also predispose to osteoarthritis. Clinically, the condition can be recognized by moderate reduction in movement, accompanied by crepitation. Early signs of the condition can be seen in 'spiking' of the articular margins of the patella. The quadriceps muscle may be wasted. In severe cases, there is a tendency to fixed flexion deformity. The knee will feel thickened, particularly at the joint margins. This is from the hypertrophy of the joint margins (Figure 13.3).

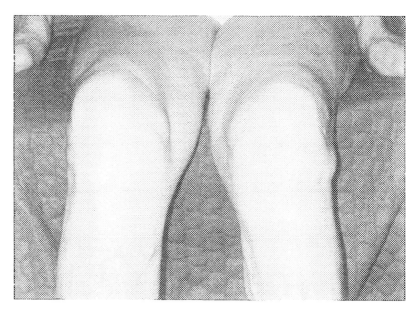

Figure 13.3 Osteoarthritis of the knee joints, showing the characteristic thickening of the articular margins as well as wasting of the quadriceps muscles.

Chondromalacia of the patella

This is typically an affection of adolescents or young adults. Here the articular surface of the patella is roughened and fibrillated. Although chondromalacia is different from patello-femoral osteoarthritis, it may be a predisposing factor. Clinically, pain and tenderness is felt behind the knee cap. This is made worse by climbing or descending stairs. Some crepitation is felt during all patello-femoral movements.

Osteochondritis dissecans

This is another knee condition which is seen in adolescents and young adults. Although the cause is unknown, the mechanism resulting in the condition is a local impairment of blood supply. Necrosis of a small area results in a loose body. The patient experiences discomfort and pain in the knee after exercise, with intermittent swelling. Locking can also be a feature.

Tears of the menisci

These are perhaps among the most common of the injuries sustained on the sports field. The medial meniscus is torn much more commonly than the lateral.

Clinically, the patient will report a sudden twisting injury with immediate pain at the joint margin. The knee immediately stiffens and it is almost impossible to straighten fully. The following day the knee swells and, with rest, returns to normal within 2 weeks. A subsequent twisting trauma, however, can give rise to sudden giving way of the knee. Swelling soon follows. Similar incidents occur repeatedly. True locking of the knee is said to be the inability to extend fully. The flexion range is retained. This characteristic is not always present, as extension can often be achieved if performed slowly. Clinical features of a torn lateral meniscus are broadly similar. The picture is often less well defined. The history may be vague. Pain is in the lateral rather than the medial side of the joint. Many types of tears can be defined within the structure of the menisci. The practitioner, however, should be concerned just to identify the presence of a tear, leaving its exact location to be sought by the orthopaedic colleague.

A *cyst* of the meniscus can be identified as a solid swelling at the level of the joint. Usually on the lateral side. These cysts arise spontaneously. Clinically, there is a history of night pain in the joint and a tender point. The cyst is usually very tense and cannot be fluctuated.

Sometimes, however accurate the patient is in recounting her story, and however detailed the practitioner's history taking, it can seem impossible to isolate the exact cause of the presenting problem. Isolating the exact aetiology of joint locking can be the most frustrating exercise in evaluating a knee joint.

In principle it is a mechanism which has either resulted in the formation of a loose body or the development of a loose structure within the joint, as seen in certain types of menisci tears. The causes of the loose body may be osteoarthritis, osteochondritis, chip fracture of a joint surface or synovial chondromatosis. Having at least established a history of a loose body, refer the patient for further orthopaedic examinations.

Extra-articular disorders of the knee

Most cases of knee pain have their origin in or very near the joint itself. In some cases, however, pain in the knee can be the predominant feature of problems of the hip. This is particularly the case in arthritis of the hip or slipped epiphysis. Less commonly, a disc lesion in the upper lumbar areas can give rise to pains in the hip.

Recurrent dislocation of the patella

Trouble usually starts during adolescence or in early adult life. Often both knees are affected and there is a clinical picture of sudden pain in the front of the knee, when the patient is flexed or semi-flexed. This is followed by inability to straighten the knee and the patellar displacement is clearly seen.

This condition is often associated with general laxity of ligaments. It is more likely to present as part of an overall history, rather than a primary condition. Some children, particularly those who take part in sporting physical activities, can present with sharp pains of the tibial tubercle. This self-limiting condition, commonly known as Osgood–Schlatter disease, is an apophysitis of the tibial tubercle. It is caused by a strain of the tubercle from the pull of the patellar tendon.

Bursitis of the knee

This is commonly found, particularly among people who spend long periods of time kneeling. The most commonly known form, and the one with the highest incidence clinically, is the pre-patellar bursitis. A soft and fluctuant swelling is found in front of the lower part of the patella ('housemaid's knee'). The swelling is clearly demarcated.

Baker's cyst

This is another commonly found swelling at the back of the knee. This is simply a herniation of the synovial cavity of the knee, with formation of a fluid-filled sac which extends backwards and downwards. This is not a primary condition, but is always a state secondary to a disorder of the knee with a resultant persistent synovial effusion, such as rheumatoid arthritis or osteoarthritis.

Ligament strain

Both lateral and medial ligaments can easily be strained, particularly in sporting activity. The pain is localized to the attachments of the ligaments onto the bone and is usually due to local inflammatory reaction, as a result of periosteal lifting at the site of attachment. The pain can be reproduced clinically by gapping the knee, that is applying a separating force, either medially to gap the knee to test the medial ligament (Figure 13.4) or laterally to gap the knee to test the lateral ligament.

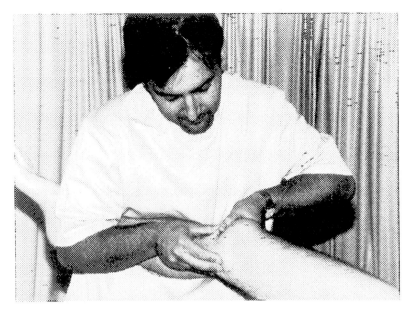

Figure 13.4 Clinically testing the medial ligament of the knee. A separating force is applied to the lateral side of the knee which results in stretching of the medial ligament.

Referred pain and nerve root pain

From time to time patients are seen whose main complaint is pain in the knee, but, local thorough examination reveals no satisfactory explanation for it. In such cases one must consider the possibility of pain being referred from a disorder distant from the knee. As previously indicated, the commonest source of such pain is a disorder of the hip. The pain is referred along the course of one of the nerves, especially the obturator nerve, which takes a large share of the innervation of the hip.

Pressure on the nerve roots of the lumbar or sacral plexus, especially from prolapsed inter-vertebral discs, may cause symptoms which are felt in the region of the knee. It is almost always the case that these symptoms are associated with other symptoms in the back, buttock or thigh.

THE LEG, ANKLE AND FOOT

Complaints of pains in the leg, ankle and foot may not be primary reasons for seeking advice, but form a large number of associated problems. Indeed, patients who present in practice with other problems are often all too keen to mention their painful legs, ankles, feet or a combination of the three!

The prevalence of such complaints may have several causes. Excessive body weight throws an increased burden on the feet, and they may be unable to withstand the stress without ill effects, especially if the intrinsic muscles are poorly developed. The wearing of ill-fitting shoes is a common cause of foot disorders. Many types of shoes are totally incompatible with the mechanics of the foot.

Most cases of symptoms in the leg, ankle and foot can be explained by local abnormality. This is markedly different from the upper limbs, where symptoms in the hand frequently have no local cause but are referred from a more proximal source.

EVALUATION OF THE PAINFUL FOOT

A thorough knowledge of the anatomy of the foot and ankle makes it possible for the structures to be examined manually. This can easily expose any joint dysfunction and sites of pain. The phalanges can be tested individually by fixing the proximal phalanx and moving the more distal joint (Figure 13.5).

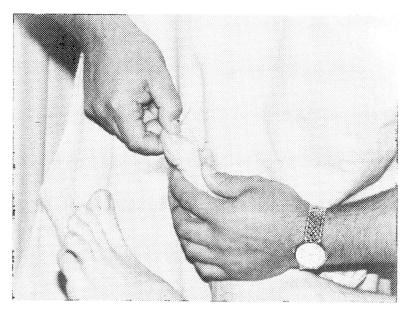

Figure 13.5 Clinically testing the individual phalanges by fixing the proximal phalanx and moving the more distal joint.

The normal foot must conform to certain important criteria:

- It must be mobile and pain free.
- It must have balanced muscle action.
- It must not show any contractures.
- The heel must be central.
- The toes must be straight and mobile.

History

The precise distribution of pain should be ascertained. The occupation and habits of the patient, or a previous injury, may be significant.

Observation

This should include the condition of footwear, comparing the two sides and looking out for the sites of greatest wear. The influence of weight-bearing stress can easily be observed when the patient stands evenly on both feet. Observe the general shape of the ankle, foot and toes. The longitudinal arch is observed and the position of the navicular is closely assessed. Close approximation of the navicular region to the ground indicates a pes planus; higher than normal indicates a pes cavus. The intrinsic muscles are tested by making the toes press hard against the ground. A crucial test for the calves is for the patient to stand on the affected leg and to raise the heel from the ground.

The patient's gait is especially helpful in showing abnormal posture of the feet, such as turning in (intoeing) or turning out, or drop foot.

Palpation

The palpation should feel for skin temperature changes, bone contours, soft tissue contours and local tenderness. The following *'pulses'* should be examined: dorsalis pedis; posterior tibial; popliteal, and femoral. This is done to test for any narrowing or occlusion of a vessel. Clinically compare the pulses and note any difference.

Movement

Both the *active* and *passive* ranges of movements should be compared with the normal side. Test for:

- At the toes: flexion and extension.
- At the mid-tarsal joint: inversion-adduction/eversion-abduction.
- At the subtalar joint: inversion-adduction/eversion-abduction.
- At the ankle joint: plantarflexion/dorsiflexion.

The muscle power is tested against the practitioner and, lastly, the integrity of the ligaments is tested.

The majority of painful conditions of the feet originate directly from their soft tissues. In most cases the problem can be identified by examining thoroughly the local muscles, ligaments, tendons, nerves and the tissues in the joint spaces. The majority of cases arise following a physical trauma or from physical stress.

The static, weight-bearing foot is self-supporting via a system of ligaments which complement a complex bony architecture. There is no supporting muscular activity from the muscles. The muscular function is employed during movement to prevent excessive forces being imposed upon the ligaments. The only deviation of function occurs when the muscles are weakened from disease or damage.

This fact can be utilized during the initial stages of evaluation. In the absence of historical evidence of neuro-muscular disease or damage, we must look to the local structures of the feet for pain causation. A history of nerve root or trunk damage, however, from either mechanical or pathological disease, together with associated signs in the examination of the peripheral and central nervous system, will lead us toward a more more widespread assessment of the patient's general state before focusing on a local area.

Local causes of foot pain

Acute foot strain

This is a common sequel to the sudden strain of an unaccustomed activity. The most common example is the corpulent individual who takes up jogging to lose weight. The repeated strain on the already distressed foot causes ligamentous inflammation with resultant pain.

Chronic foot strain

Chronic foot strain will follow the above if left unattended or the offending stress is not addressed. The mechanical effect on the structures will begin with strain and end with deformation. Persistent strain will cause ligamentous elongation and even some degeneration. Persistent joint irritation can ultimately result in damage to the joint surface, and degenerative arthritis develops. The stress inflames the joint capsule which causes further pain. Ultimately there is a bony overgrowth which further deforms the joint.

The initial symptom will be a deep ache, which is felt in the deep tendons and ligaments of the foot. Changes in mechanical pull on the calcaneum will lead to stress on the plantar fascia, which in turn becomes tender. Other ligaments which become inflamed include the calcaneo-navicular, as well as the ligaments which link the metatarsals. There is a resultant metatarsalgia (see below).

Excessive weight gain or a new occupation which requires prolonged standing, after years of sitting, may be contributing factors.

Various sequences of events have been postulated to explain how symptoms arise in the leg. In brief the prolonged, untreated chronic foot strain will lead to imbalance of the pronating muscular mechanism. When the muscular action which controls pronation is overwhelmed, the stress is conveyed to the ligaments, the joint capsules and ultimately the joint surfaces. Again, deformed joints will contribute to the complex symptom picture. Owing to their anatomical position, the posterior tibial tendon as well as anterior tibial muscle become tender and inflamed. Eventually the toe extensors change their alignment and become evertors as well as extensors. In prolonged stress the evertors may become inflamed and tender. Local, firm palpation can confirm the presence of pain in the above areas.

Metatarsalgia

Metatarsalgia is a common condition, particularly in elderly patients. Primarily, the pain and tenderness is felt on the plantar heads of the metatarsals. This is a common sequel to the loss of the transverse arch, following excessive weight-bearing upon the second, third and fourth metatarsal heads. The normal weight-bearing foot will bear five-sixths of the weight on the first and fifth metatarsals which are padded [139].

Altered gait and abnormal stress will cause the weight to be transferred to the second, third and sometimes fourth metatarsal head. These are not padded for the function and thus become tender.

There are many variations of stress imbalance resulting in unaccustomed weight bearing on ligaments and joint surfaces. Although they often develop along a characteristic course, the practitioner must be aware of any deviations. In each case it is important to identify the altered function and the resultant alteration in weight-bearing.

There are *two* frequently arising conditions which can be easily mistaken for variations of foot strain.

March fracture

This has a clinical presentation of a deep nagging pain in the foot. Tenderness is often felt during flexion or extension of the toes. Occasionally, pain is noted after a long march, hence its name. The metatarsal shaft can suffer a fracture which is hairline and no displacements of fragments are seen. This may not even show up on initial X-ray pictures. Later, a callus forms around the fracture.

Interdigital neuritis

The most common form is Morton's neuroma found mainly in middle-aged women. Characteristically they find relief in taking off their shoes rather than relieving the weight-bearing. This is because the offending and painful neuroma (a fusiform swelling of a digital nerve) is compressed between the metatarsal heads.

Compressing the metatarsal heads may produce numbness in the toes as well as turning the deep ache into a sharp pain.

The painful heel

Conditions above the heel: Achilles tendonitis; Achilles bursitis; rupture of Achilles tendon

The Achilles tendon may become tender. Inflammation of the loose connective tissue can arise from trauma or stress. The tendon is tender when squeezed and may appear thickened or swollen. Pain is aggravated by acute stretching from forceful dorsiflexion of the foot. Running, jumping or dancing may aggravate Achilles tendonitis.

Similar symptoms may be experienced when one of the bursae around the tendon becomes inflamed. The usual cause of inflamed bursae around the Achilles is ill-fitting shoes. Commonly a retrocalcaneal bursitis is the first to form. This is caused by the bursae between the skin and the Achilles tendon.

Complete or partial rupture of the Achilles tendon can be an agonizing experience. The patient classically complains of a shooting sensation, which causes a fall to the ground. The history, the severity of the pain and inability to rise up on the toes are a clear confirmation of a rupture.

Conditions beneath the heel: calcaneal spur, plantar fasciitis, painful heel pad

Occasions will arise when the site of pain spreads over a wide area, so crossing many bones and joint lines. Pain and tenderness found under the heel, spreading along the length of the foot, can be attributed to a calcaneal spur, with associated plantar fasciitis. These conditions are common in individuals whose occupation requires long periods of infrequent walking. Plantar fasciitis may be a forerunner of calcaneal spur. A calcaneal spur can also occur in isolation from plantar fasciitis and is not necessarily clearly evident on X-ray. Plantar fasciitis is a common problem for people who take up jogging without any previous sporting history and have the added disadvantage of having pronated feet.

The plantar fascia which attaches by tendinous insertion to the periosteum of the calcaneum is stretched or torn. The avulsion of the periosteum causes subperiosteal inflammation. The repair process forms calcium deposits, ultimately forming a spur. Initially the discomfort is probably due to the soft tissue inflammation. In the later stages the pain is due to the spur irritating the calcaneal pad. These pads can become a source of pain without the presence of a calcaneal spur. They are fatty and fibro-elastic tissue, liable to lose their elasticity and shock-absorbing property with age. The site becomes inflamed and painful on weight-bearing.

Painful abnormalities of the toes

Many problems can arise in the feet. Their origin can be divided into two major groups: those arising as a result of injury or structural deformities of the toes themselves or those arising from more generalized conditions. The latter are often seen during a clinical examination. As they are at the extremity of the blood flow they can be subject to circulatory deficiency and the usual signs of deficient blood supply can be observed. The mild cases are seen as pale and cold feet. The more advanced conditions of ulcerated and generally deprived feet are sometimes seen in cases where patients present with problems that may or may not be associated with the lack of blood supply. Other systemic conditions, such as diabetes and gout, all have their own characteristic signs.

Conditions resulting in damage to the nerve tissue of the lower limbs can give rise to signs and symptoms in the feet. These may present as subjective feelings in the feet, for example 'pins and needles' from nerve root entrapment, numbness and loss of feeling and control of the foot from nerve root damage, and loss of spatial co-ordination and balance from more sinister degenerative conditions of the central nervous system.

Among the more common, non-mechanical conditions which are seen in practice is Raynaud's phenomenon. This is a condition in which there is spasm of small blood vessels, especially of the fingers. The patient may observe intermittent attacks of sudden pallor or even actual blanching of the fingers. The acute pallor episode may be followed by cyanosis. The condition is attributed to arterial spasm, a manifestation of vasomotor instability. It is usually triggered by emotional stress or cold [142]. Symptoms are also felt in the hands.

Hallux valgus

This is a common and sometimes painful condition. It is particularly painful when the bursa over the medial aspect of the metatarso-phalangeal joint is enlarged and swollen (Figure 13.6). This condition is commonly known as a bunion. This symptomatic condition is found mostly in older people with a history of pronated feet with a broadened forefoot and depressed metatarsal arch. The basic hallux valgus is considered to be a congenital condition.

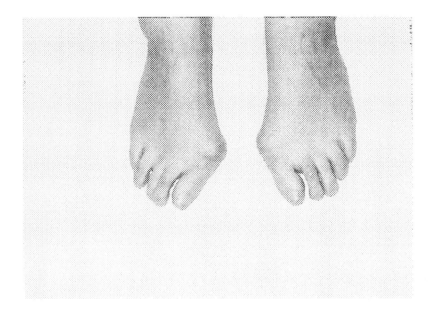

Figure 13.6 Hallux valgus. A painful bursa has also developed over the medial aspect of the metatarso-phalangeal joint, thus giving rise to a bunion.

Hallux rigidus

This is present when the big toe becomes limited in its range of extension. This also causes other foot problems, as the patient attempts to avoid stressing that joint by walking on the outer border of the foot with increased toe-in gait and thus places more stress upon the fifth metatarsal. This gait is tiring and also causes joint and callus discomfort in the outer aspect of the forefoot.

Hammer toe

This is a fixed flexion deformity of the inter-phalangeal joint, with hyperextension of the metatarso-phalangeal joint. It can be congenital or acquired. Once again it is the callus formation that usually causes most of the pain.

Although several of the above clinical situations can be identified as individual conditions, there are many combinations of clinical findings where the integrity of a normal foot has been altered, with resultant painful episodes. The osteopath aims to find the exact alteration to the normal mechanical state of the foot in order to establish the degree of change in function. This change in function may result in a confined and localized problem. On other occasions the resultant change is distant and far reaching.

How does the practitioner identify the 'knock-on' effects of a painful foot? Gait analysis is probably the most accurate method. The patient is asked to walk a few unaided steps across the room and repeat this several times. The practitioner should be able to spot any deviations from normal movement. Close attention is paid to the ankle movement, knee torsion and hip joint behaviour. This pattern is closely compared to the unaffected side. The rest of the body movements are then closely scrutinized for any change. Occasions may arise when an even closer and more detailed analysis of the foot is needed. On such occasions the help of a podiatrist is employed.

In summary, the lower limb must be considered both as an individual source of pain and the reflector of pain from another source. Although the symptoms are often experienced in one part of the lower limb, the cause of pain may come from another part of the limb. Taking pain in the knee as an example, it may be referred from the hip, or come from the spine as seen in L3/4 nerve root entrapment. Alternatively, the pain can come from within the knee, for example, osteoarthritis of the joint itself. Equally, one must recognize that foot dysfunction may give rise to knee pain, hip pain or lower back pain.

The alert practitioner must always consider the possibility of two or more causes of pain in the same area. For example, it is not unusual for an elderly patient to be suffering with degenerative changes in the knee with some contribution of pain coming from an equally degenerate hip joint. The altered gait may also give rise to spinal pain from altered weight bearing.

Finally, it is essential to keep in mind the close inter-relationship between the source of pain, the resultant adaptations made by the rest of the lower limb *and* any adaptations that the overall body posture may have undergone. This is commonly crucial to the treatment of specific problems in the lower limb.

References

1. Still, C. (1991) Frontier doctor–medical pioneer, in *The Life and Times of A.T. Still and his Family*, Thorne Jefferson University Press, Kirksville.
2. Martinke, D. J. (1991) The Philosophy of Osteopathic Medicine, in *An Osteopathic Approach to Diagnosis and Treatment*. New York, JB Lippincott.
3. Selye, H. (1978) *The Stress of Life*. McGraw Hill, New York.
4. Korr, I. M., Wright, H. M. and Chase, J. A. (1964) Cutaneous patterns of sympathetic activity in clinical abnormalities of the musculo-skeletal system. *Journal of Neural Transmission*, **25**, 589.
5. Korr, I. M. (1976) The spinal cord as an organiser of disease processes: some preliminary perspectives. *Journal of the American Osteopathic Association*, **76**, 35.
6. Dove, C. I. (1967) A history of the osteopathic vertebral lesion. *British Osteopathic Journal*, **3**, (3).
7. Korr, I. M. (1947) The neural basis of the osteopathic lesion. *Journal of the American Osteopathic Association*, **47**, 191.
8. DiGiovanna, E. L. (1991) Somatic dysfunction, in *An Osteopathic Approach to Diagnosis and Treatment* (eds DiGiovanna, E. L. and Schiowitz, S. JB Lippincott, New York, p. 9.
9. Porterfield, J. A. and Derosa, C. (1991) *Mechanical Low Back Pain – perspectives in functional anatomy*, Saunders, Philadelphia.
10. Van Buskirk, R. L. (1990) Nociceptive reflexes and the somatic dysfunction; a model. *Journal of the American Osteopathic Association*, **90**(9), 792.
11. Cavanaugh, J. (1995) Neural mechanisms of lumbar pain. *Spine*, **20**(16), 1804.
12. Yamashita, T. *et al.* (1993) Effects of substance P on the mechano-sensitive units in the lumbar facet joint and adjacent tissues. *Journal of Orthopaedic Research*, **11**, 205.
13. Coderre, T. J., Katz, J., Vaccarino, A. I. and Melzack, R. (1993) Contribution of central neuroplasticity to pathological pain: review of clinical and experimental evidence. *Pain*, **52**, 259.
14. Gillette, R. G., Kramis, R. C. and Roberts, W. J. (1993) Characterization of spinal somato-sensory neurones having receptive fields in lumbar tissues of cats. *Pain*, **5**, 85.
15. Grieve, P. G. (1981) *Common Vertebral Joint Problems*, Churchill Livingstone, London, pp.189–96.
16. Kerr, F. W. L. (1975) Neuroanatomical substrates of nociception in the spinal cord. *Pain*, **1**, 325–56.
17. Mooney, V. and Robertson, J. (1976) The facet syndrome. *Clinical Orthopaedics and Related Research*, **115**, 149.

18. Basmajiam, J. V. and De Luca, C. J. (1985) *Muscles Alive*, 5th edn, Williams and Wilkins, London.

19. Stoddard, A. (1969) *Manual of Osteopathic Practice*, Hutchinson Medical, London.

20. Korr, I. M. (1978) Sustained sympathicotonia as a factor in disease, in *The Neurolobiologic Mechanisms in Manipulative Therapy* (ed. I. M. Korr), Plenum, New York, pp. 229–86.

21. Patterson, M. M. and Steinmetz, J. E. (1986) Long-lasting alterations of spinal reflexes: a potential basis for somatic dysfunction. *Manual Medicine*, **2**, 238.

22. Mayer, D. J. and Liebeskind, J. C. (1974) Pain reduction by focal electrical stimulation of the brain: an anatomical and behavioural analysis. *Brain Research*, **68**, 73.

23. Fields, L. H. and Anderson, S. D. (1978) Evidence that raphe-spinal neurones mediate opiate and mid-brain stimulation produced analgesics. *Pain*, **5**, 333.

24. Melzack, R. and Wall, P. D. (1965) Pain mechanisms: a new theory. *Science*, **150**, 971.

25. Korr, I. M. (1975) Proprioceptors and somatic dysfunction. *Journal of the American Osteopathic Association*, **74**, 638.

26. Tondury, G. (1948) Beitrag zur Kenntnis der kleinen Wirbelgelenke. *Zeitschrift fur Anatomische Entwicklungsgeschichte*, **110**, 568.

27. Kos, J. (1968) Contribution a l'étude de l'anatomie de la vascularisation des articulations intervertebrales. *Bulletin de l'Association des Anatomistes*, **53**, 1088.

28. Kos, J. and Wolf, J. (1972) Die 'Menisci' der Zwischenwirbelgelenke und ihre mogliche Rolle bei Wirbelblockierung. *Manuelle Medizin*, **10**, 105.

29 Janda, V. (1978) Muscles, central nervous motor regulation and back problems, in *The Neurolobiologic Mechanisms in Manipulative Therapy* (ed. I. M. Korr), Plenum, New York, pp. 27–41.

30. Arkuszewski, Z. (1986) Involvement of the cervical spine in back pain. *Manual Medicine*, **2**, 126.

31. Kunert, W. (1965) Functional disorders of internal organs due to vertebral lesions. *Ciba Symposium*, **13**, 85.

32. Ghosh, P. (1990) Basic biochemistry of the intervertebral disc and its variation with ageing and degeneration. *Manual Medicine*, **5**, 48.

33. Adams, M. A. and Hutton, W. C. (1983) Mechanical function of the lumbar apophyseal joints. *Spine*, **80**, 327.

34. Lawrence, J. S. (1969) Disc degeneration and its relationship to symptoms. *Annals of the Rheumatic Diseases*, **28**, 121.

35. Wyke, B. D. (1985) Articular neurology and manipulative therapy, in *Aspects of Manipulative Therapy*, 2nd edn (eds E. F. Glasgow, L. T. Twomey, E. R. Scull, A. M. Kleyhans and R. M. Idczak), Churchill Livingstone, Edinburgh, pp. 72–80.

36. Threlkeld, A. (1992) The effects of manual therapy on connective tissue. *Physical Therapy*, **72**(12), 893.

37. Nies, N. and Sinnott, P. (1991) Variations in balance and body sway in middle-aged adults. *Spine*, **16**(3), 325.

38. Asmussen, E. and Klausen, K. (1962) Form and function of the erect human spine. *Clinical Orthopaedics and Related Research*, **25**, 55.

39. Morris, J. M., Brewer, G. and Lucas, D. B. (1962) An EMG study of intrinsic muscles of the back in man. *Journal of Anatomy*, **96**, 509.

40. Anderson, G. B. J. and Ortengren, R. (1974) Myoelectric back muscle activity during sitting. *Scandinavian Journal of Rehabilitation Medicine. Supplement*, **3**, 73.
41. Barlow, W. (1952) Postural homeostasis. *Annals of Physical Medicine*, **1**, 77.
42. Porter, R. W. and Miller, C. G. (1986) Back pain and trunk list. *Spine*, **11**(6), 596.
43. Johnston, W. L. (1983) Hip shift: testing a basic postural dysfunction, in *Postural Balance and Imbalance* (ed. B. Peterson.) American Academy of Osteopathy, Newark, Ohio, pp. 109–12.
44. Nathan, B. (1995) Philosophical notes on osteopathic theory, Part 3. Non-procedural touching and the relationship between touch and emotion. *British Osteopathic Journal*, **17**, 30.
45. Hartman, L. (1996) *Handbook of Osteopathic Technique*, Stanley Thornes, Cheltenham, UK.
46. Roston, J. B. and Haines, R. W. (1947) Cracking in the metacarpo-phalangeal joint. *Journal of Anatomy*, **81**, 165.
47. Unsworth, A., Dowson, D. and Wright, V. (1972) Cracking joints: a bioengineering study of cavitation in the metacarpo-phalangeal joint. *Annals of the Rheumatic Diseases*, **30**, 348.
48. Herzog, W., Conway, P. J., Kawchuk, G. N., Zhang, Y. and Hasler, E. M. (1993) Forces exerted during spinal manipulative therapy. *Spine*, **18**, 1206.
49. Lewit, K. (1991) *Manipulative Therapy in Rehabilitation of the Locomotor System*, 2nd edn, Butterworth Heinemann, Oxford.
50. Korr, I. M. (1975) *Physiological Basis of Osteopathic Medicine*, Insight, New York.
51. Cyriax, J. (1970) *Textbook of Orthopaedic Medicine 1*, 5th edn, Ballière, Tindall & Cassell, London.
52 Mitchell Jr, F. L., Moran, P. S. and Pruzzo, N. A. (1979) *An Evaluation and Treatment Manual of Osteopathic Muscle Energy Procedures*, Valley Park, Missouri.
53. Bourdillon, J. F. (1987) *Spinal Manipulation*, Heinemann Medical, Oxford.
54. Jones, L. H. (1981) *Strain and Counterstrain*. American Academy of Osteopathy, Colorado Springs.
55. Upledger, J. E. and Vredevoogd, M. F. A. (1983) *Cranio-sacral Therapy*, Eastland Press, Seattle.
56. Magoun, H. I. (1966) *Osteopathy in the Cranial Field*, Printing Co., Kirksville.
57. Stone, C. (1992) *Viscera Revisited*, Tigger Publishing (available from Osteopathic Supplies, Hereford).
58. Barral, J. and Mercier, P. (1988) *Visceral Manipulation*, Eastland Press, Seattle.
59. Terrett, A. G. J. (1987) Vascular accidents from cervical spine manipulation. Report on 107 cases. *Journal of Australian Chiropractors Association*, **17**(1), 15.
60. Terrett, A. G. J. (1990) It is more important to know when not to adjust. *Chiropractic Technique*, **2**(1), 1.
61. Hartman, L. (1996) *Handbook of Osteopathic Technique*, Stanley Thornes, Cheltenham, UK.
62. Kleyhans, A. M. and Terrett, A. G. J. (1985) The prevention of complications from spinal manipulative therapy, in *Aspects of Manipulative Therapy* (eds E. F. Glasgow, L. T. Twomey, E. R. Scull, A. M. Kleyhans and R. M. Idczak), Churchill Livingstone, Edinburgh, pp. 161–75.
63. Hirsch, C., Inglemark, B. E. and Miller, M. (1963) Anatomical basis for low back

pain. Studies on the presence of sensory nerve endings in ligaments, capsules and intervertebral structures in the human lumbar spine. *Acta Orthopaedica Scandinavica*, **33**, 1.

64. McCall, I., Park, W. M. and O'Brien, J. P. (1979) Induced pain referral from posterior elements in normal subjects. *Spine*, **4**, 441.

65. Dwyer, A. P., Aprill, C. and Bogduk, N. (1990) Cervical apophyseal joint pain patterns. *Spine*, **15**(6), 454.

66. Dreyfuss, P., Tibiletti, C. and Dryer, S. J. (1994) Thoracic zygapophyseal joint pain patterns. A study in normal volunteers. *Spine*, **19**(7), 807.

67. Fortin, J. D., Dwyer, A. P., West, S. and Pier, J. (1994) SI pain maps in asymptomatic volunteers. *Spine*, **19**(13), 1475.

68. Bogduk, N., Tynan, W. and Wilson, A. S. (1983) The innervation of lumbar intervertebral discs. *Journal of Anatomy*, **132**, 39.

69. Swash, M. (1989) *Hutchinson's Clinical Methods*, Baillière Tindall, London.

70. Stone, C. (1992) *Viscera Revisited*, Tigger Publishing (available from Osteopathic Supplies, Hereford).

71. Barral. J. and Mercier, P. (1988) *Visceral Manipulation*, Eastland Press, Seattle, WA.

72. Butler, D. S. (1991) *Mobilisation of the Nervous System*, Churchill Livingstone, London.

73. Goddard, M. D. and Reid, J. D. (1965) Movements induced in the lumbo-sacral roots, nerves and plexus, and in the intra-abdominal portion of the sciatic nerve. *Journal of Neurology, Neurosurgery and Psychiatry*, **28**, 12.

74. Mooney, V. T. (1977) Facet pathology, in *Proceedings of the Third Seminar of the International Federation of Orthopaedic Manipulative Therapists IFOMT*, Hayward, CA (ed. B. Kent).

75. King, J. S. (1977) Randomised trial of the Reas and Shealy methods for the treatment of back pain, in *Approaches to the Validation of Manipulation Therapy* (eds A. A. Buerger and J. S. Toby), Thomas, Springfield, IL, p. 70.

76. Farhni, W. H. (1966) Observations on SLR with reference to root adhesions. *Canadian Journal of Surgery*, **9**, 44.

77. Thelander, U., Fagerlund, M., Friberg, S. and Larson, S. (1992) Straight leg raising test versus radiologic size, shape, and position of lumbar disc hernias. *Spine*, **17**(4), 395.

78. Hudgkins, W. R. (1977) The crossed straight leg raising test. *New England Journal of Medicine*, **297**, 1127.

79. Farhni, W. H. (1976) *Backache and Primal Posture*, Musqueam Publishers, Vancouver.

80. Travell, J. G. and Simons, D. G. (1983) *Myofascial Pain and Dysfunction – the trigger point manual*, Williams and Wilkins, Baltimore.

81. Ruge, D. and Wiltse, L. (1977) *Spinal Disorders, Diagnosis and Treatment*, Lea & Febiger, Philadelphia.

82. Murdoch, G. (1959) Scoliosis in twins. *Journal of Bone and Joint Surgery*, **41B**, 736.

83. Bick, E. M. (1961) Vertebral growth: its relation to spinal abnormalities in children. *Clinical Orthopaedics and Related Research*, **21**, 43.

84. Nachemson, A. (1968) A long-term follow-up study of non treated scoliosis. *Acta Orthopaedica Scandinavica*, **39**, 466.

85. Crawford Adams, J. (1983) *Outline of Orthopaedics*, 9th edn, Churchill Livingstone, Edinburgh.

86. Vidal, P. P., Graf, W. and Berthoz, A. (1986). The orientation of the cervical vertebral column in unrestricted awake animals. I. Resting position. *Experimental Brain Research*, **61**, 549.

87. Jofe, M. H., White, A. A. and Panjabi, M. M. (1983) Physiology and biomechanics, in *The Cervical Spine* (eds The Cervical Spine Research Society), JB Lippincott, Philadelphia, pp. 23–33.

88. Graf, W., Vidal, P. P. and Evinger, C. (1986). Biomechanical properties of the head movement system, in *The Control of Head Movement Abstracts*. Satellite Symposium of XXX IUPS Congress, Whistler, BC, pp. 190–21.

89. Kingston, B. (1996) *Understanding Muscles*, Chapman & Hall, London.

90. Kapandji, I. A. (1976) *The Physiology of Joints*, vol. 3. *The Trunk and the Vertebral Column*, 2nd edn, Churchill Livingstone, New York, pp. 218–43.

91. Cavaziel, H. (1977) Acute torticollis: clinical features and treatment. *Manual of Medicine*, **4**, 58.

92. Hurwits, E., Aker, P., Adams, A., Meeker, W. and Shekelle, P. (1996) Manipulation and mobilization of the cervical spine: a systematic reviw of the literature. *Spine*, **21**(15), 1746.

93. Stevens, B. J. and McKenzie, R. A. (1988) Mechanical diagnosis and self treatment of the cervical spine, in *Physical Therapy of the Cervical and Thoracic Spine* (ed. R. Grant). Churchill Livingstone, Edinburgh, pp. 127–289.

94. McKenzie, R. A. (1990) *The Cervical and Thoracic Spine. Mechanical Diagnosis and Therapy*, Spinal Publications (NZ), Waikanae.

95. Mertz, H. J. (1985) Anthropomorphic models, in *The Biomechanics of Trauma* (eds A. M. Nahum and J. Melvin), Appleton-Century-Crofts, Norwalk, CN, pp. 31–60.

96. Sances *et al.* (1981) Bioengineering analysis of head and spine injuries. *CRC Critical Reviews in Bioengineering*, **6**, 79.

97. Herlihy, W. F. (1949) Sinu-vertebral nerve. *New Zealand Medical Journal*, **48**, 214.

98. Cailliet, R. (1981) *Neck and Arm Pain*, 2nd edn, F. A. Davis, Philadelphia.

99. Downing, C. H. (1981) *Principles and Practice of Osteopathy*, 2nd edn, Tamor Pierston Publishers, Isleworth, Middlesex.

100. Bannister, R. (revised by) (1981) *Brain's Clinical Neurology*, 5th edn, Oxford University Press, Oxford.

101. Adams, C. (1983) *Outline of Orthopaedics*, Churchill Livingstone, Edinburgh, p. 232.

102. Nachlas, I. W. (1942) Scalenus anticus syndrome or cervical foraminal compression? *Southern Medical Journal*, **35**, 663.

103. Macleod, J. (ed.) (1983) *Davidson's Principle and Practice of Medicine*, 13th edn, Churchill Livingstone, Edinburgh, p. 226.

104. Cawson, R. A., McCracken, A., Marais, P. and Letz, J. (eds) (1982) *Pathological Mechanisms and Human Disease*, CV Mosby, Missouri.

105. Hughes, R. L. (1979) Does abdominal breathing affect regional gas exchange? *Chest*, **76**, 288.

106. Ballentine, R. M. (1979) *Science of Breath: a practical guide*, Himalayan Institute, Honesdale.

107. Ogilvie, C. (1980) *Chamberlain's Symptoms and Signs in Clinical Medicine*, 10th edn, p. 161.

108. McNaught, A. B. and Callender, R. (1975) *Illustrated Physiology*, 4th edn, Churchill Livingstone, Edinburgh.

109. Epstein, B. S. (1969) *The Spine: a radiological text and atlas*, 3rd edn, Lea & Febiger, Philadelphia.

110. Lum, L. C. (1976) The syndrome of habitual hyperventilation, in *Modern Trends in Psychosomatic Medicine* (ed. O. W. Hill), Butterworth, London, pp. 6–25.

111. Huey, S. R. and Sechrest, L. (1981) Hyperventilation syndrome and psychopathology. Center for Research on the Utilization of Scientific Knowledge, Institute of Social Research, University of Michigan. Manuscript.

112. Doran, D. M. L. (1969) Mechanical and postural causes of chest pain. *Proceedings of the Royal Society of Medicine*, **62**, 876.

113. Adams, M. A. and Hutton, W. C. (1980) The effect of posture on the role of the apophyseal joints in resisting intervertebral compressive force. *Journal of Bone and Joint Surgery*, **62B**, 358.

114. Farfan, H. F. (1973) *The Mechanical Disorders of the Lower Back*, Lea and Febiger, Philadelphia.

115. Kirkaldy Willis, W. H. (1988) *Managing Low Back Pain*, 2nd edn, Churchill Livingstone, London.

116. Stodolny, J. and Mazur, T. (1989) Effects of post-isometric relaxation exercises on the ilio-psoas muscles in patients with lumbar discopathy. *Journal of Manual Medicine*, **4**(2), 52.

117. Borenstein, D. G. and Wiesel, S. W. (1989) *Low Back Pain. Medical diagnosis and comprehensive management*, WB Saunders, Philadelphia.

118. Porter, R. W. (1986) *Management of Back Pain*, Churchill Livingstone, London.

119. Mooney, V. (1987) Where is the pain coming from? *Spine*, **12**, 754.

120. Mixter, W. J. and Barr, J. S. (1934) Rupture of the intervertebral disc with involvement of the spinal canal. *New England Journal of Medicine*, **211**, 211.

121. Hitselberger, W. E. and Witten, R. M. (1968) Abnormal myelograms in asymptomatic patients. *Journal of Neurosurgery*, **28**, 204.

122. Holt Jr, E. P. (1968) The question of lumbar discography. *Journal of Bone and Joint Surgery*, **50A**, 720.

123. Wiesel, S. W., Tsourmas, N., Feffer, H. L. and Citrin, C. (1984) A study of computer assisted tomography: 1 The incidence of positive CAT scans in an asymptomatic group of patients. *Spine*, **9**, 549.

124. Boden, S. D., Davis, D. O., Dina, T. S., Patronas, N. and Wiesel, S. W. (1990) Abnormal magnetic-resonance scans of the lumbar spine in asymptomatic subjects: a prospective investigation. *Journal of Bone and Joint Surgery*, **72A**, 403.

125. Sprangfort, E. V. (1972) The lumbar disc herniation: a computer aided analysis of 2504 operations. *Acta Orthopaedica Scandinavica* (Suppl. 142) 1.

126. Porter, R. W., Wicks, M. and Hibbert, C. (1978) The size of the lumbar spinal canal in symptomatology of the disc lesion. *Journal of Bone and Joint Surgery*, **60B**, 485.

127. MacNab, I. (1972) The mechanism of spondylogenic pain, in *Cervical Pain* (eds C. Hirsch and Y. Zotterman), Pergamon, New York, pp. 89.

128. Smyth, M. J. and Wright, V. (1958) Sciatica and the intervertebral disc: an experimental study. *Journal of Bone and Joint Surgery*, **40A**, 1401.

129. Helbig, T. and Lee, C. K. (1988) The lumbar facet syndrome. *Spine*, **13**(1), 61.

130. Nachemson, A. (1989) Lumbar discography – where are we today? *Spine*, **14**, 555.

131. Delauche-Cavallier, M., Budet, G., Laredo, J,-D. *et al.* (1992) Lumbar disc herniation computed tomography scan changes after conservative treatment of nerve root compression. *Spine*, **17**(8), 927.

132. Fryholm, R. (1971) The Clinical Picture, in *Cervical Pain* (eds C. Hirsch and Y. Zotterman), Pergamon, Oxford, p. 5.

133. Getty, C. J. M., Johnson, J. R., Kirwan, E. O. G. and Sullivan, M. F. (1981) Partial undercutting facetectomy for bony entrapment of the lumbar nerve root. *Journal of Bone and Joint Surgery*, **63B**, 330.

134. Gary, A., Schneiderman, M. D., Robert, F. *et al.* (1995) The pars defect as a pain source. *Spine*, **20**, (16), 1761.

135. Fredrickson, B. G., Baker, D., McHolick, W. J. and Lubicky, J. P. (1984) The natural history of spondylolysis and spondylolisthesis. *Journal of Bone and Joint Surgery*, **66A**, 699.

136. Schwarzer, A. C. *et al.* (1994) The relative contributions of the disc and apophyseal joint in chronic low back pain. *Spine*, **19**(7), 801.

137. Gaenslen, F. G. (1927) Sacroiliac arthrodesis. *Journal of the American Medical Association*.

138. Coventry, M. B. and Tapper, E. M. (1972) Pelvic instability. *Journal of Bone and Joint Surgery*, **55A**, 83.

139. Caillet, R. (1982) *Soft Tissue Pain and Disability*, F. A. Davis, Philadelphia.

Index